DRUGS AND PHARMACOLOGY
FOR NURSES

Drugs and Pharmacology for Nurses

BY

S. J. HOPKINS, F.P.S.

GROUP PHARMACIST
UNITED CAMBRIDGE HOSPITALS

FIFTH EDITION
(*Reprint*)

CHURCHILL LIVINGSTONE
EDINBURGH AND LONDON
1973

First Edition	.	.	.	1963
Second Edition	.	.	.	1965
Third Edition	.	.	.	1966
Fourth Edition	.	.	.	1968
Reprinted	.	.	.	1970
Fifth Edition	.	.	.	1971
Reprinted	.	.	.	1973

ISBN 0 443 00773 X

Made and Printed in the British Commonwealth

PREFACE TO THE FIFTH EDITION

THIS Edition follows the pattern set by previous editions, but some sections have been re-arranged to permit easier reference. Developments in therapeutics are reflected in the notes on a number of new drugs of importance, including amantadine and levodopa for the treatment of parkinsonism, practolol and oxprenolol, β-receptor blocking agents used in cardiac arrhythmias, trimethoprim, a new antibacterial compound, and pancuronium, a muscle relaxant. New antibiotics are represented by cephalexin, flucloxacillin and rifampicin.

The Table of Drug Interactions has been revised and extended and indicates the risks of therapeutic incompatibilities that may follow multiple treatment with some of the potent drugs now in frequent use.

This multiplicity of available drugs also means that some degree of selection has been essential in this book to limit its size, but the omission of the name of any proprietary drug does not reflect in any adverse way on the value of the product concerned, and is merely an indication of the wide choice of drugs now available to the physician.

In the text, drugs in Schedules I and IV of the Poisons List, and those controlled by the Therapeutic Substances Act, are distinguished (in the main references) by a dagger thus †, and dangerous drugs are identified by a star thus *. The abbreviation (q.v.) indicates that the drug concerned is referred to again on another page.

Thanks are again due to those readers and reviewers who have been kind enough to suggest improvements. Although designed primarily for nurses, the book has achieved a wider readership, as medical representatives, dispensing assistants, pharmacists and others concerned more or less directly with the use of drugs have found the book of value.

S. J. HOPKINS.

CAMBRIDGE, 1971.

PREFACE TO THE FIRST EDITION

THIS book owes its origin to a series of lectures given at Addenbrooke's Hospital, Cambridge, and is designed to provide nurses with a basic knowledge of pharmacology, and a survey of drugs in current use. Such a basic knowledge will not only clarify many present forms of therapy, but will help the nurse to appreciate the value and limitations of new drugs that may become available in the future.

Each section of the book is introduced by a brief general review, followed by a consideration of the individual drugs of the class concerned, which are referred to under the Approved Name. Many nurses express surprise at the multiplicity of names for drugs, and it must be admitted that such variety can be very confusing. The reason is that most new drugs have a brand or trade name, and a non-proprietary or Approved Name. This Approved Name, which is often derived from the chemical name of the drug, can be used by anyone, but the brand or trade name refers to the particular product of a manufacturer. Occasionally, when more than one manufacturer is interested in marketing a drug, it may be available under several brand names. In this book the Approved Name is used as the main heading for each monograph on drugs, and some brand names are given later. An extended list of Approved Names and corresponding brand names is given in Appendix I.

As a general rule, the doses of drugs are expressed in the metric system, but in the case of some older drugs, which continue to be prescribed in terms of the imperial system, doses are given in terms of both systems. The abbreviations B.N.F. and B.P.C. refer to the British National Formulary and the British Pharmaceutical Codex respectively.

For an explanation of those medical and pharmacological terms used but not defined in the text, nurses are advised to consult one of the nursing reference books such as Livingstone's *Dictionary for Nurses*.

My thanks are due to Miss F. I. Tennant, Principal Sister Tutor, Addenbrooke's Hospital, who kindly read the manuscript and made many helpful suggestions, and to Mr C. Macmillan and Mr W. A. Macmillan of E. & S. Livingstone Ltd. for their encouragement and advice.

S. J. HOPKINS.

ADDENBROOKE'S HOSPITAL,
CAMBRIDGE.

CONTENTS

CHAPTER I

INTRODUCTION

DRUGS AND PHARMACOLOGY

A DRUG can be defined as any substance used for the treatment, relief or prophylaxis of disease, and pharmacology is the study of the mode of action of such substances. Therapeutics refers to the use of drugs in the treatment or alleviation of disease in the light of their pharmacological action.

The history of drugs is almost as old as the history of man, as from the earliest times leaves, barks, fruits and roots have been used for medicinal purposes. Some ancient peoples acquired a surprisingly high degree of knowledge of vegetable drugs, and were aware of the value of opium, senna and aloes, drugs that are still in use to-day.

Real medicine, however, began with that remarkable civilisation to which European culture owes so much, namely the Greeks, and Hippocrates (c. 400 B.C.) has justly been termed ' the Father of Medicine.' Greek medicine was naturally empirical in character, and therapy was directed mainly towards the relief of symptoms. This empirical approach to disease persisted to the latter part of the nineteenth century, when advances in experimental pathology and pharmacology began to place therapeutics on a rational basis.

Since that time advances in therapeutics have been rapid, in recent years bewilderingly so, and to-day the physician has at his command an almost embarrassing range of therapeutically active substances. The whole subject of therapeutics is one of expanding horizons, which can fascinate by its immense potentialities, or perplex by its apparent anomalies. Out of this complexity one or two simplifying generalisations can be made. Thus all drugs may be divided into a few main groups according to their origin —i.e. vegetable drugs, mineral salts, animal products and synthetic drugs—or they may be classified according to their pharmacological action. To a more limited extent some drugs may be classified according to their chemical structure.

I

Crude or Vegetable Drugs

This is the oldest group of drugs, and includes natural products such as leaves, roots, seeds and barks. The importance of this group has declined with the development of synthetic drugs, although digitalis leaf still holds a high place in the treatment of cardiac conditions. Many plants still require investigation as the source of medicinal substances, and future research on vegetable drugs may well prove rewarding.

The therapeutic value of a vegetable drug is frequently due to a single constituent, often termed an active principle, which may be an alkaloid, such as atropine (from belladonna) or a glycoside, as digoxin (from the Austrian foxglove). Alkaloids are basic substances that can combine with acids to form salts, *e.g* atropine sulphate, morphine tartrate; glycosides contain an active fraction combined with a sugar. These sugars influence the solubility and rate of absorption of the active fragment, but have no action of their own. Alkaloids and other active principles are usually more satisfactory than preparations of the crude drugs, because they are of constant composition, and their action is more consistent and reliable.

Mineral Salts

These are metallic compounds such as sodium chloride (common salt), potassium chloride, sodium bicarbonate, ferrous sulphate and calcium gluconate. Some mineral salts are of very great physiological importance, and are present in certain intravenous solutions used in the treatment of shock, and to restore the electrolyte balance of the body.

Animal Products

Although this group enjoyed considerable popularity in the past (the witches' scene in ' Macbeth ' gives an indication of the variety of animal parts once used in medicine), few products of animal origin are in use to-day. Yet these few are of great therapeutic value, as the group includes drugs such as insulin, hormone products such as ACTH, heparin and hyaluronidase.

Synthetic Drugs

Most of the powerful modern medicaments are chemical compounds which do not occur in nature, but are built up from simpler substances by the organic chemist. This group of synthetic compounds is of outstanding importance and includes hypotensive drugs, tranquillisers and antidepressants, morphine substitutes, spasmolytics, sulphonamides, orally active anticoagulants and hypoglycaemic agents.

Antibiotics

Antibiotics can be described as antimicrobial substances produced during the growth of certain fungi and associated organisms. The first of this remarkable group of substances to be discovered was penicillin and its introduction marked an entirely new approach to the treatment of bacterial infections. Penicillin is effective chiefly against Gram-positive organisms, but other antibiotics, such as the tetracyclines, have a wider range of activity that includes Gram-negative organisms. Penicillin is one of the least toxic of modern drugs, and has a wide margin of safety, but some other antibiotics, such as neomycin, are too toxic for systemic use, except in special circumstances. These more toxic compounds, however, may be useful in the treatment of infected skin conditions, often in association with an anti-inflammatory steroid. Nystatin and amphotericin are antibiotics with a selective action of value in fungal infections.

Absorption and Distribution of Drugs

Many factors influence the absorption of drugs, but the most important single factor is the route of administration. The oral route is the most common, most convenient and least expensive method of giving a drug and has much to recommend it. Few drugs, with the notable exception of alcohol, are absorbed to any great extent in the stomach, as absorption of orally administered drugs occurs mainly in the small intestine. This absorption is subject to considerable variation, owing to changes in the intestinal contents, and the degree of mobility of the gastro-intestinal tract. Many drugs are broken down by digestive enzymes before they can be absorbed, others, even in solution, may fail to pass through the intestinal mucosa, and so have only a local action on the bowel. An occasional alternative to oral administration is to give drugs under the tongue. Many drugs are readily absorbed from the mucous lining of the mouth, and sublingual administration avoids the destructive effects of gastric juice, or inactivation in the liver before reaching the general circulation. Glyceryl trinitrate, isoprenaline and testosterone are examples of drugs that are often given by the sublingual route.

As an alternative to oral administration, or where an injection is undesired or not available, drugs may be given rectally by suppository (page 15). This form of medication is sometimes useful when nausea and vomiting are present, or if the drug is a gastric irritant. Aminophylline and indomethacin are examples of irritant drugs that can be given in adequate doses as suppositories.

However, for certainty of absorption and promptness of action, administration of a drug by injection is often the method of choice. The dose can be determined with more accuracy, and all the uncertainties of other methods of administration are eliminated.

After absorption most drugs become fairly generally distributed throughout the body tissues, and may be either metabolised by enzymes into other and often inactive susbtances or excreted unchanged. The rapidity with which the tissues bind, modify or eliminate a drug determines the duration of action and frequency of dose, and when a new drug is introduced a knowledge of its distribution and fate in the body is an important factor in assessing its therapeutic value. The great majority of drugs are rapidly metabolised or detoxified to form inert substances before they are eliminated and this may be of considerable clinical importance. Thus many sulphonamides are combined with acetic acid in the body and excreted, in part at least, in an inactive form. These inactivated forms are of no value in the treatment of infections of the urinary tract, and in such cases a drug is required that is excreted in an unmodified and active state.

Other drugs may be relatively inactive in the form in which they are given, but are changed in the body to more active substances. Chloral hydrate, for example, is broken down after absorption to trichlorethanol, to which the sedative action is finally due. Similarly, phenacetin is metabolised to p-acetamidophenol, or paracetamol, which has the analgesic action of the parent drug, but is less toxic.

It should be remembered that while most drugs are excreted in the urine and faeces, others may appear to a greater or lesser extent in other body secretions. Some drugs, such as paraldehyde, are excreted in part by the lungs, others are excreted by the sweat glands, and may cause skin irritation. In pregnancy, drugs may cross the placental barrier and affect the foetus, a fact that was highlighted by the thalidomide disaster. Many antibiotics, and drugs which influence the central nervous system, may pass into the foetal circulation and as foetal enzymes are poorly developed, the metabolism of such drugs is correspondingly slow, and their effects may be prolonged. Thus pethidine given during labour to the mother may delay the onset of breathing in the new-born infant, and for that reason a mixture of pethidine with the respiratory stimulant nalorphine (Pethilorfan) is preferred. During lactation, many drugs may be excreted in part in the milk (*i.e.* penicillin, sulphonamides, salicylates, barbiturates). The amount of drug that reaches the infant may not be very great, on the other hand it may well be undesirable, and no drug should be used during pregnancy and lactation unless its use is essential.

The Dose of Drugs

The therapeutic dose of a drug is based on the smallest amount that will elicit a response, and the largest dose that can be tolerated without excessive side-effects. The accepted range of dose used clinically is thus a compromise, and the dose prescribed will vary to some extent with the weight and sex of the patient. A heavy individual will require a larger dose than a light or small patient, and the dose of some potent drugs is based on the body weight. The dose may also vary according to the condition to be treated. Some tranquillisers for example that have anti-emetic properties are given in much larger doses for psychiatric conditions than when used for the treatment of nausea and vomiting.

The route of administration also influences the size of dose given. Doses by injection are usually smaller than those given orally, and intravenous doses smaller than those given by intramuscular injection. Frequency of dose is also important, and with long-acting drugs, care must be taken to avoid over-dosage, as the drug may then accumulate in the body, and cause toxic side-effects. Although relatively large doses of a drug may be needed initially to obtain the required blood-level, the subsequent maintenance doses should be at a lower level that balances the rate of elimination or breakdown.

Idiosyncrasy and Hypersensitivity

The clinical response to most drugs used therapeutically can be predicted with a fair degree of certainty, based on past experience, but as patients do not react to drugs with machine-like precision, some individual variation in response is met with from time to time. Other patients may exhibit an unusual response to a drug, and such a reaction is known as an idiosyncrasy. These reactions may be associated with a genetic abnormality, as the haemolytic anaemia that sometimes follows the use of antimalarials of the primaquine group is due to the deficiency of a specific enzyme (glucose-6 dehydrogenase).

Hypersensitivity to drugs is much more serious. It is usually allergic in nature, and frequently indicates that the patient has become sensitised to the drug, so that subsequent treatment evokes an excessive response. Acetylsalicylic acid (aspirin) may precipitate a severe asthmatic attack in hypersensitive patients, especially those with a history of allergic disease. Penicillin, even in very small doses, may precipitate an anaphylactic shock (*q.v.*) in a sensitised patient, causing bronchoconstriction, low blood pressure and collapse. Many other drugs can occasionally cause a similar reaction, and the prompt intramuscular injection of adrenaline solution (1 ml.) may be life-saving. Other hypersensitivity reactions that may occur with a very wide range of drugs include skin reactions, or urticaria and the so-called ' drug fever ' is a pyrexial reaction similar to serum sickness (*q.v.*). Disturbances of the blood-forming system such as aplastic anaemia, and agranulocytosis may also be the result of a drug sensitivity. Haemolysis or the breakdown of already-formed blood cells may also be brought about by drugs such as the sulphonamides. Reliable tests to detect hypersensitivity have yet to be devised.

Side-effects

Hypersensitivity reactions to drugs must be distinguished from side-effects. Few drugs have a single, clear-cut and selective action on a particular organ of the body, and a side-effect is an unwanted pharmacological response that cannot be separated from the main action of the drug (although it may sometimes be reduced by combined therapy with other drugs). Thus morphine is a powerful analgesic by virtue of its depressant effect on the sensory area of the brain, but it also has a stimulant effect on the vomiting centre. This stimulation is the cause of the nausea and vomiting that may follow an injection of morphine, and which is a potential danger after operations such as cataract removal or gastrectomy. Other examples of side-effects of drugs include the dryness of the mouth and disturbances of vision that may occur when atropine and other anticholinergic drugs are given as antispasmodics and the drug-induced symptoms resembling parkinsonism that may result from extended treatment with tranquillisers of the phenothiazine group.

A knowledge of the side-effects of drugs is of great importance, and when a new compound has been synthesised by the organic chemist, it always undergoes a prolonged testing scheme before it is used clinically. These tests are first carried out in animals to assess activity, potency and toxicity, but there is always some difficulty in translating results obtained in such animal tests to the treatment of human illness. The tests are constantly being revised as the knowledge of side-effects increases, and the thalidomide disaster in recent years has heightened awareness of the dangers of inadequate testing.

Thalidomide was introduced as a safe hypnotic and less dangerous alternative to the barbiturates, a statement which was true in the light of knowledge at that time.

The original tests carried out with thalidomide in animals had shown that the drug had no adverse effect on development, and the drug was considered safe to use clinically. Unhappily, it was later discovered that if given during the early weeks of pregnancy, it could cause gross foetal abnormalities, and many children were born with deformed limbs due to thalidomide taken by the mother. This unusual toxic effect has led to a much more rigorous scheme of testing new drugs and the use of a wider range of test animals.

The introduction of any new drug thus carries very definite risks, but if no risks were taken, no therapeutic advance would be possible. The preliminary tests are therefore designed to obtain as much information about the drug as possible, so that the risks are reduced. In spite of exhaustive tests, some side-effects may not be revealed until the drug is used therapeutically on a wide scale, sometimes for a considerable time. Hepatic reactions, for example, are difficult to detect, either during preliminary testing or clinical trial, owing to the low incidence of such reactions, and the nurse can play a valuable and important part in detecting drug reactions by noting and reporting any unusual or unanticipated response to treatment with either a new or established product.

A Committee on Safety of Drugs now exists to investigate

and publicise all new reactions to drugs, and this increased awareness of potential dangers is in itself a valuable safety measure.

Drug Interactions

The introduction of more powerful drugs and the increasing
use of multiple therapy with two or more drugs has brought to
light a new problem, that of drug interaction. When two potent
drugs are given together, the action of one drug upon the other
may lead to an increase, reduction or modification of effect, sometimes with serious results. Some reactions may be unexpected,
such as the hypertensive crisis in a patient receiving an antidepressant of the monoamine oxidase inhibitor type after foods
containing pressor amines, i.e. cheese, broad beans, Marmite,
Bovril and chianti.

Many drugs, once absorbed, become more or less firmly bound
for a time to the plasma proteins. Slow diffusion into the circulation and tissues is followed by gradual metabolism or excretion of
the drug. This plasma binding is sometimes of therapeutic value,
as the long-acting sulphonamides owe much of their usefulness to
the high degree of plasma binding that occurs with these drugs.
The degree and firmness of binding varies very considerably from
drug to drug, and this difference can cause difficulties when two
or more drugs are prescribed together.

For example, the oral anticoagulants are extensively but not
firmly bound to plasma proteins, and the drugs are released from
the binding sites as the circulating drug is metabolised. But the
rate of release may be accelerated if a second drug with greater
plasma-binding power, such as phenylbutazone, is given. The
second drug will then displace the first, leading to a higher blood
level of the anticoagulant, with consequent risk of haemorrhage.
Many drugs are metabolised by the body enzymes, and some may
increase the amount of drug-metabolising enzymes in the liver,
and so not only increase the rate of their own breakdown, but also
that of other drugs. Some barbiturates increase enzyme activity,
and if given with an anticoagulant, may cause a more rapid breakdown, and in consequence the dose of anticoagulant will have to
be increased. A similar adjustment of dose in the reverse direction will be necessary when the barbiturate is withdrawn, otherwise an excessive response, with possible haemorrhage, may occur.

The monoamine oxidase inhibitors are another source of
danger, as they potentiate the effects of pressor drugs, central

nervous system stimulants and many other drugs. Some of the more important drug interactions are summarised in the following tables, but the best way to minimise drug reactions is to avoid combined therapy as much as possible.

	Drugs	Effects of Combination
Alcohol	C.N.S. depressants	The sedative effects of most central depressant drugs, are increased by alcohol, and in high doses may cause severe respiratory depression.
Anticoagulants (excluding heparin)	Chloral, glutethimide, griseofulvin, pheno-barbitone	Phenobarbitone in common with some other drugs, increases the production of certain drug-metabolising enzymes by the liver, and this activity may require the administration of larger doses of anticoagulants. Withdrawal of the sedative may result in a rise in the anticoagulant response, with possible haemorrhage.
	Clofibrate, phenylbuta-zone, phenytoin, salicylates	These drugs increase the effects of anticoagulants on the clotting time of the blood by the displacement of the anticoagulant that is bound to the plasma protein.
	Rifampicin	Rifamycin decreases the activity of oral anticoagulants, and combined therapy requires adjustment of dose.
Antihistamines	Alcohol and other C.N.S. depressants (*q.v.*)	
Barbiturates	Alcohol and other C.N.S. depressants (*q.v.*) Anticoagulants (*q.v.*) Griseofulvin, Phenytoin	Phenytoin is given with phenobarbitone in the treatment of epilepsy, but the increased production of drug-metabolising enzymes induced by phenobarbitone may reduce the duration of action of the phenytoin. Phenobarbitone can also reduce the blood level of griseofulvin.
Central stimu-lants of the amphetamine type	Monamine-oxidase inhibitors (*q.v.*) Hypotensive drugs (*q.v.*)	

	Drugs	Effects of Combination
Chloral	Anticoagulants (*q.v.*)	
Chlorpromazine and related drugs	Alcohol and other C.N.S. depressants (*q.v.*) Hypotensive agents (*q.v.*)	
Clofibrate	Anticoagulants (*q.v.*) Oral anti-diabetic agents (*q.v.*)	
Digitalis	Thiazide diuretics (*q.v.*)	
Griseofulvin	Anticoagulants (*q.v.*)	
Hypotensive agents	Monoamine oxidase inhibitors (*q.v.*) Thiazide diuretics (*q.v.*) Antidepressants Pressor drugs	Tricyclic antidepressants may antagonise the action of guanethidine and other antihypertensive drugs. Sympathomimetic drugs, by their pressor action, have a similar effect.
Monoamine oxidase inhibitors	Alcohol Antihistamines Amphetamines and other pressor drugs Benzhexol and other drugs used in Parkinsonism Hypotensive drugs (*q.v.*) Insulin L-dopa Narcotic analgesics Oral anti-diabetic drugs Thiazide diuretics (*q.v.*) Tricyclic antidepressants	The monoamine oxidase inhibitors may increase or modify the action of a wide range of unrelated substances. The action of any C.N.S. stimulant will be increased, sometimes markedly so, and the effects of narcotic analgesics, tricyclic antidepressants, hypotensive drugs and thiazide diuretics may also be potentiated. Monoamine oxidase inhibitors increase hepatic glycolysis and potentiate the action of oral anti-diabetic drugs. The pressor effects of tyramine, present in foods such as cheese, broad beans, Marmite and chianti will also be increased by the monoamine oxidase inhibitors.
Morphine, pethidine and similar narcotics	Monoamine oxidase inhibitors (*q.v.*)	
Oral anti-diabetic drugs	Barbiturates (*q.v.*) Clofibrate (*q.v.*) Salicylates Sulphonamides Monoamine oxidase, inhibitors (*q.v.*)	The action of oral antidiabetic drugs may be increased by displacement from plasma binding, or by increasing the activity of liver enzymes.

Drugs		Effects of Combination
Penicillin	Chloramphenicol and tetracyclines	Chloramphenicol and the tetracyclines are bacteriostatic in action, whereas penicillin is bactericidal. In general, combination should be avoided, as mixtures of bacteriostatic and bactericidal antibiotics may have an antagonistic action.
Phenylbutazone and related compounds	Anticoagulants (*q.v.*) Long-acting sulphonamides	These suphonamides can be displaced from plasma binding by other drugs, such as phenylbutazone. Such displacement modifies both duration of action and tissue concentration of the sulphonamide.
Phenytoin	Anticoagulants (*q.v.*)	
Propranolol and related beta-adrenergic blocking agents	Ether, chloroform	Effects of the anaesthetic may be potentiated.
Salicylates	Anti-coagulants (*q.v.*) Oral antidiabetic drugs (*q.v.*) Insulin Methotrexate	Salicylates increase the uptake and use of glucose by the tissues, thus increasing the effects of insulin. Salicylates also increase the action of methotrexate by displacement from binding sites.
Thiazide diuretics	Digitalis Hypotensive drugs (*q.v.*) Monoamine oxidase inhibitors (*q.v.*)	The loss of potassium caused by the thiazide diuretics may increase the sensitivity of the heart to digitalis.
Tubocurarine and other muscle relaxants	Neomycin and related antibiotics Neostigmine and similar anticholinesterases	These antibiotics also have some curare-like properties, and may extend the relaxant action of tubocurarine and delay restoration of muscular function. Neostigimine inhibits the breakdown of acetylcholine at nerve endings and such inhibition reverses the action of curare-form muscle relaxants. This effect is made use of in surgery to promote prompt return of muscle function after operation. (Suxamethonium is not reversible by neostigmine.)

Presentation of Drugs

It is one thing to extract or synthesise an active compound, but to present it in a form acceptable to the patient is another. Unless a patient actually takes the prescribed medicament in the correct dose, diagnosis and therapy are both in vain, and consequently the art of preparing medicinal substances in a form suitable for administration is of considerable importance. Many factors govern the final form of presentation. In making an acceptable preparation of a drug it is essential to retain the therapeutic activity, and successful formulation demands a wide knowledge of chemical structure, pharmacology, solubility, stability and activity of the drug.

Thus it is of little use to prepare a coated tablet to conceal the bitter taste of a drug if the coating fails to disintegrate in the alimentary tract, or to sterilise an unstable drug without considering the addition of a stabilising agent to limit or prevent decomposition during sterilisation. The choice of containers and closures may also play a significant but often forgotten part in ensuring that the product will retain its activity during storage under widely different climatic conditions.

Many preparations of drugs now on the market exhibit considerable ingenuity in the means employed to increase acceptability or prolong the action of the drug, but basically the preparations of drugs used in therapeutics can be divided into three main groups —*i.e.* oral preparations, applications and injections. Each group may be further subdivided, and examples of most forms of presentation will be found in the British National Formulary (B.N.F.). Oral preparations include the following :—

Mixtures.—Mixtures are aqueous solutions or suspensions of drugs in water, together with flavouring or suspending agents. They were once the most popular form of drug presentation, but have been largely replaced by tablets.

Mixtures, however, are not to be despised, as they are still of value in selected circumstances, even if given merely as a placebo, and it is worth noting that some fifty different mixtures are described in the British National Formulary. The standard dose of mixtures in the B.N.F. is 10 ml. and Kaolin and Morphine Mixture (Mist *: Kaolin : et Morph :) is a familiar example.

* As Latin was once the language used in prescription writing, the Latin names of a number of old preparations still survive, *e.g.* ' Mist.' for mixture, ' Gutt ' for eye drops, ' Ung. ' for ointment. Traces of this Latin influence also persist in the names of various metallic salts. Thus sodii refers to sodium, argentii to silver, ferri to iron, hydrargyri to mercury and cupri to copper.

Draught.—Strictly speaking, a single dose of a drug administered in an aqueous vehicle ; Paraldehyde Draught, B.P.C. is an example.

Infusions.—Infusions are aqueous solutions of the active principles of crude drugs. Like tea, an infusion is prepared by adding boiling water to the drug, and the liquid, when decanted and cooled, forms the infusion. They were once used extensively as the basic, aqueous constituents of many mixtures, *e.g.* Infusion of Gentian in Gentian and Alkali Mixture (Mist : Gent : Alk :). Infusions do not keep well, and a preservative, such as spirit of chloroform, is usually added to mixtures containing infusions.

Elixirs.—Flavoured and sweetened solutions of drugs, usually those of bitter taste, *e.g.* Cascara Elixir and Ephedrine Elixir, B.N.F.

Tinctures.—Tinctures are alcoholic solutions of the active principles of crude drugs, *e.g.* Belladonna Tincture. Tinctures keep well, and retain their activity for a considerable period. The term once included alcoholic solutions of other substances, and the well-known tincture of iodine is a surviving example of this older use.

Emulsion.—A term applied to mixtures of oils and water, rendered homogeneous by the addition of other substances known as emulsifying agents. Liquid Paraffin Emulsion, B.P.C., is an example of an oil-in-water emulsion and contains methyl cellulose as the emulsifying agent. The natural gum acacia has similar properties, and is an effective emulsifying agent for a variety of oils. Water-in-oil emulsions, *e.g.* Oily Cream B.P., (Ung. Aquos :) contain derivatives of lanolin or wool fat as the emulsifying agent.

Linctus.—A sweet, syrupy preparation of a drug used in the treatment of cough, *e.g.* Codeine Linctus, Simple Linctus, B.P.C.

Tablets.—One of the most satisfactory and reliable forms of oral medication. They have the great advantage over mixtures of affording an accurate dose, but the ease with which they can be taken sometimes leads to indiscriminate self-medication by many patients. The frequent and often excessive use of aspirin and other analgesic tablets is a familiar example. Tablets are prepared either directly from the drug itself, as with aspirin or, in the case of potent drugs of low dose, by first diluting the drug with an inert powder such as lactose, to obtain a suitable bulk to form a tablet of convenient size. The powder thus obtained is mixed with a small amount of starch, and then formed into granules, which are subsequently compressed into tablets. The starch is added to ensure disintegration when the tablets are swallowed. Many tablets are now coated to improve stability and appearance. In cases where the drug is a gastric irritant or is broken down by gastric acid, a so-called ' enteric ' coating may be used. Such coating is designed to permit the tablet to pass unchanged into the intestine, where absorption takes place. Some long-acting tablets contain the drug in the interstices of a porous plastic core, from which the active compound is slowly leached out as the tablet passes along the alimentary tract.

Cachets.—Small boxes made of rice flour, used for giving drugs that have a bitter or nauseous taste, and which are prescribed in doses larger than those that can easily be given in tablet form, *e.g.* cachets of PAS (para-aminosalicylic acid).

Capsules.—Small containers made of hard gelatin, resembling a cylindrical box with a very deep lid. They are useful as a means of administering bitter drugs such as the barbiturates, *e.g.* amylobarbitone capsules, and are also popular as containers for orally-active antibiotics, *e.g.* ampicillin capsules. Flexible gelatin capsules are also used occasionally, particularly for small doses of unpleasant liquids such as tetrachlorethylene.

Pills.—Pills are small spheres containing active constituents massed together with inert additives and gum. They are now rarely used, as tablets are much more satisfactory and reliable.

Preparations for Local Application

This group comprises a wide range of products intended for local application to the body, some with a general, others with a restricted use, and include the following :—

Lotions.—Solutions or suspensions of drugs for application to the skin, wounds or mucous membranes, *e.g.* Aluminium Acetate Lotion B.N.F., and Calamine Lotion (Lotio Calaminae). Eye lotions are still occasionally prescribed as collyria, *e.g.* Collyr : Sodii Bicarb.

Liniments.—Thin creams or oily preparations of drugs, applied to the skin by rubbing, *e.g.* White Liniment, and Methyl Salicylate Liniment.

Ointments.—Semi-solid preparations intended for application to the skin, *e.g.* Zinc Ointment (Ung : Zinc :). The base in which the active medicament is incorporated may vary considerably according to the drug and condition under treatment. Greasy bases contain soft paraffin, aqueous bases may contain emulsifying waxes, and others may contain wool fat. Eye ointments are prepared with a base of yellow soft paraffin, liquid paraffin and wool fat.

Creams.—These are semi-solid emulsions, and differ from ointments in containing a high proportion of water. Cetrimïde cream and chlorhexidine cream are examples of aqueous creams containing emulsifying waxes. Zinc cream is an oily cream containing wool fat as the emulsifying agent.

Pastes.—Stiff ointments, often containing a large amount of zinc oxide ; *e.g.* Coal Tar Paste (Pasta Picis Carb :), Zinc Oxide and Salicylic Acid Paste (Lassar's Paste, B.N.F.).

Suppositories.—Solid products prepared for rectal administration. The medicament is incorporated in a fatty or glycogelatin base that melts about body temperature, and may have a systemic or a local action.

Pessaries.—Medicated solid products prepared for vaginal administration and intended to have a local effect.

Injections

An injection is a sterile solution of a drug intended for parenteral administration by intramuscular, intravenous or subcutaneous injection, or less frequently by intradermal, intrathecal or intra-articular administration. The intramuscular route is employed for most injections, as absorption is fairly rapid and even potentially irritant solutions of drugs may be tolerated by this route. Subcutaneous injections are absorbed more slowly, and are less well tolerated.

Drugs which are too irritant to be given intramuscularly can often be given, after suitable dilution, by slow intravenous injection or by intravenous drip infusion.

Intradermal injections are used mainly for diagnostic tests, and intrathecal injections are occasionally employed when the drug concerned does not penetrate the blood-brain barrier easily, and direct injection into the c.s.f. is necessary. In the treatment of meningitis for example, a high and localised concentration of an antibiotic in the c.s.f. can be obtained by intrathecal injection. Intra-articular injection refers to the injection of a solution or suspension of a drug into a joint. Injections are best dispensed as ampoules, which are sealed glass containers containing a single dose. Multiple-dose containers are also used but are less satisfactory. These are rubber-capped bottles, designed to permit successive doses to be withdrawn by a syringe. All solutions supplied in multiple-dose containers must contain a preservative to guard against the risk of accidental bacterial contamination of the contents.

Inhalations

The older types of inhalation, occasionally referred to as vapours, are products containing aromatic and antiseptic substances of a volatile nature. In use, a small amount of the preparation is added to a quantity of boiling water, and the steam and volatile constituents of the product are then inhaled. Menthol, often in association with Compound Tincture of Benzoin, is frequently inhaled in this way.

In recent years the oral inhalation of certain drugs, particularly bronchodilators such as isoprenaline (q.v.), has been developed extensively with the introduction of the aerosol. These aerosols, exemplified by the Medi-haler and similar products, contain the drug in solution in a pressurised container, with an inert gas as the propellant. When the pressure is temporarily released by depressing the valve of the aerosol, the medicament is discharged as an exceedingly fine spray. These spray particles are so fine that if inhaled, they are carried deep into the lungs, where absorption is so rapid that the response is comparable with that following an injection. Any large particles would be trapped in the upper part of the respiratory tract, and so fail to be absorbed. These aerosol products are usually supplied with a metering valve, so that only a measured dose is released for each inhalation. In the treatment of asthma and bronchospasm, these aerosol products permit a dose to be given quickly at the time of need, and evoke a rapid and effective response. Their chief danger is the risk of overdosage and consequent cardiac stimulation that may occur if the drug is inhaled too frequently by over-anxious patients. With proper use, this danger can be markedly reduced, and explicit instructions concerning frequency of dose should be given to all patients using these bronchodilator aerosols.

CHAPTER II

DRUGS ACTING ON THE CENTRAL NERVOUS SYSTEM

DRUGS which act on some part of the central nervous system represent the largest and most important group of therapeutic agents. They can be divided into two main groups—the central nervous system (C.N.S.) stimulants and the central nervous system depressants. The latter is by far the larger and more important group, and can be further divided and classified in general terms as anaesthetics, narcotics, hypnotics, sedatives, tranquillisers, antidepressants, anticonvulsants, and analgesics.

GENERAL ANAESTHETICS

These are substances which bring about a loss of consciousness. They vary widely in composition from simple gases to complex organic chemicals, but fall easily into two main groups—those given by inhalation, and those given by intravenous injection. Surgical anaesthesia is characterised by loss of both consciousness and pain, and an adequate degree of relaxation of muscle. Three main stages are recognised : STAGE I—A stage in which the perception of pain is reduced, or almost suppressed, but the patient is still conscious, although very detached. STAGE II—A very variable stage in which consciousness is lost, but irrational acts of an excited nature can occur. This stage is not common with intravenous anaesthetics. STAGE III—Full anaesthesia. In this stage the irregular breathing of Stage II becomes steady, reflexes are abolished, and a progressive degree of muscular relaxation occurs as anaesthesia deepens.

Before the introduction of intravenous anaesthetics and muscle relaxants, adequate relaxation could be achieved only by full amounts of anaesthetic, with undesired toxic side-effects. To-day, by suitable premedication and the use of short-acting or long-acting relaxants, relaxation can be secured under a light plane of anaesthesia, thus reducing shock and trauma, permitting a more rapid return to consciousness and enabling major operations to be carried out in the elderly that were once considered impossible.

INHALATION ANAESTHETICS

Chloroform

A clear heavy liquid with a characteristic sweetish odour. It is of some historical interest as one of the first inhalation anaesthetics, being introduced by Simpson in 1847. Unlike ether the vapour is not inflammable. The induction of anaesthesia is smooth, muscular relaxation is good, and the vapour does not irritate the bronchi. Chloroform, however, has some serious disadvantages. It may cause a fall in blood pressure and a potentially dangerous depression of respiration. Sudden death from cardiac arrest may occur during chloroform anaesthesia. This is due to an increased sensitivity of the heart to adrenaline, which may cause ventricular fibrillation, but can be minimised by adequate premedication with atropine. The drug has a toxic effect on the liver, and for this reason chloroform should not be given to patients with hepatic disease as jaundice may occur during the post-operative period. These toxic effects have led to a marked decline in the use of chloroform, as with new apparatus its advantages may be achieved with safer drugs.

Cyclopropane

This anaesthetic is an inflammable gas, and is supplied in metal cylinders, which are orange-coloured for identification. It is a powerful, non-irritant, volatile anaesthetic, with which induction is prompt, recovery rapid, and post-operative vomiting slight. Cyclopropane is therefore often preferred in chest surgery. It may cause a marked depression of respiration in some patients, but its most serious disadvantage is its tendency to cause cardiac irregularities. This risk is increased by adrenaline and many similar drugs. Cyclopropane, however, can be given with large amounts of oxygen, and is therefore sometimes preferred for patients with heart disease. It is expensive and should be used in closed-circuit apparatus.

Ether

A clear, colourless, inflammable liquid. It decomposes slowly on exposure to light and air, and anaesthetic ether is therefore supplied in amber bottles. It has long been used as an anaesthetic, as it causes less depression of respiration and lowering of blood pressure than chloroform, and has no toxic effects on the heart.

When ether is used as the sole anaesthetic the induction period is slow, and the stage of excitement is prolonged, but this may be overcome by using an ether-nitrous oxide mixture, and also by previous medication with hypnotics. An increase in the flow of saliva and mucus occurs during ether anaesthesia, owing to the irritant effect of the drug on the bronchial tract, but this can be reduced by premedication with atropine. This irritant action may also cause coughing or occasional laryngeal spasm, but this passes off as the bronchial muscles relax with the deepening anaesthesia. Ether has a wide margin of safety, and there is little risk of ventricular fibrillation, the most dangerous complication being ether convulsions. These are not common and are more likely to occur during deep anaesthesia in children who have a raised temperature due to infection. In such circumstances the anaesthetic should be stopped and a small dose of an intravenous barbiturate given ; oxygen may also be necessary for the deepening respiratory depression that follows.

Ethyl Chloride

This is a gas at ordinary temperatures, but liquefies so easily that it is supplied in bottles with special spray nozzles. As an anaesthetic its use is limited as the vapour is irritant to the bronchial tract, but it may be used for short operations as recovery from light ethyl chloride anaesthesia is rapid. Nausea is uncommon, but headache may occur. Ethyl chloride for anaesthetic use contains eau-de-Cologne to mask the somewhat unpleasant odour of the gas.

Halothane

A clear colourless liquid with a chloroform-like odour. It is a volatile anaesthetic of high potency with which induction of anaesthesia is smooth and rapid. A fall in blood pressure and a slowing of the pulse may occur during halothane anaesthesia, but the latter can be relieved by an injection of atropine. Halothane increases the relaxant effects of tubocurarine. Jaundice and liver damage have sometimes followed halothane anaesthesia, but it has not been proved that halothane is the cause of the hepatic dysfunction. The drug is powerful but expensive, and is best given by apparatus specially designed for its use. It has the considerable advantages of not being inflammable, or forming explosive mixtures with air or oxygen. Methoxyflurane (Penthrane) is an anaesthetic similar in general properties to halothane. *Brand name:* Fluothane.

Nitrous Oxide

The oldest and safest of the inhalation anaesthetics. It is a gas at ordinary temperatures, but for anaesthetic purposes it is compressed and supplied in metal cylinders, which are painted blue as an aid to identification. When pure nitrous oxide is inhaled for half a minute or so, a light degree of anaesthesia is produced which lasts about forty seconds. Recovery is rapid and complete in two to three minutes, and after-effects are uncommon. If inhalation of the pure gas is continued, cyanosis develops very quickly owing to lack of oxygen and full nitrous oxide anaesthesia is limited to dental extractions and other brief operations. With mixtures of nitrous oxide and oxygen, anaesthesia may be prolonged without difficulty, and if supplemented by ether or other anaesthetic, a deeper plane of anaesthesia can be achieved.

Trichloroethylene

A liquid with an odour recalling that of chloroform, and for anaesthetic use it is usually tinted blue to aid identification. It is less powerful than ether or chloroform, but induction of anaesthesia is smooth and rapid. Trichloroethylene is useful for short operations, as it does not produce deep anaesthesia or full muscular relaxation. For extended operations anaesthesia may be induced with trichloroethylene, and maintained with more potent drugs. It should never be used in closed-circuit apparatus, as the soda-lime in such apparatus may decompose the drug and form a toxic by-product. Adrenaline should never be given during anaesthesia with trichloroethylene, as there is then a risk of ventricular fibrillation. *Brand name:* Trilene.

Vinyl Ether

A clear colourless liquid with some of the properties of ether and ethyl chloride. Vinyl ether is much more powerful than ether, and is more rapid in action, but recovery is equally rapid. Nausea and vomiting are not common, but salivation may be troublesome. It is considered by some anaesthetists to be one of the safest of all anaesthetics, particularly for dental anaesthesia in children, as recovery is more rapid than after halothane, and there are fewer side-effects. *Brand name:* Vinesthene.

INTRAVENOUS ANAESTHETICS

These drugs are, with very few exceptions, short-acting barbiturates in the form of the sodium salts. These sodium salts are soluble in water, and in suitable strength can be injected directly into a vein. Such solutions are very alkaline, and great care must be taken that none of the injection solution escapes into the surrounding tissues. Any such leakage may cause severe tissue or nerve damage. If accidentally injected intra-arterially instead of intravenously, severe and extremely painful arterial spasm is caused, followed by thrombosis which may lead to subsequent gangrene or even the loss of the arm. The injection of such barbiturate solutions therefore requires considerable care, and fractional doses are given very slowly at first so that the effect can be assessed. The induction phase characteristic of inhalation anaesthesia is absent, and surgical anaesthesia occurs very quickly without excitement.

Hexobarbitone Sodium †

This substance was the first of the intravenous barbiturates, introduced under the name Evipan. It is used as a 10 per cent. solution, which should be freshly prepared and given slowly at the rate of 1 ml. in fifteen seconds. Unconsciousness occurs in about thirty seconds, and anaesthesia may be maintained by subsequent doses. The drug has now been largely replaced by thiopentone sodium, which gives greater muscle relaxation. *Brand name :* Cyclonal Sodium.†

Thiopentone Sodium †

Thiopentone sodium is a widely used intravenous anaesthetic, and is given as a freshly prepared 2·5 per cent. solution, in doses of 100 to 150 mg., with further doses at intervals if anaesthesia is to be prolonged. A 5 per cent. solution may also be used, but is more likely to cause venous thrombosis. The anaesthetic effect is apparent within thirty seconds, and there is no stage of excitement. Depth of anaesthesia is determined by the degree of depression of respiration, as the usual eye signs are unreliable. Such respiratory depression, although relatively transient, may be severe. The drug produces some fall in blood pressure, and care is necessary in patients with hypertension, cardiac disease or impaired liver function. Thiopentone may also be used in association with the muscle relaxants, and the combination enables the dose of thiopentone to be reduced whilst permitting full muscular relaxation for major abdominal operations. *Brand names :* Intraval Sodium † ; Pentothal.†

Other soluble barbiturates used as intravenous anaesthetics include thialbarbitone sodium (Kemithal †), and methohexitone sodium (Brietal †). Methohexitone sodium is a very quick-acting drug, but its chief advantage is that recovery of consciousness is prompt. It is therefore useful for minor procedures in out-patient and casualty departments.

Propanidid

Many attempts have been made to find non-barbiturate intravenous anaesthetics with less marked respiratory and circulatory depressant effects, and propanidid has many of the required properties. Propanidid is given by intravenous injection as a 2·5 per cent. solution in doses of 5 to 10 mg. per kg. body weight, and it induces a smooth anaesthesia which lasts about three to five minutes. It may be used in association with volatile anaesthetics if a longer action is required. Recovery from propanidid is rapid and may be complete in five to ten minutes, so the drug is very suitable for out-patient use. Cardiac irregularities are uncommon with propanidid, an effect that may be linked with its local anaesthetic action (see lignocaine, page 91). *Brand name:* Epontol.

BASAL ANAESTHETIC

Bromethol †

Bromethol is sometimes referred to as a basal anaesthetic, *i.e.* one that produces a light plane of anaesthesia, and with which other drugs are required to produce full surgical anaesthesia. It has been used in general surgery and to control the spasms of tetanus, but owing to irregular absorption and frequent respiratory depression its use has declined. It is still used occasionally in eclampsia, and in the production of obstetric amnesia. The standard dose of bromethol is 0·1 ml. per kg. body weight, diluted with warm water to make a 2·5 per cent. solution, and given by slow rectal infusion. The solution should be freshly prepared, and tested before use with congo red indicator. Any solution giving a blue colour, indicating decomposition, must be discarded. Paraldehyde (*q.v.*) as an 8 per cent. solution, is also given rectally as a basal anaesthetic. *Brand name :* Avertin.†

LOCAL ANAESTHETICS

Drugs which prevent the transmission of impulses along sensory nerves, so that the impulse does not reach the central nervous system to be felt as pain, are known as local anaesthetics. As a group they are of considerable importance, and can be divided into those compounds which are applied to the skin and mucous membranes, and those which are injected around nerve trunks. The distinction is not complete as some compounds can be used both topically and by injection. Those drugs used to produce regional anaesthesia by intraspinal injection will be considered separately.

Cocaine *

Cocaine is the alkaloid obtained from coca leaves and is the oldest of the local anaesthetics. It has powerful anaesthetic properties, both when applied locally or when injected, but as there is considerable individual variation in the sensitivity to cocaine, and to its toxic effects, the drug has been largely replaced by safer compounds.

Cocaine hydrochloride still has a place in ophthalmology, as it also dilates the pupil of the eye as well as producing a marked anaesthetic effect. Solutions of 2 per cent. strength are commonly used. Limited amounts of stronger solutions are sometimes used for application to the nose and throat.

Cocaine also has a stimulant action on the central nervous system, and the marked euphoric effects thus produced have led to addiction to the drug. This is a serious social problem, and for that reason cocaine is now little used therapeutically, but many other drugs are also capable of causing addiction. The only safe rule is never to take any potent drug unless it has been prescribed for a particular need.

A large number of synthetic local anaesthetics have been introduced from time to time, and whilst few have so wide a range of anaesthetic activity as cocaine, they have very useful applications, and the very considerable advantage of reduced toxicity. Representative synthetic compounds include the following :—

Benzocaine

Benzocaine is virtually insoluble in water, and in consequence it is used mainly for topical application as ointment (10 per cent.) or dusting powder, or as the anaesthetic constituent of various antiseptic lozenges. The drug is soluble in oils and fats, and suppositories of benzocaine (500 mg.) are used for painful haemorrhoids.

Procaine Hydrochloride †

At one time procaine hydrochloride was the most widely used of the cocaine substitutes, as it is amongst the least toxic of the local anaesthetics. Originally introduced as Novocain, it has now been replaced to a great extent by lignocaine (*q.v.*). Procaine is of no value as a topical anaesthetic, as it is not absorbed, but when injected as a 1 to 2 per cent. solution, anaesthesia is rapidly produced. Adrenaline or noradrenaline may be added in a strength of 1-50,000 to 1-200,000, to localise the distribution of the anaesthetic, thus permitting a prolonged action. Such combined solutions have been widely employed for infiltration anaesthesia in minor surgery, regional nerve blocks, in dentistry and to relieve the pain of sprains and minor fractures. They should not be used for the anaesthesia of fingers or toes, as the prolonged vasoconstrictor effects may reduce blood flow so much that tissue damage may occur. The once wide use of procaine is an indication of its low toxicity, but hypersensitivity to the drug is not unknown.

Cinchocaine †

Cinchocaine is of interest as one of the most powerful of local anaesthetics. It is more toxic than cocaine, but the greater potency permits lower doses, and the drug has an increased margin of safety. Cinchocaine has a range of activity similar to that of cocaine but it is used mainly by local application as an ointment (1 per cent.). Suppositories are also available. *Brand names:* Nupercaine, Nupercainol.

Lignocaine †

Originally introduced as Xylocaine, this compound is one of the most active and widely used of the local anaesthetics. It produces a local anaesthesia similar to procaine, but the action is more rapid, intense and prolonged. It is widely employed in dentistry as a 2 per cent. solution, together with a vasoconstrictor such as adrenaline or noradrenaline to localise the action; in regional anaesthesia 0·5 to 1 per cent. solutions are used. Lignocaine is also of considerable value for peridural and epidural anaesthesia during thoracic surgery (see also spinal anaesthetics). Like cocaine, lignocaine is effective when applied topically, and may be used as ointment, eye drops (2 per cent.) and throat spray (4 per cent.). Xylodase is a cream containing lignocaine and hyaluronidase, for application to mucous areas. A gel containing 1 to 2 per cent. lignocaine is widely used as a urethral anaesthetic before instrumentation. In the U.S.A. the drug is known as lidocaine. The use of lignocaine in the treatment of cardiac arrhythmia is referred to on page 91. *Brand names :* Xylocaine, Xylotox, Lidothesin.

A number of other local anaesthetics of the cocaine type are also available such as amethocaine † and prilocaine † (Citanest †) but are used less extensively.

SPINAL AND EPIDURAL ANAESTHESIA

Amethocaine, cinchocaine and some related drugs may be used by intraspinal and epidural injection to produce a localised anaesthesia. For a full consideration of the subject the standard textbooks of anaesthesia should be consulted, but briefly it should be noted that anaesthesia of the lower limbs and abdomen may be obtained by injecting specially prepared local anaesthetic solutions into the subarachnoid space. Such solutions, which must be injected below the first and second lumbar vertebrae to avoid injury to the spinal cord, produce their effects by anaesthetising the spinal nerves at their junction with the spinal column. Spinal anaesthetics produce great muscular relaxation, and may be used in conditions and patients where other methods might be less safe. The area and degree of anaesthesia can be controlled by modifying the specific gravity of the solution and altering the position of the patient so that the solution flows over the appropriate nerves. Disadvantages of the method include the increased risk of infection by bacteria reaching the cerebrospinal fluid, the fall in blood pressure that may occur, and the frequency of post-operative headache.

Epidural anaesthesia is a development of spinal anaesthesia, and is carried out by injecting the anaesthetic solution into the space outside the dura (the epidural space). As the solution takes time to diffuse and reach the nerves the onset of action is slow, but in skilled hands the method has certain advantages. It is used chiefly in obstetrics.

SEDATIVES AND HYPNOTICS

Sedatives are drugs that reduce mental activity, and thus predispose to sleep, whereas hypnotics are sleep-inducing drugs. There is no sharp distinction between the groups, as many sedatives, in full doses, have a hypnotic action, and small doses of some hypnotics have useful sedative properties. Insomnia is a common problem, and before drugs are used it should be remembered that simple measures, such as adequate physical relaxation and absence of stimulants, will often promote sleep. When insomnia is due to pain, sedatives and hypnotics are useless if given alone, and in such cases it is essential to give an analgesic as well, when the relief of the pain will reinforce the action of the hypnotic.

It should be borne in mind that although drug-induced sleep may appear to resemble natural sleep, the two are far from being identical. Natural sleep has two main phases, referred to as the orthodox or slow wave phase, and the paradoxical or R.E.M. (rapid eye movement) phase. Hypnotic drugs may suppress the R.E.M. phase, and also influence the orthodox phase. The latter plays an important part in the growth and restoration of body tissues, but the R.E.M. phase is linked with the restorative activities of brain tissue. Thus although hypnotic drugs are of great value in short-term treatment, their extended use may have hitherto unsuspected disadvantages.

Carbromal † (dose, 0·3 to 1 G.)

Carbromal is one of the older non-barbiturate sedative and hypnotic drugs. As it is not very soluble, it should be taken with a hot drink about half an hour before bed-time. Continual use over long periods may cause purpuric eruptions and severe depression. It is present with pentobarbitone sodium in Carbrital. *Brand name :* Adalin.†

Ethchlorvynol † (Arvynol,† Serenesil †), ethinamate † (Valmidate †) and bromvaletone † (Bromural) † are examples of other hypnotics of medium activity.

Chloral Hydrate † (dose, 0·3 to 2 G.)

A crystalline substance with a characteristic odour and bitter taste. It is rapidly absorbed when given orally, and within thirty minutes produces a condition resembling natural sleep, which may last for several hours. In standard doses it is a useful and safe hypnotic, of particular value in nervous insomnia and mania. Prolonged use of chloral may produce tolerance and dependence, but otherwise the drug has few side-effects in ordinary doses. As it is well tolerated by infants, chloral hydrate is often used for infantile convulsions. Paediatric Chloral Elixir (200 mg. in 5 ml.) is a suitable preparation and may be given in doses of 2·5 to 7·5 ml. Chloral hydrate should be given well diluted, as otherwise it may cause gastric irritation and for that reason the drug is not available in tablet form. If combined with phenazone to form dichloralphenazone, as in Welldorm,† the irritant properties of chloral are reduced, and the product is therefore suitable for administration as a tablet. Each Welldorm † tablet is equivalent to 0·6 G. of chloral hydrate.

Chloral is altered in the body to trichloroethanol, and the sedative effects are finally due to that compound. The phosphoric acid derivative of trichloroethanol (triclofos †) has the sedative action of the parent drug without the side-effects, and the compound is available as Tricloryl † in tablets, containing 0·5 G. and as a syrup (100 mg. per ml.).

Somilan † is a similar product containing chloral-betaine.

Glutethimide † (dose, 250 to 500 mg.)

Glutethimide has an action very similar to that of the short-acting barbiturates, and is useful when a non-barbiturate sedative and hypnotic is required. Prolonged administration has caused toxic psychoses, and addiction has been reported following its use in mental stress and depression. *Brand name :* Doriden.†

Methaqualone † (dose, 75 to 300 mg.)

Methaqualone is a widely used sedative and hypnotic, and also has some anticonvulsant properties. As a day-time sedative, doses of 75 mg. may be given, but as a hypnotic a dose of 150 to 300 mg.

is required. Doses of 100 to 300 mg. daily have been used in epilepsy in association with other anticonvulsants. Methaqualone is present with diphenhydramine in Mandrax.† *Brand name :* Melsedin.†

Methylpentynol † (dose, 250 to 1000 mg.)

A clear liquid similar in physical properties to paraldehyde. It is a very mild hypnotic with a very brief action, and its chief therapeutic use is the temporary relief of nervous tension and apprehension. For this purpose it is given in doses of 250-500 mg., usually as capsules. Methylpentynol carbamate has a longer action, and is given in doses of 200 to 400 mg. In larger doses of 500 to 1000 mg. it may be given as a mild hypnotic. *Brand names :* Oblivon,† Somnesin.† Oblivon-C † is a longer-acting modification.

Methyprylone † (dose, 200 to 400 mg.)

A compound similar to glutethimide in action, and useful as an alternative to the barbiturates. It is an effective day-time sedative in anxiety and stress, or in larger doses as an hypnotic for insomnia. *Brand name :* Noludar.†

Nitrazepam † (dose, 5 to 20 mg.)

Most hypnotics have a general depressant action on the brain, particularly on the so-called 'reticular formation' which is adjacent to the hypothalamus. Nitrazepam, which is related chemically to tranquillisers such as chlordiazepoxide, has a different action, and by reducing the susceptibility of the hypothalamus to external stimuli, has sleep-inducing properties of a new type. The sleep induced by nitrazepam appears to resemble natural sleep more closely than that induced by barbiturates and other central nervous system depressants, and arousal and return to sleep also follow a more natural pattern.

Nitrazepam is given in doses of 5 to 10 mg., which may be increased in some cases to 20 mg. The effects of the drug begin within thirty to forty-five minutes, and sleep usually lasts up to eight hours. The full response may not be invoked immediately in patients who have taken barbiturates for long periods. The toxicity of the drug is low, and very large doses have been given experimentally without harmful effects. Its introduction marks a new approach to the old problem of insomnia. *Brand name :* Mogadon.†

Paraldehyde † (dose, 2 to 8 ml.)

Paraldehyde is a colourless liquid with a characteristic odour and burning taste. It is one of the safest hypnotics available, resembling chloral hydrate in action, being rapidly absorbed and inducing sleep within about fifteen minutes. Like other volatile substances it is excreted in part by the lungs, and imparts an unpleasant odour to the breath. Paraldehyde is used mainly in mental disorders, in cardiac conditions (as it has little depressant effect on the heart) and in the treatment of tetanus. It may be given in mixture form as Paraldehyde Draught, and doses of 15 to 30 ml. mixed with arachis oil or saline may be given as an enema. Paraldehyde may be given by intramuscular injection (which may be painful) in doses of 5 to 10 ml. for violent patients, or in status epilepticus. Paraldehyde decomposes slowly on exposure to light and air with the formation of toxic break-down products, and it should be stored in small bottles in a cool, dark place. Addiction to the drug is not unknown.

Potassium Bromide (dose, 1 to 6 G. daily in divided doses)

This substance was once widely employed in the treatment of epilepsy before anticonvulsants were available, but it now survives only as a very mild sedative of doubtful value. If given for long periods bromides tend to accumulate in the body, as urinary elimination is incomplete, and a condition of mental confusion, known as ' bromism ', may occur, often accompanied by a rash resembling acne.

BARBITURATES

The barbiturates are an extremely important and very widely used group of hypnotics and sedatives. They are all derivatives of barbituric acid, and are usually classified according to their duration of action. Differences in degree and nature of their activity are related both to the variations in their structure and to their fate in the body.

Thus the longer-acting compounds are slowly absorbed and excreted largely unchanged in the urine, whereas the medium and rapid-acting compounds are broken down in varying degree by the liver and muscles, or are removed from the circulation by temporary storage in the body fat. The barbiturates have a general depressant action on the central nervous system at all levels, and the degree of effect varies according to dose. In normal doses they have little action on blood pressure or respiration when taken alone, but respiratory depression may be markedly increased if much alcohol is also taken. Alcohol also has sedative and hypnotic properties, and if taken with barbiturates the effect of both drugs is increased. Patients should be warned of this danger when taking barbiturates, as coma and death have occurred from the severe respiratory depression caused by the combined effects of the hypnotic and alcohol. Tolerance to the barbiturates may occur but psychic dependence is more common in mentally unstable patients. Barbiturate reactions sometimes occur but are usually allergic in character, and are more common in patients with a history of urticaria, asthma or similar conditions.

As barbiturates are now widely and sometimes excessively prescribed, the effect of combined therapy with other drugs should be considered. This is of particular importance when anticoagulant drugs are also given. The subject is referred to more fully in the section on ' drug interactions ' on page 9.

Barbitone Sodium † (dose, 300 to 600 mg.)

Barbitone sodium was introduced as Medinal† in 1903 and is still in use. It has a prolonged action, and drowsiness may occur next day. It is excreted largely unchanged in the urine, so that the drug may accumulate in the tissues if treatment is prolonged, or if renal function is impaired. Shorter-acting barbiturates are now usually preferred.

Phenobarbitone † (dose, 30 to 120 mg.)

Phenobarbitone and phenobarbitone sodium have a more general sedative action than barbitone, and are of value in a wide range of nervous and tension states, and in hypertension, angina and some cardiac conditions. Apart from its sedative and hypnotic effects, phenobarbitone has anticonvulsant properties, and it is widely employed in the treatment of epilepsy, often with other drugs.

The sedative effects of phenobarbitone are more marked when the drug is given by intramuscular injection, and it is sometimes valuable in calming over-excited, agitated or violent patients. Ampoules containing 200 mg. of the drug in a special solvent are available.

Other barbiturates can be grouped into *medium-acting compounds*, exemplified by :

Amylobarbitone (Amytal †).
Amylobarbitone Sodium † (Sodium Amytal †).
Butobarbitone (Soneryl) †.

And *short-acting compounds* including :

Cyclobarbitone,†
Pentobarbitone Sodium (Nembutal †)
Quinalbarbitone Sodium (Seconal †).

This classification is subject to considerable individual variation, but is a useful working guide.

TABLE OF BARBITURATES

Approved Name	Brand Name	Dose
Amylobarbitone	Amytal	100 to 200 mg.
Amylobarbitone Sodium	Sodium Amytal	100 to 200 mg.
Barbitone	Veronal	300 to 600 mg.
Barbitone Sodium	Medinal	300 to 600 mg.
Butobarbitone	Soneryl	100 to 200 mg.
Cyclobarbitone	Phanodorm	200 to 400 mg.
Heptobarbitone	Medomin	50 to 400 mg.
Nealbarbitone	Censedal	60 to 200 mg.
Pentobarbitone Sodium	Nembutal	100 to 200 mg.
Phenobarbitone	Gardenal	30 to 120 mg.
	Luminal	30 to 120 mg.
Phenobarbitone Sodium	Gardenal Sodium	30 to 120 mg.
	Luminal Sodium	30 to 120 mg.
Quinalbarbitone Sodium	Seconal Sodium	100 to 200 mg.

The barbiturates are of no value in the insomnia due to pain. In such cases, the addition of an analgesic is necessary to relieve the pain, when the sedative effect can come into force. Sonalgin † and Tercin † are examples of products containing a barbiturate and an analgesic, formulated for such combined action.

In cases of barbiturate poisoning, measures must be taken to increase the elimination of the absorbed drug, and stimulants may be needed to counteract the respiratory depression and fall in blood pressure that occurs. The subject is discussed in more detail on page 49.

TRANQUILLISERS

This term is sometimes more easily understood than defined, as it refers to a highly varied group of drugs of widely different chemical structure used in the treatment of anxiety, tension, agitation and other forms of mental illness. Temporary anxiety and depression, such as that caused by grief, is a natural reaction to an emotional stress, and in normal individuals the mental balance is soon restored. In psychotic and psychoneurotic patients this balance is markedly disturbed, and severe anxiety, tension, agitation or mania may occur.

For many years barbiturates remained the standard treatment for many psychiatric conditions, but they have the disadvantage of causing a general sedation, and the introduction of the major tranquillisers of the chlorpromazine type marked a great advance in the treatment of mental illness. Other drugs with a more specific action on certain tissues of the brain have also been discovered, and a number of selective anti-depressant drugs such as imipramine (q.v.) are now available.

The chlorpromazine group of drugs (which are derivatives of phenothiazine) have a distinctive action on the subcortical tissues of the brain, and induce a calm state of mind without clouding of consciousness, reduce tension and agitation without somnolence, and relieve stress and psychomotor over-activity without depression. Many of these compounds also have other forms of central activity, and auxiliary effects include the potentiation of anaesthetics, analgesics and sedatives, reduction in the perception and reaction to pain, and an anti-emetic action. Some newer compounds have a more powerful and selective action.

Therapeutically these drugs are used in a wide range of psychiatric conditions including schizophrenia, chronic and acute psychoses, anxiety and tension states, and in the treatment of drug addiction. Side-effects that occur from time to time include jaundice, blood disorders such as agranulocytosis, rash and tremor. In many cases the milder side-effects disappear with a reduction in dose.

Chlorpromazine † (dose, 75 to 500 mg. in divided doses daily ; 25 to 50 mg. by injection)

Chlorpromazine, introduced as Largactil, was the first of the

Approved Name	Brand Name	Main Actions	Products
Fluphenazine †	Moditen	Tranquilliser	Tablets, 1, 2·5, 5 mg. Elixir, 2·5 mg./5 ml. Ampoules, 25 mg.
Fluphenazine † decanoate	Modecate	Tranquilliser	Ampoules, 12·5 mg.
Methotrimeprazine †	Veractil	An alternative to chlorpromazine in psychiatric disorders. Not for elderly patients	Tablets, 5, 25, 100 mg. Ampoules, 25 mg.
Pericyazine †	Neulactil	Tranquilliser, anti-schizophrenic	Tablets, 2·5, 10 mg. Syrup, 2·5 mg./5 ml. Syrup Forte, 10 mg./5 ml. Ampoules, 10 mg.
Perphenazine †	Fentazin	Tranquilliser and anti-emetic of high potency	Tablets, 2, 4, 8 mg. Syrup, 3 mg./5 ml. Ampoules, 5 mg.
Prochlorperazine †	Stemetil	Central sedative and anti-emetic. The high dose products are for psychiatric treatment	Tablets, 5, 25 mg. Syrup, 5 mg./5 ml. Syrup Forte, 25 mg./5 ml. Suppositories, 5, 25 mg. Ampoules, 12·5, 25 mg.
Promazine †	Sparine	Tranquilliser and anti-emetic. The 'Latab' product is a long-acting tablet	Tablets, 25, 50, 100 mg. Latab, 50 mg. Suspension, 50 mg./5 ml. Ampoules, 50, 100 mg.
Thiethylperazine †	Torecan	Anti-emetic and anti-vertigo	Tablets, 10 mg. Suppositories, 10 mg. Ampoules, 10 mg.
Thiopropazate †	Dartalan	Tranquilliser and anti-emetic	Tablets, 5, 10 mg.
Thioridazine †	Melleril	Tranquilliser. Drug has no anti-emetic properties	Tablets, 10, 25, 50, 100 mg. Syrup, 25 mg./5 ml.
Trifluoperazine †	Stelazine	Tranquilliser and anti-emetic. The 'Spansule' is a sustained release form	Tablets, 1, 5 mg. Spansules, 2, 15 mg. Syrup, 1 mg./5 ml. Ampoules, 1 mg.
Trimeprazine †	Vallergan	Mainly used in pruritus, and for premedication	Tablets, 10 mg. Syrup, 7·5 mg./5 ml. Syrup Forte, 6 mg./ml. Ampoules, 50 mg.

major tranquillisers, and it has a remarkable and diverse action on the central nervous system.   It has a powerful calming effect on aggressive schizophrenic patients, and those in the manic-depressive state.   It relieves senile agitation, and withdrawn patients become more alert and co-operative.   Chlorpromazine is also widely employed for premedication before anaesthesia to reduce apprehension and potentiate the effects of other drugs, and its powerful anti-emetic action is another advantage.   It is also used in surgery, in association with muscle relaxants and other drugs, to potentiate the effects of anaesthetics, and thus permit a reduction in dose.   This combined treatment is a useful method of reducing surgical hazards in poor-risk patients.   Chlorpromazine also causes a decreased awareness of pain, or an emotional indifference, which is of great value in the treatment of severe and continuous pain, permitting adequate relief without undue sedation or excessive doses of analgesics.

The average oral dose of chlorpromazine is 25 mg., but in severe mental conditions much larger doses may be required. Syrup and suppositories of chlorpromazine are available, and the drug may also be given by intravenous drip infusion, slow intravenous injection, or by deep intramuscular injection.   Mild side-effects such as dryness of the mouth may occur early in treatment, but if jaundice and agranulocytosis occur later the drug must be withdrawn.   Recovery from liver damage by chlorpromazine is usually good if the drug is withdrawn promptly.   Care should be taken in cardiovascular disease, as chlorpromazine may cause a fall in blood pressure, and in cases of overdose general supportive treatment is required, as there is no specific antidote.   Chlorpromazine solutions are potentially irritant to the skin, and may cause a severe dermatitis in susceptible cases.   Nurses and others who may handle solutions should wear rubber gloves.   *Brand name :* Largactil.†

Analogous Compounds

A number of compounds chemically related to chlorpromazine are now available.   Most of these have a basically similar action, but the changes in structure may be reflected in a reduced dose, an extended action, or in a more specific therapeutic application. Representative compounds are given in the table on page 33.

OTHER TRANQUILLISERS

A tranquillising action is found in many drugs unrelated to chlorpromazine, and the range of available drugs is increasing. The following notes refer to representative compounds, but the list is necessarily incomplete as the whole subject is one of rapidly expanding horizons.

Chlordiazepoxide † (dose, 30 to 100 mg. daily)

Anxiety and tension are the natural accompaniment of much illness, and the relief of mental stress is sometimes as necessary as the specific treatment of the disease. There are also many occasions when no organic disease can be found to account for the symptoms, and such conditions are known as functional disorders. In such cases, relief of anxiety and tension is a powerful therapeutic measure, and here, as well as in psychosomatic disorders such as some skin conditions, which are associated with stress, symptomatic relief can be achieved by various tranquillising drugs. Chlordiazepoxide is widely used in the treatment of functional disorders, as it is effective in a variety of conditions associated with anxiety and stress, in menopausal states, and alcoholism. It is also of value in the treatment of depression when anxiety and tension are also present. Chlordiazepoxide also has muscle relaxant properties, and in association with an anticholinergic drug (as in Libraxin), it is useful in gastro-intestinal disorders. The standard dose in functional disorders is 10 mg. three times a day, but larger doses are necessary in severe anxiety and tension. *Brand name :* Librium.†

Chlorprothixene † (dose 30 to 300 mg. daily)

Chlorprothixene is an antidepressant drug, useful in the treatment of depressive states complicated by anxiety and agitation, and in confusional conditions. In more severe conditions such as acute schizophrenia doses of 300 mg. daily or more may be necessary, but in depressive states doses of 30 to 90 mg. may be adequate. Chlorprothixene has a rapid action, and symptomatic improvement often occurs soon after treatment is commenced. In common with many other drugs of this type, chlorprothixene may potentiate the action of a wide range of other therapeutic agents which influence the central nervous system. *Brand name :* Taractan.†

Diazepam † (dose 4 to 40 mg. daily)

Diazepam is chemically related to chlordiazepoxide, and is used to reduce anxiety in agitated and neurotic patients. In such psychiatric conditions it may be given in doses of 2 mg. three times a day, increased in more severe conditions according to need and response. Diazepam also has a relaxant effect on skeletal muscle, and is useful in relieving physical and emotional tension ; also the muscle spasm and pain of arthritic conditions. When given by intravenous or intramuscular injection, the muscle relaxant effects are more marked, and diazepam has been used with success in association with other drugs in the treatment of tetanus. *Brand name :* Valium.†

Droperidol † (dose 5 to 10 mg. by injection, 10 to 20 mg. orally)

Droperidol is a neuroleptic drug, and produces a state of mental detachment and indifference to the environment, yet permits communication when required. It is used in association with phenoperidine (*q.v.*) when an operative procedure is necessary during which the patient must be co-operative, aware of others, yet is free from pain and anxiety, and is mentally detached from the surrounding circumstances. Droperidol is also used for pre-medication, and in psychiatry for the treatment of schizophrenia. The drug is given orally in doses of 10 to 20 mg., and in doses of 5 mg. intravenously, or 10 mg. by intramuscular injection, and is well tolerated. It has little action on the cardiovascular system, and does not cause respiratory depression. *Brand name:* Droleptan.†

Haloperidol † (dose, 1·5 to 10 mg. daily)

Haloperidol is a psychotrophic agent, chemically unrelated to the promazine group of drugs, but possessing similar tranquillising properties. It is used in the treatment of schizophrenia and other psychotic disorders, and in mania and other states may be given by intramuscular or intravenous injection in doses of 5 mg., repeated at six-hourly intervals. Orally, haloperidol may be given in doses of 1·5 mg. four times a day, or treatment may be commenced with low doses of 0·75 mg., doubling every fourth day according to need. Haloperidol is also given as a pre-anaesthetic drug, and is useful as an anti-emetic. *Brand name :* Serenace.†

Meprobamate † (dose, 1200 mg. daily)

This compound has mild muscle-relaxant properties similar to those of mephenesin (*q.v.*), but it is used mainly as a tranquillising drug in nervous tension, anxiety and alcoholism. It exerts its action by depressing nerve impulses in the spinal cord, and it affords relief in anxiety and tension states without causing much drowsiness. Occasionally meprobamate treatment has the reverse effect of stimulation and not sedation, and skin rash may also occur in susceptible patients. Although meprobamate has little hypnotic power, its relaxant action assists the induction of natural sleep. *Brand names :* Equanil,† Mepavlon,† Miltown.†

Methylpentynol † (dose, 250 to 1000 mg.)

Methylpentynol was originally introduced as a mild quick-acting hypnotic (see p. 28), but is now used mainly to allay apprehension and nervous tension, and as a mild pre-operative sedative. A longer-acting form is available as Oblivon-C.† *Brand names :* Oblivon,† Somnesin.†

Reserpine † (dose, 0·25 to 2 mg. daily)

Reserpine is an alkaloid obtained from the Indian plant Rauwolfia. It has a depressant action on the central nervous system and is used in agitated states such as senile psychoses and schizophrenia and also in mild anxiety states. The action is slow and benefit may not be experienced for two or three weeks if reserpine is used alone. Care must be taken with full doses as a severe mental depression may occur. Even in lower doses drowsiness, nasal congestion, and gastric disturbances may be experienced. Reserpine also has hypotensive properties, and is useful in the treatment of early hypertension. The effect is slow in onset and variable in intensity and the dose must be adjusted to suit the individual patient. In severe hypertension, other drugs with a more specific action and fewer side-effects are now preferred. *Brand name :* Serpasil.†

ANTIDEPRESSANTS

In a state of health, depression due to external conditions, as a natural reaction to grief or disappointment, is relatively mild and self-limiting, but depression may also occur without apparent cause, and may be severe and prolonged.

In such a condition, referred to as endogenous depression, sedatives and stimulants are of little value, but in recent years a number of new drugs have been synthesised which have a specific and selective antidepressant action. The mode of action is distinct from that of tranquillisers and sedatives, and these compounds are sometimes referred to as thymoleptic drugs. It should be noted that they differ from the monoamine oxidase inhibitors, and should not be given with any member of that group of antidepressant drugs.

Imipramine † (dose, 75 to 150 mg. daily)

Imipramine is one of the best known of the purely anti-depressant drugs, and although the mode of action is still not clear it is of great value in endogenous depression. It is given in doses of 25 mg. three times a day, but in elderly patients lower initial doses of 10 mg. should be given. The effect is slow in onset, and may not be apparent for two or three weeks, but is characterised by an unblocking of the fixed depressive mood, a reduction in obsession, and an improvement in approachability and social contact. Extended treatment is often necessary to ensure full remission of symptoms, and therapy should be continued as long as necessary. In the neurotic or reactive type of depression, imipramine is less effective, and in such conditions a monoamine oxidase inhibitor is preferred.

Imipramine is well tolerated, but atropine-like side-effects may occur with some patients, and a parkinsonism type of tremor may also be noted. *Brand name:* Tofranil.†

Amitriptyline † (dose, 75 to 150 mg. daily)

Amitriptyline has both antidepressant and anti-anxiety properties, and is used in a wide range of psychiatric conditions, including schizophrenia, neurotic and reactive depression, anxiety hysteria and melancholia. The average adult dose is 25 mg. three times a day, but double doses may be necessary initially to control the symptoms. Subsequent maintenance doses should be adjusted to the level that gives the optimum response, but prolonged treatment is necessary to achieve full remission of symptoms. Side-effects are linked with the anticholinergic properties of the drug, and dryness of the mouth and blurring of vision may occur.

Glaucoma and urinary retention are contra-indications. *Brand names* : Laroxyl,† Saroten,† Tryptizol.†

Desipramine † (dose, 50 to 200 mg. daily)

The latent period before the effects of imipramine become apparent is thought to be due to the slow conversion of the drug in the body to desipramine, to which compound the antidepressant effect of imipramine is finally due. This metabolite has now been synthesised, and is used therapeutically when a drug with a more rapid action than imipramine is required.

Improvement may occur within four to seven days of commencing treatment, but if lifting of the depression has not been achieved after about three weeks, further treatment is unlikely to be successful. *Brand name* : Pertofran.†

Doxepin hydrochloride (dose 30 to 300 mg. daily)

Doxepin is a tricyclic tranquillising agent, of use in a range of psychoneurotic disorders where either anxiety or depression may be, or appears to be, the predominant symptom. The drug is also useful in treating the insomnia and apprehension associated with these anxiety-depressive states. The rapidity and degree of response varies with each patient, but mild cases may respond in one to two weeks to doses of 30 to 50 mg. daily. Patients with more severe symptoms may require doses of 75 to 150 mg. daily; where the depression is severe, doses of 300 mg. daily may be necessary. In common with related drugs, doxepin should not be used in association with monoamine oxidase inhibitors. *Brand name* : Sinequan.†

Iprindole † (dose, 15 to 60 mg.)

Iprindole is an antidepressant which basically resembles imipramine in action but may have less atropine-like side-effects : Long treatment is necessary in severe depression. *Brand name:* Prondol.†

Nortriptyline † (dose, 20 to 100 mg. daily)

Nortriptyline has the antidepressant properties of imipramine, but it also has some tranquillising action. It is useful in a wide range of psychiatric conditions, including depression, anxiety and tension states, psychosomatic disorders, and in the treatment of enuresis. Average doses are 20 to 100 mg. daily, but larger initial doses may be necessary in some cases. Side-effects are similar to those experienced with amitriptyline. *Brand names :* Allegron,† Aventyl.†

Protriptyline † (dose, 15 to 60 mg. daily)

Protriptyline has the specific antidepressant action associated with the imipramine group of drugs, but the response to treatment is more rapid. The drug is also effective in lower doses, and is useful in patients who have failed to respond to other antidepressants. Protriptyline is indicated in a wide range of depressed conditions, from the mildly neurotic state to conditions of severe withdrawal, and has the advantage of not having any sedative effect. Where the depression is associated with anxiety or agitation, combined therapy with a tranquilliser may be necessary. Protriptyline is not a monoamine oxidase inhibitor, and so is free from the dangers of combined treatment associated with that group of drugs. *Brand name :* Concordin.†

Trimipramine † (dose, 75 to 300 mg. daily)

Trimipramine is related to imipramine, and is used for similar purposes. It has the advantage of being effective in anxiety and agitation, and so is useful in a wider range of psychiatric conditions. The maintenance dose must be adjusted according to need to suit the individual patient, and long treatment may be necessary to evoke the maximum response and adequate remission of symptoms. *Brand name :* Surmontil.†

Lithium carbonate (dose 0·5 to 2 G. daily)

Although lithium bromide was once used as a sedative, it is only in recent years that the value of lithium carbonate in the treatment of the manic phase of manic-depressive psychoses has been discovered. As lithium carbonate is a simple inorganic compound, this therapeutic action is surprising, but may be linked with changes in the pattern of electrolyte balance between intracellular and extracellular fluid. Lithium carbonate is given in doses of 500 mg. three or four times a day for a week, reduced later to a maintenance dose of 500 mg. daily. An excessive intake of lithium may cause vomiting and drowsiness, and withdrawal of treatment one day each week has been suggested as a safety measure. *Brand names :* Camcolit, Priadel.

MONOAMINE OXIDASE INHIBITORS

When drugs related to isoniazid were introduced for the treatment of tuberculosis, some patients experienced a marked feeling of well-being or euphoria. Investigation indicated that quite apart from any anti-tubercular activity, these drugs inhibited the action of the enzyme monoamine oxidase. That enzyme controls the level of adrenaline, noradrenaline and serotonin in brain tissue

TABLE OF MONOAMINE OXIDASE INHIBITORS

Approved Name	Brand Name	Products
Iproniazid	Marsilid	Tablets, 25 mg.; 50 mg.
Isocarboxazid	Marplan	Tablets, 25 mg.; 50 mg.
Mebanazine	Actomol	Capsules, 5 mg.
Nialamide	Niamid	Tablets, 25 mg.; 100 mg.
Phenelzine	Nardil	Tablets, 15 mg.
Tranylcypromine	Parnate	Tablets, 10 mg.

and its inhibition appeared to have a stimulant effect by allowing the concentration of serotonin and adrenaline to rise, and had obvious therapeutic possibilities in the treatment of depression.

Whether in fact this is the basis of the therapeutic action of these monoamine oxidase inhibitors is still not clear, but in practice they have proved of great value in the treatment of exogenous or reactive depression particularly when complicated by anxiety. The action is slow, and treatment may have to be continued for two to four weeks before any response occurs. The enzyme monoamine oxidase also occurs in the liver and inhibition of the enzyme can affect liver function, so that care must be taken if these powerful drugs are used in cases of hepatic damage. The table above indicates the range of available products.

It must be remembered that these inhibitors are not only powerful drugs in themselves but they can also increase the action of many other drugs, particularly analgesics and pressor drugs. Alarming hypertensive reactions may follow combined use, and pethidine, adrenaline and other pressor drugs, imipramine and related compounds, should never be given to patients receiving monoamine oxidase inhibitors, or within ten to fourteen days of ceasing such treatment. Even certain foods such as cheese, yeast extracts and broad beans may cause a dangerous rise in blood pressure, and should be avoided.

This problem is of importance to the anaesthetist, who may have to deal with a patient receiving a monoamine oxidase inhibitor, yet who also requires a narcotic analgesic. A delay of 10-14 days before an operation can be carried out with safety is not always practicable, and a test has been devised to indicate those patients likely to show an excessive sensitivity to analgesics or pressor drugs. The test is carried out by first noting blood pressure, pulse and respiration, and then giving 5 mg. of pethidine or 0·5 mg. of morphine by injection. Response is recorded at 5-10 minute intervals for one hour. If no rise in blood pressure occurs, a 10 mg. dose of pethidine or 1 mg. of morphine is given, with a 40 mg. dose of pethidine or 4 mg. of morphine after another hour. If there is no reaction, the fourth injection may be regarded as a premedication dose.

These effects have drawn attention to the increasing number of drug reactions, particularly when new and powerful drugs are prescribed together. The mode of action of many new compounds is still not clear, so that the possibility of reactions cannot always be predicted. Nurses, who see more of a patient than the doctor, should be alert to the risk of reactions with new drugs, and should report any unexpected effects, even if seemingly trivial at the time, in order that the risk may be assessed against the benefits received. The Table of Drug Reactions on pages 9 to 11 indicates some of the more common effects of combined therapy.

ANTICONVULSANTS

These drugs are used in the treatment of epilepsy. This disease, once called "the falling sickness," may be manifested as a general convulsion or grand mal, popularly known as a fit, or as a momentary loss of consciousness without any convulsion (petit mal), or as psychomotor epilepsy, in which convulsions are absent, but psychological disturbances and irrational behaviour occur.

For many years the standard drug in the treatment of epilepsy has been phenobarbitone (q.v.). Given in doses of 30 to 120 mg., it has both a specific anticonvulsant action and a general sedative effect, and is of particular value in grand mal. Long-continued treatment extending over a period of years may be necessary to maintain control of symptoms in grand mal, and if the sedative effects of phenobarbitone in effective doses are too marked, the dose of phenobarbitone may be reduced, and phenytoin or primidone given as supplementary treatment. Phenobarbitone is less effective in psychomotor epilepsy, and of little value in petit mal. Other barbiturates used in epilepsy include methylphenobarbitone (Prominal) and phenylmethylbarbitone (Rutonal).

Phenytoin Sodium † (dose, 50 to 200 mg. daily)

Originally introduced as Epanutin, this drug is an anticonvulsant with little hypnotic power, and is mainly effective in grand mal and psychomotor epilepsy. Combined therapy with phenobarbitone may sometimes evoke an increased response. Phenytoin can be given in doses of 250 mg. by intravenous or intramuscular injection for the control of status epilepticus. Toxic side-effects with phenytoin are not uncommon, and may be severe, but dizziness, nausea and skin reactions may usually be controlled by a temporary reduction in dose. In a few patients the drug may cause a marked overgrowth of the gums. *Brand name :* Epanutin.†

Ethotoin † (dose, 1 to 3 G. daily)

Ethotoin is chemically related to phenytoin, and has similar but less potent anticonvulsant properties. It is less likely to cause side-effects than phenytoin, but combined therapy with other anticonvulsants is often necessary to obtain an adequate response. *Brand name :* Peganone.†

Methoin † (dose, 100 to 500 mg. daily)

Methoin has properties similar to those of phenytoin, and the drug may be useful in patients not responding to phenytoin, or when that drug is not tolerated. Dermatitis and toxic effects on the haematological system may occur with methoin, and blood tests are advisable during treatment. *Brand name :* Mesontoin.†

Primidone (dose, 0·5 to 2 G. daily)

Primidone has some chemical relationship to phenobarbitone, but as indicated by the dose it is less potent. It is chiefly of value in grand mal and psychomotor epilepsy, particularly when response to phenobarbitone or phenytoin is inadequate, but in general it is less effective in petit mal. Treatment is initiated with doses of 250 mg. daily, increased at intervals of three days to a daily dose of 0·5 to 2 G. according to need. Primidone occasionally causes drowsiness, but is otherwise well tolerated, and initial reactions are usually transient. *Brand name :* Mysoline.

Troxidone † (dose, 900 mg. to 1·8 G. daily)

Troxidone is more specific in action than other anticonvulsants, as it is effective mainly in petit mal. Grand mal attacks may be increased by troxidone, so the drug is of little value in a patient afflicted by both types of seizure. Unfortunately, therapy may be complicated by visual disturbances in which bright objects appear to have a 'glare,' and rashes, blood disorders and anaemia may occur. Blood tests are necessary during treatment. *Brand name :* Tridione.†

Other anti-epileptics

Several other anticonvulsant drugs are available but they are used mainly in patients not responding to treatment with the more generally effective compounds already referred to. Representative products include beclamide (Nydrane), dose 1·5 to 4 G. daily, carbamazepine (Tegretol), dose 0·5 to 1 G. daily, phensuximide (Milontin), dose 1 to 3 G. daily, paramethadione (Paradione †), dose 900 to 1800 mg. daily, ethosuximide (Zarontin), dose 0·5 to 2 G. daily, sulthiame (Ospolot), dose 200 to 600 mg. daily, and phenacemide (Phenurone †), dose 1·5 to 3 G. daily. In all cases the change from one drug to another should be made gradually, with overlapping doses, as attacks may increase if a drug is withdrawn too rapidly.

Chlormethiazole † (dose 0·5 to 1·5 G.)

This drug has anticonvulsant and sedative properties of an unusual type. It is chemically related to part of the vitamin B_1 structure, and has therapeutic applications in the treatment of eclamptic toxaemia, status epilepticus, mania and alcoholism. In toxaemia and other severe conditions, chlormethiazole is given by slow intravenous drip infusion as a 0·8 per cent. solution. Supervision is necessary during administration as the sedative effects may cause respiratory depression and airway obstruction. Oral treatment is usually adequate in alcoholism, and doses of 1·5 G. may be given four times a day initially, reduced later to 0·5 G., with a total dose of about 30 G. over nine days. *Brand name :* Heminevrin.†

TABLE OF ANTICONVULSANTS

Approved Name	Brand Name
Those effective in petit mal	
Phenobarbitone	Gardenal, Luminal
Methylphenobarbitone	Prominal
Phenylmethylbarbitone	Rutonal
Ethosuximide	Emeside, Zarontin
Paramethadione	Paradione
Phensuximide	Milontin
Troxidone	Tridione
Those effective in grand mal and other types of seizure	
Phenobarbitone	Gardenal, Luminal
Methylphenobarbitone	Prominal
Beclamide	Nydrane
Carbamazepine	Tegretol
Ethotoin	Peganone
Methoin	Mesontin
Phenacemide	Phenurone
Phenytoin	Epanutin
Primidone	Mysoline
Sulthiame	Ospolot

CENTRAL NERVOUS SYSTEM STIMULANTS

The drugs which stimulate the central nervous system show wide differences in chemical structure, mode of action and type of stimulant activity. In view of the complexity of the central nervous system, this variation in the pattern of activity of central stimulant drugs is not surprising, and their therapeutic uses exhibit a similar diversity. Some have a euphoriant action, others increase mental activity, and others raise the blood pressure or stimulate respiration. In general the therapeutic value of central stimulants is limited, as stimulation of the central nervous system cannot be continued without a subsequent compensatory depression or reduction in response.   Within these limits certain C.N.S. stimulants have some therapeutic value, and the following drugs are of interest and importance.

Caffeine (dose, 250 to 500 mg.)

Caffeine is one of the most widely used central stimulants, as it is the chief constituent of tea and coffee.   It acts mainly on the sensory cortex of the brain, increasing mental alertness and post-poning drowsiness and fatigue.   Caffeine also reduces cerebral blood flow by constricting the cerebral vessels, and the addition of caffeine to various analgesic preparations used for headache and migraine, such as Tab A.P.C. (aspirin, phenacetin and caffeine) is a therapeutic application of this effect.   The brain medulla, the respiratory centre and the myocardium are also stimulated by caffeine, and depth and rate of respiration and cardiac output are increased.   These respiratory and cardiac stimulant effects are most marked when the drug is given by injection as the soluble derivative, caffeine sodium benzoate, in doses of 250 to 500 mg.   The related drug aminophylline (q.v.) has a similar but more powerful action, and is preferred when a rapid-acting cardiac or respiratory stimulant is required.

Caffeine also has useful diuretic properties, as it increases blood flow through the kidneys, and also reduces the re-absorption of salts and water by the tubules.   This diuretic action of caffeine is discussed more fully on page 104.

Ethamivan (dose, 5 to 10 mg. per kg.)

Ethamivan is a respiratory stimulant that also has a pressor action due to the constriction of the peripheral blood vessels. This latter effect is mediated by a stimulant effect on the vaso-motor centre.   The drug is useful in respiratory depression in barbiturate poisoning, and other hypoventilatory states, but the action is brief, and to maintain continuity of action ethamivan is usually given by slow intravenous drip infusion as a 0·6 per cent. solution.   It may also be given by direct injection as a 5 per cent. solution.   Ethamivan is sometimes given orally in the treatment of neonatal respiratory distress in doses of 12·5 to 25 mg. as Ethamivan Elixir B.N.F. (50 mg. per ml.).   *Brand name :* Vandid.

Nikethamide (dose, 0·5 to 2 G.)

Originally introduced as Coramine, nikethamide has useful respiratory stimulant properties by its action on the medullary centre of the brain. It has been used in the treatment of shock, and the respiratory distress of chronic bronchitis. It has some pressor action, probably as a result of improved respiration, but for circulatory failure and traumatic shock more powerful pressor drugs are available. Nikethamide is given by intramuscular or intravenous injection, and as the action is brief, frequent repetition of the dose may be necessary to maintain the response. *Brand name :* Coramine.

Prethcamide (dose, 200 to 400 mg.)

Hypoventilation and pulmonary insufficiency lead to carbon dioxide retention and a lowering of arterial oxygen. In severe cases this may cause right ventricular failure. Prethcamide represents a new approach to the problem, as the drug stimulates respiration and improves pulmonary function, especially in bronchitic and emphysematous patients. *Brand name :* Micoren.

Amiphenazole (Daptazole), bemegride (Megimide) and leptazol (Cardiazol) represent other respiratory stimulants now used less frequently.

Amphetamine Sulphate † (dose, 5 to 10 mg.)

Amphetamine has a marked stimulant effect on the cortex of the brain, causing a temporary increase in alertness, relief of fatigue and a general euphoria. It is used in the treatment of narcolepsy and related disorders of the central nervous system but in general is of limited therapeutic value. The stimulant action of the drug has led to abuse, and students should note that although amphetamine can increase mental activity, the quality of the increase cannot be predicted. Thinking may become erratic and less controllable with loss of judgement and accuracy. Excessive doses of amphetamine sulphate may cause headache, anorexia, cyanosis, disorientation and collapse. Amphetamine also tends to reduce the appetite, presumably by increasing mental activity with a consequent reduced preoccupation with food, and it has been used in some cases of obesity. By virtue of its stimulant effects on the cortex, respiratory and vasomotor centres, it has been given by injection in the treatment of barbiturate poisoning, although methylamphetamine is often preferred.

Dexamphetamine Sulphate † (dose, 5 to 10 mg.)

This compound has a very close chemical relationship to amphetamine sulphate, and has a similar central stimulant action. It also has appetite depressant properties, and is used in conjunction with dietary restrictions in the treatment of obesity. A psychological element is often present in cases of over-eating, and the stimulant action of the drug may then be helpful. A number of long-acting forms of dexamphetamine sulphate are now available, designed to permit a smooth and extended degree of appetite control, and Dexten,† Dexedrine Spansules,† Duromine † and Durophet † are examples of such products. Phenmetrazine (Preludin †), diethylpropion (Tenuate †) and fenfluramine (Ponderax †) are other appetite depressants, but the latter has the advantage of having virtually no central stimulant effects.

Methylamphetamine † (dose, 2·5 to 10 mg. orally ;   10 to 30 mg. by injection)

Methylamphetamine resembles amphetamine in its general stimulant effects, and is used for similar purposes. When given by injection it has a more powerful and prolonged pressor action and is of value in shock and collapse, and in overcoming the fall in blood pressure that occurs during spinal anaesthesia. Methylamphetamine is also used as a central stimulant in the treatment of barbiturate poisoning. *Brand name :* Methedrine.†

Methyl phenidate † (dose, 10 mg.)

Methyl phenidate has useful central stimulant properties, but these are less marked than those of the amphetamines, and the drug is considered to have a potency between that group of drugs and caffeine. *Brand name :* Ritalin.†

Meclofenoxate † (dose, 200 to 300 mg.)

Meclofenoxate has a central stimulant action that differs sharply from that of the amphetamines, and can be described as a neuroregulator. It is used in a wide range of conditions where a mild central stimulant action is required. *Brand name:* Lucidril.†

Barbiturate Poisoning

Drugs which stimulate both the cortex of the brain and the respiratory centre have obvious value in the treatment of barbiturate and narcotic poisoning. At one time picrotoxin, a powerful central stimulant, in association with the amphetamines was the specific treatment for barbiturate overdosage and coma, and was given in doses of 6 mg. by intravenous injection every twenty minutes or so until consciousness was regained. Later bemegride (Megimide) was introduced and claimed to be a selective stimulant in barbiturate poisoning. More recently, greater reliance has been placed on increasing the elimination of the barbiturate by forced diuresis, using mannitol. This sugar is not metabolised, and when given by intravenous injection as a 20 per cent. solution, it functions as an osmotic diuretic, increasing the elimination of barbiturates, salicylates and other toxic substances. In addition to any drug treatment, the maintenance of a good air-way, with ventilatory assistance when required, remain essential measures in all cases of barbiturate poisoning.

CHAPTER III

NARCOTICS, ANALGESICS AND RELATED DRUGS

THE problem of pain has long puzzled both physicians and theologians, and as pain is a feature of many diseases and brings the patient to the doctor more quickly than any other symptom, its relief has always been of considerable importance. The more potent analgesic or pain-relieving drugs are usually regarded as narcotics, and are powerful drugs which both relieve pain and induce sleep. They differ from anaesthetics as the sleep follows, and does not precede, the relief of pain. Analgesic drugs are those that relieve pain without causing sleep. Opium, the oldest and one of the most certain remedies for pain, is the best-known narcotic and acetylsalicylic acid (aspirin) is the most widely used analgesic.

Opium * (dose, 25 to 200 mg.)

Opium is the dried juice obtained from the seed-capsules of the opium poppy, which is grown extensively in Turkey, Persia and India, and the method of collection is much the same as that described by Dioscorides some 2000 years ago. It is a brown powder with a characteristic smell, and contains morphine, codeine, papaverine and many other alkaloids. The narcotic action is due mainly to the morphine, and it is as that drug by injection that opium is usually employed. Opium also reduces peristalsis, and is of value when given orally for the treatment of diarrhoea and other intestinal disorders. It is usually given with astringents such as catechu in Chalk and Opium Mixture B.N.F.

PREPARATIONS

Tincture of opium (laudanum *) B.P. (Dose, 0·25 to 2 ml.; equivalent to about 3 to 20 mg. morphine.)

Camphorated tincture of opium † (paregoric). (Dose, 2 to 10 ml.)

Papaveretum * (dose, 10 to 20 mg.)

Papaveretum is a mixture of the main alkaloids of opium, and contains about 50 per cent. morphine ; it is given mainly by injection, often in association with hyoscine. Omnopon * is a proprietary product of similar composition. Powder of ipecacuanha and opium (Dover's powder), dose 0·3 to 0·6 G., contains 1 per cent. morphine and is occasionally used as a diaphoretic, often with acetylsalicylic acid.

Morphine * (dose, 10 to 20 mg.)

Morphine is one of the most powerful of analgesics in common use, and the effect is mediated by a depression of the sensory nerves of the brain. The drug has a two-fold action, as it not only lowers the sensitivity to pain, but also allays apprehension and anxiety, and this combined action is of great value in severe pain and the accompanying mental distress. Morphine is therefore of outstanding value in myocardial infarction, in painful neoplastic disease, in coronary thrombosis, dyspnoea of heart failure, internal haemorrhage and acute febrile conditions. In biliary colic, morphine will relieve the pain without reducing the spasm, and combined use with atropine may give greater relief. Morphine reduces cough by a depressant action of the cough centre of the brain medulla, and by a similar action on the respiratory centre it causes the respiration to become slower. For this reason morphine should not be used in asthma or other chest conditions where breathing is already inefficient. In some patients medullary stimulation may precede depression, and as a result nausea and vomiting may occur. For pre-operative use morphine is usually given by subcutaneous or intramuscular injection, and it is frequently combined with atropine in order to reduce respiratory depression, vomiting and bronchial secretion. In severe pain, morphine not only affords relief, but also frequently brings about a change in the mental attitude to pain, and permits a degree of detachment that is often of great help to the patient. This mental change increases the total analgesic action, and is probably linked to the euphoric action of the drug, which in some respects is the most dangerous side-effect of morphine.

This euphoria, or sense of well-being, may easily lead to morphine addiction with all the miseries and mental, moral and physical degeneration that are associated with drug addiction. Morphine should therefore never be given for long periods, except in the severe pain of incurable disease, where the problems of tolerance, increased doses and risk of addiction are of less importance than the relief of pain.

Toxic Effects.—The toxic dose of morphine varies considerably, and in susceptible patients even therapeutic doses may cause vomiting, restlessness, tremor and confusion. With larger doses respiration is depressed, cyanosis develops and a comatose condition with pin-point pupils may occur. Pin-point pupils that do not react to light are a diagnostic sign of morphine poisoning (but must be distinguished from that caused by cerebral haemorrhage or concussion). Children and the aged are particularly susceptible to morphine, and for such patients the dose should be adjusted to need and response.

Diamorphine * (dose, 5 to 10 mg.)

Diamorphine, also known as heroin, is prepared from morphine and has a similar but more powerful analgesic action. It also has a greater depressant effect on the respiration, but causes less gastric disturbance and constipation. It is more soluble than morphine, and is of greatest value when increasing doses are required by injection for the control of severe pain in the terminal stages of carcinoma. It is very liable to cause addiction, and for that reason should be used only when less dangerous drugs are ineffective. Diamorphine is also a powerful depressant of the cough centre, and is sometimes used as a linctus in severe and intractable cough.

Pethidine * (dose, 50 to 100 mg. orally ; 25 to 100 mg. by intramuscular injection, 25 to 50 mg. intravenously)

Pethidine is a synthetic drug which has certain of the properties of both morphine and atropine, and has analgesic, antispasmodic and sedative actions. Although it lacks the hypnotic effects of morphine, it is of great value in severe pain, and has the advantage over morphine of causing less depression of respiration, constipation, and other unwanted side-effects. In biliary and renal colic associated with stone, the antispasmodic properties of pethidine may reinforce the analgesic effect, and so give greater relief. Pethidine is most effective when given by intramuscular injection, when relief may occur in less than fifteen minutes, and persist for two to five hours according to the severity of the pain. Pethidine may also be given intravenously, but is less well tolerated and may cause a fall in blood-pressure due to vasodilatation and respiratory depression. The response to oral therapy is less intense. It is widely used as an obstetric analgesic, as it reduces pain without markedly reducing uterine contractions. To offset the depression of respiration which may occur, pethidine is often given with small doses of levallorphan (*q.v.*), which minimises the effects on respiration without influencing the analgesic potency. Pethilorfan * is a preparation of pethidine and levallorphan designed for this purpose. Prolonged use of the drug should be avoided as addiction, as severe as morphine addiction, may occur.

Methadone * (dose, 5 to 10 mg.)

A powerful synthetic analgesic resembling morphine in general activity, but with less sedative or euphoric potency. It is well absorbed orally, and the effect, which comes on in about forty-five minutes, may last about four hours. A more rapid action follows intramuscular or subcutaneous injection. Methadone is very useful when relief of pain without sedation is required, and it is also valuable as a powerful cough-centre depressant for the control of useless cough in malignant conditions. It is not suitable for routine treatment as methadone is a drug of addiction. Metha-done linctus contains 2 mg. per 5 ml., and is intended for adult use. Deaths have occurred following the administration of this linctus to children. Methadone is also used as an alternative to morphine in the withdrawal treatment of drug addiction. *Brand name :* Physeptone.*

Dipipanone * (dose, 25 to 50 mg.)

Dipipanone is a synthetic analgesic of considerable power, but unlike methadone it has sedative properties and is useful when both analgesia and sedation are required. It is given by intramuscular or subcutaneous injection, and is valuable when severe pain is no longer controlled by morphine or pethidine. The action is rapid and lasts four to six hours, and is accompanied by less respiratory depression than comparable doses of morphine. Dipipanone should be used with care in renal damage, as the action of the drug may then be prolonged. Nausea and vomiting may occur with dipipanone, owing to medullary stimulation, but may be reduced by the administration of an anti-emetic. Diconal is an oral product containing dipipanone and cyclizine, designed to reduce these side-effects. *Brand name :* Pipadone.*

Pentazocine (dose, 30 to 60 mg.)

Many attempts have been made to find a synthetic analgesic as potent as morphine but free from the liability to cause addiction. Pentazocine represents a major advance in this field, as it is a clinically effective, non-addicting analgesic. The average adult dose is 30 mg. by subcutaneous, intramuscular or intravenous injection. The effect has been compared with that of 10 mg. of morphine, and pentazocine is used in the relief of severe pain of widely varied origin. The onset of action is rapid, and side-effects are few. Pentazocine is also useful in obstetrics as it has little effect on uterine contractions, and no adverse effects on the foetus. The drug may also be given orally in doses of 25 to 100 mg. but the analgesic response is less powerful than that following administration by injection. *Brand name :* Fortral.

Phenazocine ★ (dose, 1 to 3 mg. by intramuscular injection ; 5 mg. orally.)

Phenazocine is a synthetic analgesic with general properties of morphine. It causes fewer side-effects, and has the advantages of greater analgesic potency, quicker action, longer duration of effect, and slower development of tolerance. It is effective orally as well as by injection, and is a valuable alternative to morphine. *Brand name :* Narphen.★

Levorphanol ★ (dose, 1·5 to 4·5 mg. orally ; 2 to 4 mg. by intramuscular injection, 1 to 1·5 mg. intravenously)

A synthetic compound with morphine-like analgesic properties, but with less sedative effect, and is most useful as a daytime analgesic. It is a relatively long-acting compound, with the advantage of being equally effective by mouth as by injection. *Brand name :* Dromoran.★

Fentanyl ★ (dose, 0·1 to 0·6 mg.)

Fentanyl is an analgesic similar to phenoperidine (*q.v.*) but of considerably higher potency. In doses of 0·1 to 0·2 mg. intravenously, with supplementary doses later if required, adequate analgesia with spontaneous respiration is obtained. For surgical analgesia with controlled respiration, initial doses of 0·2 to 0·6 mg. are used. It should not be given to patients taking the monoamine oxidase inhibitor type of antidepressant.

Fentanyl is also used in association with droperidol (*q.v.*) to promote anaesthesia in children and the aged, and to induce a state of detachment with analgesia during certain diagnostic procedures. *Brand name :* Sublimase.

Phenoperidine * (dose, 0·5 to 5 mg.)

Phenoperidine is a powerful analgesic of the pethidine type, but it possesses additional and unusual properties. For use as an analgesic, doses up to 2 mg. may be given by intramuscular injection. As an adjunct to anaesthesia, the drug is given by intravenous injection in doses of 1 mg., but in chest surgery, or other operations requiring controlled respiration, larger initial doses of 2 to 5 mg. may be necessary.

In conjunction with droperidol (*q.v.*) phenoperidine produces a state of mental detachment and analgesia referred to a neurolepto-analgesia. This mental indifference to the environment is of particular value where certain procedures, such as pneumoencephalography, have to be carried out where analgesia is essential but co-operation from the patient is also required. Phenoperidine is also useful as an analgesic for cardiac catheterisation. The action may be neutralised if required by a morphine antagonist such as nalorphine (*q.v.*). The drug should not be given to patients receiving treatment with monoamine oxidase inhibitors. *Brand name :* Operidine.*

Dextromoramide* (Palfium*) oxycodone* (Proladone*) are other examples of potent synthetic morphine-like analgesics. In general they cause less depression of respiration than morphine, and are useful as alternatives when morphine is less effective, or is poorly tolerated.

Codeine† (dose, 10 to 60 mg.)

Codeine is one of the alkaloids present with morphine in opium. It has only about one-sixth of the analgesic potency of morphine, but it does not cause so much respiratory depression. The value of codeine as an analgesic is limited, but it is less constipating than morphine, and is sometimes useful in the treatment of abdominal pain. Codeine is used mainly as the phosphate in association with acetylsalicylic acid and phenacetin as in Compound Codeine Tablets and it is a constituent of many proprietary analgesic tablets, although the analgesic value of the small dose of codeine in

3

these products is questionable. Codeine also has a depressant action on the cough centre, and is widely employed as Linctus Codeine in the treatment of dry and useless cough.

Dextropropoxyphene † (dose, 30 to 65 mg.)

An analgesic resembling codeine in potency, and often given in association with aspirin or paracetamol. It is used in rheumatic disorders, and in a wide range of chronic or recurring painful conditions, but unlike codeine, it has no cough-relieving properties. *Brand name :* Doloxene.†

Dihydrocodeine † (dose, 30 to 60 mg.)

A derivative of codeine with increased analgesic potency. It is much more powerful than the salicylates, but less powerful than the opiates, and is valuable in the treatment of a variety of painful conditions where the use of opiate analgesics is not justified. Side-effects such as nausea are less prominent than with some more potent analgesics, but as dihydrocodeine liberates histamine in the body, care should be taken if the drug is given to asthmatics. *Brand name :* D.F. 118.†

Pholcodine (dose, 5 to 15 mg.)

Pholcodine is a derivative of morphine which has no analgesic power, but is considered here as it has cough-suppressant properties similar to those of codeine. It is used as Linctus Pholcodine for the treatment of dry and useless cough in both children and adults. Such cough is exhausting to the patient, and may interfere with sleep. In pleural conditions the act of coughing may cause severe pain, and suppression of coughing may in itself be a valuable therapeutic measure. Morphine is effective, but has obvious disadvantages as a cough suppressant, and pholcodine is now the standard drug. Many proprietary cough preparations have pholcodine as the main constituent.

Narcotic Antagonists

Certain synthetic compounds are known that have the power to reduce or suppress some of the effects of morphine and related drugs.

Nalorphine and levallorphan are compounds of this type, and they have applications in the treatment of overdose or excessive response to morphine-like analgesics, particularly the respiratory depression. Following the intravenous injection of nalorphine, respiration is stimulated, the pulse is improved, and coma is relieved. Levallorphan has a similar action, and is frequently used together with pethidine in labour to reduce neonatal asphyxia.

The effect of these drugs is the specific one of antagonising the action of the morphine group of analgesics. In consequence they are of no value in reducing the respiratory depression caused by other drugs such as the barbiturates.

Brand names : Lethidrone † (nalorphine) (dose, 5 to 10 mg.), Lorfan (levallorphan) (dose, 0·2 to 2 mg.). Pethilorfan * is a mixture of pethidine and levallorphan in proportions designed to produce adequate analgesia in labour without neonatal distress.

MILD ANALGESICS, ANTI-RHEUMATIC AND URICOSURIC DRUGS

Several mild analgesics are available which are very useful in alleviating minor painful conditions which do not call for treatment with powerful drugs. Some of these analgesics also have a marked anti-inflammatory action that is of considerable value in rheumatoid conditions, as they relieve pain and increase mobility of inflamed joints. This anti-rheumatic effect is distinct from the analgesic action, and may be due, in part at least, to an increased mobilisation of fluid from the inflamed tissues. (The anti-inflammatory action of the corticosteroids is referred to on page 180. It should not be forgotten that pain may at times be a very useful aid to diagnosis, and for that reason analgesics should not be given indiscriminately. The milder drugs are sometimes referred to as the coal-tar analgesics, and the following compounds are of interest.

Acetylsalicylic Acid, Aspirin (dose, 0·3 to 1 G.)

Introduced in 1899, aspirin is one of the most valuable and widely used of the mild analgesics. It is the principal constituent of a variety of popular pain-relieving preparations, and is often combined with phenacetin and other drugs. Aspirin is rapidly absorbed and rapidly excreted, so that administration every four or six hours is necessary for maintenance of effect. It is used to relieve the pain of headache, neuralgia, influenza, and its analgesic and anti-inflammatory properties are of value in various rheumatic and muscular conditions.

The drug also has an antipyretic action, *i.e.* it lowers an elevated body temperature by increasing the heat loss. This is brought about by dilatation of the skin blood vessels and sweating, and the drug is useful in a variety of feverish conditions. Aspirin is in general well tolerated, but it can cause nausea, indigestion, gastric irritation and gastric haemorrhage in susceptible patients. This blood loss may occur to a significant extent in patients who take aspirin for prolonged periods, and may be the cause of an unsuspected anaemia. Many of the side-effects of aspirin can be minimised by taking the drug after meals, or in association with an alkali such as sodium bicarbonate or chalk (calcium carbonate) which renders the aspirin soluble. Disprin and similar products contain aspirin in association with calcium carbonate, and represent a form of soluble aspirin.

Excessive doses of aspirin and other salicylates cause nausea, tinnitus, dizziness and confusion. Cardiovascular collapse and respiratory failure may follow toxic doses. Treatment of salicylate poisoning includes gastric lavage, intravenous sodium bicarbonate or lactate to reduce the marked acidosis, and respiratory stimulants.

Idiosyncrasy to aspirin is not uncommon, and quite small doses may precipitate an asthmatic attack, or cause other allergic symptoms in sensitive patients. In patients with stomach ulcers, the gastric irritant effects of aspirin may cause local bleeding, and it should also be noted that large doses of salicylates may lower the prothrombin level of the blood. Purpura is an occasional side-effect of prolonged salicylate treatment.

Sodium Salicylate (dose, 0·6 to 2 G.)

Sodium salicylate has the general properties of salicylates as referred to under aspirin, but is more irritant. The analgesic action is less powerful than that of aspirin, and the drug is mainly used in rheumatic conditions. It also has a specific effect in acute rheumatic fever, and is given in large doses, up to 12 G. daily, which are followed by rapid relief of pain, a reduction of the swelling of the affected joints, and a lowering of the temperature and pulse-rate. Cardiac damage in rheumatic fever is also considered to be reduced by adequate salicylate therapy. As sodium salicylate is rapidly excreted, three-hourly doses are usual, adjusted later so that adequate blood-levels are obtained with a minimum of side-effects. Response to treatment is prompt, but the drug should be continued in adequate doses until symptoms have fully subsided. Sodium salicylate also increases the excretion of uric acid, and when given in the higher dose range the drug has proved useful in the treatment of chronic gout.

Methyl Salicylate

Methyl salicylate is included here only for completeness, as it is too toxic for systemic use. It is a clear, pale yellow liquid, with characteristic odour, and is used as Liniment and Ointment of Methyl Salicylate for the relief of lumbago, sciatica and rheumatism. Methyl salicylate, sometimes referred to as oil of wintergreen, is very toxic if taken orally, and may cause convulsions, pneumonia and respiratory failure, especially in young children.

Phenacetin (dose, 0·3 to 0·6 G.)

Phenacetin was introduced about 1890, and remained for many years one of the most widely prescribed of the mild analgesics. It is often used in association with aspirin and is present in a wide range of proprietary analgesic tablets. Phenacetin lowers the sensitivity of the nerve centres to pain, and is useful in headache, neuralgia and muscle and joint pain, but is not powerful enough to be of any value in severe pain. Phenacetin also has some antipyretic action, *i.e.* can lower an elevated body temperature by its action on the temperature-regulating centre in the hypothalamus and is of some use in fever. It may occasionally cause methaemoglobinaemia after full doses or in susceptible patients. In recent years it has been noted that prolonged treatment with high doses of phenacetin may cause kidney damage, ('phenacetin nephritis') and the routine use of phenacetin has declined. It may well be that prolonged treatment with any analgesic may cause kidney damage, and the condition is better described as analgesic nephropathy.

Paracetamol (dose, 0.5 to 1 G.)

The analgesic action of phenacetin is not due to the drug as given but to a metabolite now known as paracetamol. This metabolite has the analgesic properties of the older drug, but appears to be free from the occasional side-effects associated with phenacetin. Paracetamol was introduced as Panadol, and is now available under many other trade names.

Phenazone (dose, 0·3 to 0·6 G.)

Phenazone has the general analgesic properties of phenacetin, but it is more likely to cause side-effects such as nausea and skin rash, and agranulocytosis may follow prolonged use. The drug is now rarely prescribed, but it should be noted that it is present in Welldorm (*q.v.*).

Anti-rheumatic Drugs

Phenylbutazone † (dose, 200 to 400 mg. daily)

In recent years many drugs have been introduced for the treatment of rheumatoid and arthritic conditions. These drugs have analgesic properties, but they also have an anti-inflammatory action that is of value in arthritic and rheumatoid disorders. They relieve pain and inflammation, improve grip strength, and do much to alleviate the limitations imposed by the arthritic state. Phenylbutazone was the first of this type of drug, and is given in initial doses of 200 to 400 mg. daily, but this dose should be reduced as soon as possible to the lowest effective maintenance dose, as the drug is not always well tolerated. It may cause nausea, stomatitis and other side-effects, may reactivate latent peptic ulcers, and blood disorders such as agranulocytosis may occur. Blood-counts should be taken at intervals during phenylbutazone treatment. Suppositories of phenylbutazone are available if gastric disturbance is severe. *Brand name :* Butazolidin.†

Flufenamic acid † (dose, 400 to 600 mg. daily)

The search for drugs with both analgesic and anti-inflammatory properties has led to the investigation of many new groups of substances, and the fenamates are drugs of interest and value. Mefenamic acid (*q.v.*) was the first of this group to be used therapeutically, and more recently flufenamic acid has been introduced as an anti-inflammatory analgesic for rheumatic conditions. It is a powerful drug, relieving both pain and stiffness, and is generally well tolerated, but gastro-intestinal disturbance occasionally follows its use. These symptoms may subside with a reduction in dose, but peptic ulcer and colitis are definite contra-indications. The safety of the drug in pregnancy has yet to be proved, and caution is necessary in patients with renal disease. *Brand name :* Arlef.†

Ibuprofen (dose, 200 mg.)

A well-tolerated analgesic and mild anti-inflammatory compound. Useful when pharmacologically related compounds cause gastric disturbance and other side-effects. *Brand name :* Brufen.

Indomethacin † (dose, 25 to 50 mg.)

Indomethacin is a potent anti-inflammatory agent with analgesic and antipyretic properties. It is used in the treatment of a wide range of musculoskeletal disorders such as rheumatoid arthritis and related conditions, and its powerful action may permit a reduction in dose of corticosteroids, or even their complete replacement.

Indomethacin is given in doses of 25 mg. three times a day with food, but it may cause gastro-intestinal disturbances, and peptic ulcer is a contra-indication. Suppositories are available for use when the drug is not tolerated orally, and are also useful at night when a long action is required to reduce morning stiffness. *Brand name :* Indocid.

Mefenamic acid † (dose, 250 to 500 mg.)

Mefenamic acid is related to flufenamic acid (*q.v.*) and has a similar anti-inflammatory action. It has been suggested that a disturbance of tryptophane metabolism occurs in rheumatoid arthritis, and as mefanamic acid is related to one of the metabolic breakdown products of tryptophane, there is a possible link between the biochemical changes of rheumatoid conditions and the anti-inflammatory action of mefenamic acid and its derivatives. The standard dose is 500 mg. initially, followed by maintenance doses of 250 to 500 mg. six-hourly. Mefenamic acid is usually well tolerated, but after full doses diarrhoea may occur in some patients, and the drug should be discontinued at once. It is more effective than the mild analgesics, and may help to bridge the gap between these drugs and the more potent compounds. *Brand name :* Ponstan.†

Oxyphenbutazone † (dose, 100 to 200 mg.)

Oxyphenbutazone is closely related to phenylbutazone, as it is formed in the body and excreted in the urine when that drug is given. Like phenylbutazone, it has analgesic and anti-inflammatory properties, and is used as an alternative drug in the treatment of rheumatoid and arthritic states. Oxyphen-butazone may also be useful in the treatment of inflammatory ophthalmic conditions. *Brand name :* Tanderil.†

Uricosuric Drugs

Colchicine † (dose, o·5 to 1 mg.)

Drugs which increase the excretion of uric acid are sometimes referred to as uricosuric drugs, and are useful in the treatment of gout. Phenylbutazone has some uricosuric action in addition to its anti-inflammatory effects, and it is therefore convenient to consider here certain drugs which are not anti-inflammatory agents, but have a specific action in gout. Colchicine, the alkaloid of the autumn crocus, is one of the oldest and most valuable remedies in acute gout, and it is also useful in suppressive treatment. In an acute attack, colchicine is given in doses of o·5 to 1 mg. every two hours until relief is obtained, or until a maximum dose of 6 mg. has been given. In practice, vomiting and purging may limit the oral use of full doses. In the suppressive treatment of gout, colchicine is given in doses of o·5 to 1 mg. daily or on alternate days, but its use has declined with the introduction of more specific drugs.

Probenecid (dose, 1 to 2 G. daily)

Probenecid has a complex action on the kidney, increasing the rate of excretion of some substances, such as uric acid, but de-creasing the rate of others such as penicillin and aminosalicylic acid. The former property makes probenecid of value in the treat-ment of chronic gout, and the drug is given in doses of o·5 to 1 G. twice daily. Prolonged treatment is necessary, but during the first few weeks of treatment, attacks of gout may increase tempo-rarily as the stores of urates are mobilised. Combined admin-istration with colchicine will control these acute attacks, and the urine should be kept alkaline by giving potassium citrate or sodium bicarbonate to prevent urate crystals appearing in the urinary tract. Salicylates should not be given with probenecid, as the uricosuric effect is reduced. *Brand name :* Benemid.

Sulphinpyrazone † (dose, 200 to 500 mg. daily)

Sulphinpyrazone is related to phenylbutazone but is a much more powerful uricosuric drug. It brings about a mobilisation of urate deposits, and an increased excretion of urates in the urine, but a high fluid intake is necessary during treatment to avoid crystalluria. Sulphinpyrazone may precipitate attacks of acute gout during the early stages of treatment, so low initial doses of 50 mg. four times a day are given. These acute attacks can be controlled by combined administration of colchicine in doses of 0·5 to 1 mg. daily. Salicylates are not suitable, as they inhibit the action of sulphinpyrazone. When the initial attacks of acute gout have subsided, the dose of sulphinpyrazone may be increased to 500 mg. daily, with later maintenance doses of 200 mg. daily. *Brand name :* Anturan.†

Ethebenicid (dose, 1 G. daily)

Ethebenicid is chemically related to probenicid, and has similar uricosuric properties. It is useful in gouty arthritis and some forms of hyperuricaemia. *Brand name :* Urelim.

Allopurinol (dose, 200 to 600 mg. daily)

Allopurinol has a unique double action in the treatment of gout, as it not only promotes the dissolution and excretion of urate deposits, but also inhibits the action of an enzyme concerned with purine metabolism and so indirectly with the formation of uric acid. In this way allopurinol differs sharply from other uricosuric drugs and represents a new and effective approach to the treatment of gout. The prophylactic use of colchicine may be necessary during the initial stages of treatment to avoid precipitating an attack of acute gout, and a high fluid intake is essential throughout treatment.

Mild conditions respond to doses of 200 to 400 mg. daily : only in severe conditions should larger doses be given. Salicylates do not interfere with the action of allopurinol, and combined therapy will sometimes afford increased relief. *Brand name :* Zyloric.

MIGRAINE

Migraine is a complex of symptoms, consisting essentially of periodic recurrent pulsating headache, frequently unilateral at first, and accompanied by gastric disturbance. The attack is often heralded and followed by visual disturbances and photophobia.

The mechanism of migraine attacks is by no means clear. The preliminary stage may be associated with a constriction of the blood vessels supplying the cerebrum and retina, but the headache is due to a vascular dilatation and rigidity of the blood vessels. A steady severe ache may replace the earlier throbbing. No neurological cause for the condition has been found, and there is probably a basic constitutional tendency that is triggered off by a variety of apparently unrelated stimuli. Treatment varies from mild analgesics and tranquillisers to ergotamine, and for prophylaxis the use of serotonin antagonists has been suggested.

Ergotamine tartrate † (dose, 1 to 2 mg. orally ; 0·25 to 0·5 mg. by injection)

Ergotamine is one of the alkaloids of ergot, and like ergometrine (*q.v.*) it has some oxytocic properties. It also has a powerful constrictor action on peripheral and cerebral blood vessels, and therapeutically it is used only for the relief of migraine. The best response is obtained if the drug is taken in adequate dose before an attack has fully developed, although in an established attack an intramuscular or subcutaneous injection of 0·25 mg. of ergotamine tartrate will often bring swift relief. The dose may be repeated if necessary. As an alternative to injections, ergotamine may be given by aerosol inhalation. The Medihaler Ergotamine † device permits rapid absorption of an adequate dose, and is sometimes very effective. The optimum oral dose is best determined by experience, and should be taken at the first sign of an attack. Not more than 6 mg. should be taken in one day, or more than 12 mg. in one week. With higher doses the peripheral vasoconstriction is both powerful and prolonged, and may cause gangrene of the extremities. For this reason ergotamine is not used prophylactically. The response to oral ergotamine is improved by the use of drugs such as caffeine, which also reduce cerebral blood flow, and anti-emetics to relieve the nausea associated with migraine. Cafergot,† Ergodryl,† Migril † and Orgraine † represent mixed products formulated on that principle. Suppositories containing ergotamine tartrate 2 mg. with caffeine 100 mg. are also available. *Brand names :* Femergin,† Lingraine.†

Methysergide † (dose, 1 to 2 mg.)

It is considered that serotonin plays some part in the migraine syndrome, possibly by lowering the pain threshold. Ergotamine has some anti-serotonin properties, and when methysergide was found to have a similar but more powerful action, it was tried empirically in the treatment of migraine. The drug is of no value in the treatment of the acute attack, but is of definite value in prophylaxis. Methysergide is given orally in doses of 1 to 2 mg. three times a day, but extended treatment may be necessary before the dose can be reduced and the drug slowly withdrawn. Methysergide is also of value in other conditions associated with serotonin release, such as carcinoid disease, where it may give prompt relief of the severe diarrhoea. *Brand name :* Deseril.†

CHAPTER IV

DRUGS ACTING ON THE AUTONOMIC NERVOUS SYSTEM

THE autonomic or involuntary nervous system controls the internal functions of the body, as opposed to the external functions, which are controlled by the brain. It is therefore concerned with the activities of the gastro-intestinal tract, the heart and vascular system, the eyes, the suprarenal and other secretory glands. The autonomic nervous system maintains the physiological equilibrium of the body, yet at the same time it is not completely independent of the central nervous system, as factors which affect the higher centres may also influence some physiological function of the body. The effect of fear and anger on the pulse-rate is an example of this interdependence.

Anatomically, the autonomic nervous system consists of two parts, the sympathetic and parasympathetic nervous systems. It will be appreciated that each organ controlled by the autonomic nervous system can be stimulated or inhibited according to physiological needs, and the functions of the sympathetic and parasympathetic nervous systems can be regarded as akin to those of the spur and reins. The two parts of the system can therefore be considered as having basically opposite effects, and this difference is reflected in the anatomical details of their structure.

The sympathetic part consists of a series of short nerve fibres, running out from the thoracic and lumbar parts of the spinal cord, and a chain of attached nerve ganglia. From these ganglia other and longer nerve fibres (the post-ganglionic fibres) pass out to the smooth muscle of the visceral organs. The parasympathetic nervous fibres originate in the midbrain, medulla and sacral portions of the spinal cord, and these pre-ganglionic fibres also pass out to ganglia, from which post-ganglionic fibres link with the organs concerned. In general, the parasympathetic ganglia are near to the organs supplied, so the post-ganglionic fibres are short; whereas the sympathetic fibres are correspondingly long.

The study of the mechanism by which the nerves of this autonomic nervous system finally affect the organs of the body with which they are connected is a fascinating one, and it has led to considerable advances in therapeutics. Briefly, when an impulse passes out from the spinal cord and reaches a ganglion, a chemical is liberated, which carries the impulse across to the post-ganglionic nerve. That substance is acetylcholine, and as soon as the impulse has passed the released acetylcholine is broken down immediately by an enzyme (cholinesterase) into acetic acid and choline, and so inactivated.

The impulse continues along the post-ganglionic fibres, and in the case of parasympathetic nerves acetylcholine is released again when the impulse reaches the point where the nerve joins the organ concerned, *i.e.* the myoneural junction. The acetylcholine acts on a receptor of the organ to produce the necessary response. This response is limited in duration and intensity by the rapid destruction of the acetylcholine by the tissue enzymes, as it is when released in the ganglia.

Similar considerations apply to the sympathetic nervous system, up to the moment that the impulse reaches the myoneural junction. At that point, instead of acetylcholine, adrenaline and noradrenaline are released. These two compounds are closely related, but noradrenaline is of greater physiological importance. Chemically they are nitrogen derivatives known as amines, and when released at the sympathetic nerve endings they are inactivated by the enzyme amine oxidase.

Noradrenaline and adrenaline are also liberated into the blood stream by the medulla of the adrenal (suprarenal) glands, and thus have more general effects. The activities of these two parts of the autonomic nervous system are therefore of profound physiological importance, and some of their main effects can be summarised as follows :

Organ	Sympathetic Stimulation	Parasympathetic Stimulation
Heart	Rate increased	Rate slowed
Blood vessels . . .	Constricted	Dilated
Lungs (bronchial muscles) .	Relaxed	Contracted
Gastro-intestinal tract . .	Activity and secretion decreased	Increased
Urinary System—		
Bladder	Relaxed	Contracted
Sphincter . . .	Contracted	Relaxed
Eye	Pupil dilated	Constricted

The field of activity of the autonomic nervous system is extremely wide, and in health the two parts of the system are in dynamic balance, constantly changing according to physiological needs. Conversely, the system can be influenced by drugs at a

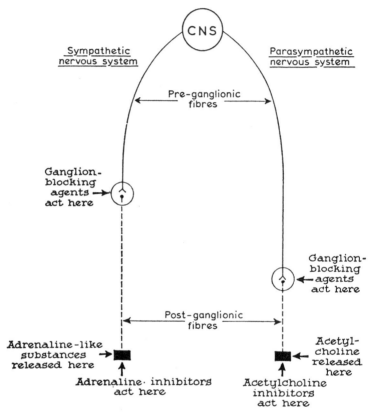

Note.—Because parasympathetic nerves liberate acetylcholine at the nerve endings, they are also known as *cholinergic* nerves. The *adrenergic* nerves are those that liberate adrenaline and noradrenaline, *i.e.* the sympathetic nerves.

number of points, and it will be appreciated that a depression of one part of the system will produce an end effect similar to that resulting from the stimulation of the other part.

Drugs which bring about changes similar or related to those caused by the normal release of adrenaline-like substances are termed sympathomimetic drugs; those that inhibit such changes are termed sympatholytic. Similar considerations apply to the parasympathetic system. Further, other drugs may prevent the transmission of impulses from the ganglia to the post-ganglionic nerves, and such drugs are known generically as blocking agents. These various factors and their points of action can be summarised graphically in the diagram on page 68.

SYMPATHOMIMETIC DRUGS

Adrenaline † (dose, o·2 to o·5 mg. by subcutaneous injection)

Sympathomimetic drugs, as already stated, are those that produce effects similar to those caused naturally by stimulation of the sympathetic nerves. One of the most powerful of such drugs is adrenaline itself, originally extracted from the suprarenal glands, but now made synthetically. When injected, it increases the force and the rate of the heart-beat, and the increased output of the heart causes a rise in the blood pressure. The peripheral blood vessels are constricted, but there is no general vasoconstriction and the rise in blood pressure caused by adrenaline is due mainly to the increase in cardiac output. Other effects include a relaxation of bronchial muscles, dilatation of the pupils, and a release of dextrose from the liver. These effects, however, are brief, as adrenaline is rapidly destroyed in the body by tissue enzymes.

Adrenaline is normally used as a 1-1000 solution in doses of o·2 to o·5 ml. by subcutaneous injection in the treatment of asthmatic attacks, bronchial spasm and in the control of allergic reactions such as serum sickness and urticaria. In status asthmaticus, where its powerful relaxant action on the bronchial muscles may be life-saving, it can be given subcutaneously in doses of o·05 ml. per minute or as a single dose of o·2 to o·5 ml. Intravenous injections of adrenaline 1-1000 are potentially dangerous, as ventricular fibrillation may result, but slow infusion of o·1 ml. per minute may give rapid relief in status asthmaticus. Very small doses have been injected directly into the heart muscle in cases of cardiac arrest. Adrenaline in strengths varying from 1-50,000 to 1-200,000 is often added to local anaesthetic solutions for its vasoconstrictor action, which limits the spread of the anaesthetic and so prolongs the effect. Stronger solutions of adrenaline are sometimes used by oral inhalation for the control of asthma.

Noradrenaline † (dose, 2 to 20 micrograms by intravenous infusion)

This compound, like adrenaline, is released when sympathetic nerves are stimulated, and the two substances are very closely related both chemically and pharmacologically. Adrenaline however may cause fear and anxiety, as well as palpitation and tremor, and to avoid any cardiac side-effects, noradrenaline is often preferred. Noradrenaline is also a powerful vasoconstrictor, but unlike adrenaline it has no stimulant effects on the heart when used systemically. The vasoconstrictor action is not selective as with adrenaline, but is exerted on the blood vessels generally, and so results in a rapid rise in blood pressure. This rise is accompanied by a compensatory slowing of the heart, and the drug is of considerable value in the treatment of shock and vaso-motor collapse. Noradrenaline is given by slow intravenous drip infusion, after diluting 2 to 4 ml. of the standard 1-1000 solution to 500-1000 ml. with saline. The rate of flow depends on the response, and treatment requires close supervision, as the blood pressure may vary markedly with small changes in the dose. Great care is also necessary to avoid the injection of any solution outside the vein, as the intense vasoconstriction produced may cause local damage. *Brand name:* Levophed† : Levophed special is a 1-10,000 solution for injection into the heart muscle in cases of cardiac arrest.

Metaraminol (dose, 2 to 10 mg.)

Metaraminol has the general vasoconstrictor properties of noradrenaline, but whilst the onset of action is rapid the increase in blood pressure is more steady, and is maintained for a longer period, and the drug thus has some of the properties of both noradrenaline and ephedrine (*q.v.*). Further, whilst the pressor effect is powerful, metaraminol does not cause the intense local vasoconstriction characteristic of noradrenaline solutions, and so the drug may be given by subcutaneous or intramuscular injec-tion, as well as by slow intravenous drip infusion. Metaraminol is used in the severe hypotension of shock, including myocardial infarction, haemorrhage, trauma and surgery, and doses range from 2 to 10 mg. (s.c. or i.m.) to 15 to 100 mg. by intravenous drip infusion, after dilution with 500 ml. of normal saline or 5 per cent. dextrose solution. *Brand name:* Aramine.

Ephedrine Hydrochloride † (dose, 15 to 60 mg.)

Ephedrine is the alkaloid of a plant used medicinally in China for thousands of years, but is now manufactured synthetically. In the main, the action of ephedrine resembles that of adrenaline, but there are important differences.   The drug is effective orally, and produces a slow but prolonged rise in blood pressure by constriction of the peripheral vessels.   It also relaxes the bronchioles, and is valuable in the treatment of bronchial asthma.   Ephedrine has a stimulant action on the central nervous system, and this may cause insomnia in asthmatics who take the drug regularly.   In such cases a mild hypnotic may be given to offset the stimulant action.   Applied locally to mucous membranes, the vasoconstrictive action of ephedrine is useful in relieving congestion, and nasal drops and sprays are used in hay fever and catarrh.   Ephedrine is occasionally given by injection to counteract the fall in blood pressure during spinal anaesthesia and also in shock, but more powerful drugs are preferred.   Ephedrine has a relaxant effect on the bladder, but it constricts the sphincter, and on that account it has been used in the treatment of enuresis.   By the same action, elderly male patients may have difficulty in micturition whilst taking ephedrine.   In view of the effect of ephedrine on the vascular and central nervous systems, it should be used with caution in cardiovascular disease, hypertension and thyrotoxicosis.

Amphetamine Sulphate † (dose, 5 to 10 mg.)

Amphetamine is a synthetic drug closely related to ephedrine, but has much more powerful central stimulant properties.   It has been used by injection in the treatment of shock and barbiturate overdosage, but when a pressor drug of this type is required methylamphetamine (*q.v.*) is preferred.   The oral use of amphetamine sulphate is referred to on page 47.

Methylamphetamine Hydrochloride † (dose, 2·5 to 10 mg.; 10 to 30 mg. by injection)

Methylamphetamine has the general properties of the amphetamine group, and is given orally for its central stimulant action in parkinsonism and narcolepsy, and by injection in psychiatry to improve rapport between doctor and patient.   It has a powerful pressor action, and when given by intravenous or intramuscular injection, is of value in restoring the blood pressure in the treatment of shock, trauma, and overdosage of barbiturates, anaesthetics and other C.N.S. depressants.

It must be remembered that in severe traumatic shock, accompanied by loss of blood, the restoration of the blood volume by transfusion, or the drip infusion of plasma or other fluids is necessary before pressor drugs can be effective. Occasionally both measures fail to restore the blood pressure, and in such circumstances the intravenous injection of hydrocortisone (*q.v.*) may be life-saving. *Brand name:* Methedrine.†

Methoxamine Hydrochloride (dose, 5 to 20 mg. by intramuscular injection; 5 to 10 mg. intravenously)

Methoxamine is a sympathomimetic drug with a powerful and prolonged constrictor effect on the peripheral blood vessels, and the advantage of having little action on the heart. It is used to restore blood pressure in shock and during surgery, and to maintain the blood pressure during spinal anaesthesia. The prompt effect of an intravenous dose may be maintained by subsequent intramuscular injections according to need. Methoxamine is also valuable as a safe pressor drug for use during cyclopropane anaesthesia. Cyclopropane may cause ventricular arrhythmia, and the use of adrenaline and associated drugs is then potentially dangerous. Methoxamine is an exception and it is also of use in arresting paroxysmal tachycardia. *Brand name:* Vasoxine.

Mephentermine Sulphate † (dose, 20 to 80 mg. by intramuscular or slow intravenous injection; 20 mg. orally)

A sympathomimetic amine with the general properties of this group of drugs. It is given by injection to raise and maintain the blood pressure in shock, myocardial infarction, during spinal anaesthesia and other conditions of hypotension. Mephentermine is occasionally given orally as a cerebral stimulant in some psychiatric conditions. *Brand name:* Mephine.†

Isoprenaline (dose, 5 to 20 mg.)

Isoprenaline is a derivative of adrenaline, and has some of the properties of the parent drug. It has a more powerful bronchodilator action than adrenaline, and although it may increase the heart rate, it has no vasoconstrictor action or pressor effect. It is given as sublingual tablets in the treatment of asthma and bronchospasm, or as an oral inhalation of a spray solution.   A wide range of proprietary anti-asthmatic products contain isoprenaline and other bronchodilator or spasmolytic drugs.   Many of these are now formulated as aerosols, and offer accuracy of dose and ease of administration.   Some care however is necessary with the use of these aerosols to obtain the maximum benefit.   The patient should place the mouthpiece well in the mouth, breathe out as much as possible, and at the moment of breathing in again, a dose of the aerosol should be released, and inhaled as deeply as possible.   In this way the full benefit of the drug will be secured, and the need for frequent supplementary ' puffs ' of aerosol will be removed.   The toxic effects ascribed to these aerosols have been due mainly to grossly excessive doses, and patients should be instructed in the proper use of these highly effective aerosols.

Salbutamol (dose, 2 to 4 mg.)

Salbutamol is chemically related to isoprenaline, but has virtually no cardiovascular action.   It is effective as a bronchodilator when given as a tablet, or by oral inhalation of an aerosol spray.   Salbutamol is inactivated by tissue enzymes less rapidly than isoprenaline, and so has a more prolonged action.   *Brand name:* Ventolin.

PARASYMPATHOMIMETIC DRUGS

The drugs that produce effects similar to those following stimulation of the parasympathetic nervous system can be divided into two groups :—

(1) Those which simulate the action of acetylcholine by a direct effect on those organs controlled by parasympathetic nerves.

(2) Those which prevent the destruction of normally released acetylcholine by the enzyme cholinesterase, and by thus allowing the concentration of acetylcholine to rise, can bring about effects similar to those of (1) above.

GROUP I

Although acetylcholine, like the corresponding adrenaline of the sympathetic system, is the natural agent, it is broken down in the body so rapidly that it is of no therapeutic value, and clinically other derivatives of choline, or related synthetic compounds, are used.

Carbachol † (dose, 1 to 4 mg. orally ; 0·25 to 0·5 mg. by sub-cutaneous injection)

Carbachol has the general pharmacological properties of acetylcholine, but is not broken down in the body by cholinesterase and is therefore more stable and also effective orally. The increased stability is reflected in its longer action, and although active by mouth, it is most effective when given by subcutaneous injection. (Intravenous injection is dangerous because of the cardiac effects.) Carbachol contracts intestinal and bladder muscles, and is valuable in the treatment of abdominal distension, post-operative intestinal atony and retention of urine. It also dilates the peripheral blood vessels, and is sometimes used in Raynaud's disease and other disorders of the peripheral circulation.

Bethanechol (dose, 5 to 25 mg. orally)

Bethanechol resembles acetylcholine and carbachol in its general properties, and is used to relieve post-operative abdominal distention and urinary retention. *Brand name:* Mechothane.

Pilocarpine Nitrate †

Pilocarpine is an alkaloid obtained from jaborandi leaves. It is mentioned here as it has some of the properties of acetylcholine, but it is now used therapeutically only as a miotic in the treatment of glaucoma. Physostigmine and other drugs used in ophthalmology are referred to in Chapter XIX.

GROUP II

Naturally released acetylcholine is rapidly destroyed by the tissue enzyme cholinesterase, and substances which suppress or inhibit the action of the enzyme are termed anticholinesterases. These drugs prolong and increase the action of released acetylcholine by preventing its destruction, and they have a number of therapeutic applications. In theory, the action of acetylcholine should be increased wherever it occurs in the body, but in practice the anticholinesterases are used mainly for their effects on the endings of the parasympathetic nerves and the associated organs.

The following drugs are of interest :

Neostigmine (dose, 0·5 to 2 mg. by subcutaneous or intramuscular injection; 15 to 30 mg. orally)

Neostigmine is a synthetic anticholinesterase, and acts chiefly on the nerve endings of skeletal or voluntary muscles. It is used like carbachol in the treatment of post-operative paralytic ileus and urinary retention, and is effective by injection in doses of 0·5 to 1 mg. Neostigmine is also used as eye drops in glaucoma, but its most important therapeutic uses are the treatment of myasthenia gravis and the reversal of the action of the muscle relaxant tubocurarine (*q.v.*). These uses of neostigmine spring directly from the increased effects of the drug on voluntary muscles.

Myasthenia gravis is a disease of the skeletal muscles, and is characterised by a progressive muscular weakness. The eyelids and muscles of the face are first affected, the limbs tire easily, and later, as the chest muscles become affected, breathing is difficult. The cause is unknown, but as the condition can be relieved by anticholinesterases it appears to be due to some breakdown at the myoneural junction in the production or use of acetylcholine. Following an intramuscular or subcutaneous injection of 0·5 mg. or more of neostigmine, a dramatic improvement occurs within an hour, but must be sustained by further treatment. Oral therapy is often effective, and doses of 15 to 20 mg. may be given four times a day, but the optimum dose must be based on need and response. In myasthenia the large doses of neostigmine required may cause some intestinal colic, but this side-effect may be controlled by atropine.

Neostigmine can also antagonise the effects of certain muscle relaxants such as tubocurarine and gallamine. This use of the drug in anaesthesia is discussed on page 84. *Brand name:* Prostigmin.

Pyridostigmine (dose, 60 to 240 mg. orally; 1 to 5 mg. by subcutaneous or intramuscular injection)

Pyridostigmine is a synthetic drug similar to neostigmine in its general properties, but the action is slower and more prolonged. It causes less intestinal disturbance than neostigmine, and is a useful alternative when a less intense action is adequate or for night-time use when a longer action is required. It is occasionally given by injection for post-operative ileus. An average dose of 60 mg. is equivalent to about 15 mg. of neostigmine. *Brand name:* Mestinon.

Edrophonium (dose, 2 to 10 mg. by intravenous injection)

Edrophonium is chemically related to neostigmine, but it is used mainly in the diagnosis of myasthenia gravis as the action is too brief for treatment of the disease. The test is carried out by giving a dose of 2 mg. intravenously, followed by a dose of 8 mg. about 30 seconds later. A patient with myasthenia gravis will experience a temporary increase in muscle power, lasting about five minutes. The drug is also useful in determining the adequacy of a dose of neostigmine. If further improvement of the myasthenic condition follows the use of edrophonium after neostigmine, the dose of the latter is inadequate, and should be increased. Conversely, an increase in muscle weakness after edrophonium is an indication to reduce the dose of neostigmine. *Brand name:* Tensilon.

Physostigmine

Physostigmine and other anticholinesterases used as miotics in the treatment of glaucoma are referred to in Chapter XIX.

SIDE EFFECTS OF ANTICHOLINESTERASES

The side and toxic effects of the anticholinesterases are reflections of their general activity. Thus the stimulation of the gastro-intestinal tract results in nausea, vomiting, colic and increased peristaltic activity. The pupils are constricted, the pulse is weak, and dyspnoea may occur from the increased pulmonary secretions. The immediate treatment is the injection of atropine in doses of 1 to 2 mg., which rapidly counteracts the toxic effects on the circulation and the lungs. The secondary toxic effects should subside as the drug is excreted. Certain organophosphate insecticides function as anticholinesterases and may cause severe poisoning, with death from respiratory failure. For specific treatment see page 299.

ACETYLCHOLINE ANTAGONISTS

A number of drugs are available which inhibit the action of acetylcholine released at nerve endings, and by virtue of that action have a number of therapeutic applications. The oldest and most widely used member of this group is belladonna, and the alkaloid atropine obtained from it, but a number of synthetic compounds are also used.

Belladonna †

The leaf of the deadly nightshade, *Atropa belladonna*. Its principal constituent is atropine (*q.v.*), but a related alkaloid, hyoscyamine, is also present. Henbane, or hyoscyamus, is a plant related to belladonna and contains atropine, hyoscyamine and hyoscine. Hyoscyamus is occasionally added to purgatives to reduce griping and colic and tincture of hyoscyamus is given with Mixture of Potassium Citrate for spasm of the urinary tract.

Atropine † (dose, 0·25 to 2 mg.; orally or by injection)

The general effect of atropine is a reduction of muscle tone and of gastro-intestinal activity. It is therefore widely used for the relief of renal, biliary and intestinal colic, and may be given by subcutaneous or intramuscular injection when a rapid action is required. The reduction of muscle tone extends to the bladder, and the drug has been used in the treatment of enuresis. Atropine is also used in the treatment of peptic ulcer, as it reduces gastric spasm and motility, and so prolongs the effects of antacid therapy, but the effects are variable. The antispasmodic action is also valuable in asthma and whooping-cough. Atropine also affects the eye, causing dilatation of the pupil and paralysis of the accommodation, and it is widely used as eye drops (1 per cent.) in ophthalmology as a mydriatic. Preoperatively, atropine is given to decrease secretions of the bronchial and salivary systems, and to prevent cardiac depression. The dryness of the mouth that follows treatment with atropine or belladonna is a familiar example of the effect of the drug on secretions. Belladonna and its alkaloids have been used in the symptomatic treatment of parkinsonism (*q.v.*).

Official Preparations—
> Tincture of Belladonna (dose, o·5 to 2 ml.).
> Tincture of Hyoscyamus (dose, 2 to 5 ml.).
> Tincture of Stramonium (dose, o·5 to 2 ml.).

Atropine Methonitrate † (dose, o·2 to o·6 mg.)

Atropine has been used for the treatment of congenital pyloric stenosis and pylorospasm in infants, but the methonitrate compound is equally effective and less toxic. It may be given as solution of atropine methonitrate (o·o1 per cent.) in doses of 2 ml., and given half an hour before food as often as seven times a day. The dose may be increased slowly to a maximum of 6 ml. Eumydrin drops are similar, but much stronger (o·6 per cent) and an average dose is two drops. *Brand name:* Eumydrin †.

Hyoscine † (dose, o·3 to o·6 mg.)

This drug, also known as scopolamine, is closely related to atropine, but differs in having a depressant and not a stimulant action on the central nervous system. When given by injection it has a powerful hypnotic action, and is useful in mania and delirium. Hyoscine is often given pre-operatively with morphine for its depressant action, and for reducing the laryngospasm associated with intravenous barbiturate anaesthesia. Its use in parkinsonism is discussed on page 80. Hyoscine also has anti-emetic properties, and is a constituent of some travel-sickness remedies. A derivative of hyoscine (hyoscine-N-butyl bromide), available as Buscopan, is used as an antispasmodic and to relax smooth muscle in peptic ulcer, colic and related conditions. It is best given by injection in doses of 10 to 20 mg., as it may be ineffective orally owing to poor absorption.

Homatropine Hydrobromide †

A derivative of atropine, used mainly in ophthalmology as a mydriatic with a more rapid and less-prolonged action than atropine. The effect is increased by the addition of cocaine, and homatropine is often used as a 2 per cent. solution in association with cocaine 1 per cent. as in cocaine and homatropine eye drops B.P.C.★

SYNTHETIC ATROPINE-LIKE COMPOUNDS

The side-effects associated with the systemic use of atropine, such as dryness of the mouth and disturbances of vision, have led to the introduction of a large number of synthetic compounds with a more selective action.   With these drugs the mydriatic and anti-salivary effects are reduced to some extent (although by no means abolished) and they therefore have certain advantages over atropine.   The following compound is representative of this group of drugs although the ideal selective atropine substitute has yet to be discovered.

Propantheline (dose, 15 to 30 mg.)

Propantheline has a marked atropine-like action in blocking the effects of acetylcholine released at the endings of parasympathetic nerves, and so is useful in intestinal hypermotility and colic, peptic ulcer, and spasms of the bladder and ureters.   It has also been used in enuresis.   *Brand name:* Pro-Banthine.

The following drugs are some of the many alternative products. In some cases, combined products with phenobarbitone are available: dicyclomine (Merbentyl;   dose, 10 to 20 mg.), oxyphenonium (Antrenyl;   dose, 5 to 10 mg.), poldine (Nacton;   dose, 2 to 4 mg.), methoscopolamine bromide (Pamine;   dose, 2·5 to 5 mg.), penthenate bromide (Monodral;   dose, 5 mg.) and dicyclomine (Wyovin;   dose, 10 to 20 mg.).

PARKINSON'S DISEASE

Originally described in 1817 as 'the shaking palsy,' Parkinson's disease is also known as paralysis agitans.   It is due to a degeneration of certain cells of the brain, and is characterised by tremor of the hands, weakness and rigidity of muscles, excessive salivation, cramp and spasm.   Most forms of the disease are progressive, and treatment is palliative and is aimed at relieving the tremor, rigidity and akinesia characteristic of parkinsonism.   In general, drugs are most effective against rigidity or tremor, as the akinesia is seldom relieved. Claims are made that some drugs relieve tremor more than rigidity, or rigidity more than tremor, but in practice, the best drug or combination of drugs for the individual

patient must be determined by the slow process of trial and acceptance or rejection. Recently, the treatment of parkinsonism has
been markedly changed by the introduction of two new drugs,
amantadine (*q.v.*) and L-dopa (*q.v.*).

Belladonna †

Belladonna and related drugs have long been used in the
treatment of parkinsonism, as by their action on the motor
centres of the brain, tremor and rigidity are reduced, posture,
gait and speech are improved, and the excessive salivation is
relieved. Large doses are essential, but the use of this group of
drugs has declined as synthetic compounds with a more selective
action and fewer side-effects have become available.

Benzhexol † (dose, 2 to 20 mg. daily)

Benzhexol has some of the anticholinergic properties of
atropine, but is used mainly for the relief of parkinsonism. It is
effective in controlling the muscular rigidity of the disease more
than the tremor, but it also has a central stimulant action, and so
has value in reducing the inertia and depression that is often
present in parkinsonism. The initial dose of 1 to 2 mg. daily is
gradually increased according to response, and maintenance doses
vary from 6 to 20 mg. or more daily. Some dryness of the mouth
and other atropine-like side-effects may occur with full doses.
Brand names: Artane,† Pipanol.†

Benztropine † (dose, 0·5 to 6 mg. daily)

Benztropine methanesulphonate is mainly effective in controlling the tremor and rigidity of parkinsonism, and the muscle
relaxation obtained reduces the discomfort and restlessness at
night. The drug does not have the central stimulant properties of
benzhexol, and is more suitable for elderly patients. Benztropine
is also useful in controlling the symptoms of drug-induced
parkinsonism. The initial dose is 0·5 to 1 mg. daily, increased
slowly to a maximum of 6 mg. daily according to response. *Brand
name:* Cogentin.†

Orphenadrine † (dose, 200 to 400 mg. daily)

Although orphenadrine is closely related to the antihistaminic
drug diphenhydramine, it has but weak antihistamine activity,
and is used mainly in parkinsonism for its spasmolytic effects on

voluntary muscle. It is sometimes effective when the response to other drugs is unsatisfactory. Orphenadrine controls rigidity more than tremor, and sometimes the tremor will be increased as the rigidity is relieved. Orphenadrine also reduces excessive salivation, and its central stimulant properties are useful in relieving the depression that is often associated with Parkinson's disease. *Brand name:* Disipal.†

Methixene † (dose, 7·5 to 60 mg. daily)

Methixene is an exceptional drug, as it reduces the tremor of parkinsonism more than the rigidity. Combined treatment with other drugs which have a greater effect on rigidity may evoke the best response. Small doses of 2·5 mg. three times a day are given initially, rising slowly until the maximum relief is obtained. *Brand name:* Tremonil.

Related Drugs

The aim of treatment in Parkinson's disease is to obtain maximum symptomatic relief with a minimum degree of side-effects, but as tolerance to an effective drug may occur, alternative or combined forms of treatment are desirable. In all cases transition from one drug to another should be gradual, as otherwise the symptoms may become exacerbated during the change-over period. Biperiden (Akineton †), chlorphenoxamine (Clorevan †), procyclidine (Kemadrin †) and phenglutarimide (Aturbane) represent other compounds used in the symptomatic treatment of Parkinson's disease. Some antihistamines such as diphenhydramine and promethazine (*q.v.*) have some value in parkinsonism, and are also used in controlling the side-effects of certain drugs used in psychiatry. Some of these side-effects resemble those of Parkinson's disease, and the condition has been referred to as ' drug-induced parkinsonism,' and may be relieved by promethazine and related compounds. A departure from conventional therapy for Parkinson's disease is the recent introduction of amantadine and levodopa, as these drugs represent a new approach to the problem.

Amantadine (dose, 100 mg.)

Amantadine is a synthetic compound, and was originally used as an antivival agent in the prophylaxis of influenza. By chance it was given to a patient with Parkinson's disease, who commented on the subsequent relief of rigidity and tremor. The drug has since been examined critically and has proved a definite advance in the treatment of parkinsonism. It has a wide range of activity, and improves mood, walking ability, stiffness, tremor and rigidity, and if required, can be combined with other forms of therapy. Amantadine is given in capsules of 100 mg. daily for one week, increased to two capsules daily if required. Response to treatment is rapid, and side-effects, such as dizziness and confusion, can be controlled by a reduction in dose. There are some similarities between the response to amantadine and that to levodopa (*q.v.*), and although the degree of benefit may be less with the former, the response is more rapid, and has fewer side-effects. *Brand name:* Symmetrel.

Levodopa (L-dopa)

Metabolic studies of the lesions present in the substantia nigra of patients with Parkinson's disease have shown that there is a relationship between these lesions and a deficiency in the amount of dopamine in the corpus striatum. Dopamine acts as a neurotransmitter in the extra-pyramidal system of the brain, and is concerned with motor function, so that parkinsonism may be regarded as a specific deficiency of dopamine.

Deficiency diseases can often be treated by supplying the deficient substance, but unfortunately dopamine does not pass the blood-brain barrier, and so is useless in the treatment of parkinsonism. The difficulty can be overcome by the administration of L-dopa, which is a precursor of dopamine; and is converted by the tissue enzyme decarboxylase to the active drug. Following the oral administration of L-dopa to parkinsonian patients, the amount of dopamine in the striatum and other brain centres rises, and in the majority of patients is slowly followed by considerable symptomatic relief. Akinesia is relieved before rigidity, but the suppression of tremor is slower and less complete. The dose varies considerably with different patients, but in any case initial doses should be small, ranging from 0·25 to 0·5 G. daily, increasing by similar amounts at weekly intervals according to response. Maintenance doses may vary from 2 to 8 G. daily. Side-effects include nausea, vomiting, anorexia, psychiatric disturbances and involuntary body movements. L-dopa should not be used with monoamine oxidase inhibitors and care should be taken with sympathomimetic drugs, tricyclic antidepressants, phenothiazine derivatives, reserpine and anti-hypertensive drugs.   Pyridoxine also antagonises the action of L-dopa.   The urine may be coloured during L-dopa treatment, but such changes are of no significance. The true place of L-dopa in the management of Parkinson's disease has still to be assessed, but there is no doubt that the introduction of the drug marks a new stage in the control of this distressing condition.   *Brand names :* Brocadopa, Larodopa.

SKELETAL MUSCLE RELAXANTS

Skeletal or striped muscle differs from smooth muscle both anatomically and physiologically.   Although acetylcholine is liberated at the nerve-endings of both types of muscle, it is only in smooth muscle that atropine functions as an acetylcholine antagonist, and has a relaxant effect.

Skeletal muscle relaxants, which differ sharply from atropine and related compounds, produce a relaxation by blocking the access of released acetylcholine to receptor sites on the muscle end-plate (see p. 68), and thus prevent the contraction that normally follows stimulation of muscle.   Certain compounds have wide applications in surgery, as they enable adequate relaxation of muscle to be achieved without deep anaesthesia.   Shock is reduced and recovery from the lower dose of anaesthetic is more rapid. Others are more useful in spastic conditions, but the mode of action differs.

Tubocurarine †

The strange stories told for hundreds of years of a remarkable arrow poison used by certain South American Indians had a foundation in fact.   The poison, obtained from various plants, was used in hunting, and killed the animals not by a general toxic effect, but by causing a complete paralysis of all muscles, including respiratory muscle.   The main constituent of the poison was the alkaloid tubocurarine, and the pure substance is now used extensively as a muscle relaxant in abdominal surgery.   The alkaloid is not effective when given orally, and it is normally administered as a 1 per cent. solution by intravenous injection. The initial dose varies from 10 to 20 mg., and the drug rapidly produces a weakness of voluntary muscles, commencing with the eyelids and spreading to the face, neck, limbs, abdomen and finally the respiratory muscles, which are the last to be affected.

The effect of the drug begins within sixty to ninety seconds after the injection, and reaches a maximum in three to five minutes. The action begins to decline after about twenty minutes, but may be maintained by supplementary doses at thirty-minute intervals. Respiratory paralysis follows full doses, and assisted respiration is then necessary until the effects of the drug have worn off. The effects of tubocurarine are increased by ether, and when ether is used as the anaesthetic the dose of tubocurarine must be reduced by at least half.

The drug is used mainly in abdominal surgery, in orthopaedic manipulations and to control the muscle spasms of tetanus.   As no significant amount of tubocurarine crosses the placenta, the drug is also used as a muscle relaxant in obstetrics.

Neostigmine reverses the action of tubocurarine, and is given intravenously in doses of 2·5 mg. or more to reduce overdosage or shorten the recovery period following tubocurarine administration. It is essential to give 0·5 to 1 mg. of atropine a few minutes before the neostigmine is injected to prevent excessive slowing of the heart-rate. *Brand name:* Tubarine.†

Alcuronium †

This synthetic compound is related to the curare alkaloids, and has similar muscle-relaxant properties but is effective in smaller doses. The relaxant effect is increased when halothane is used, as the anaesthetic also has muscle-relaxant properties. It is given in initial doses of 10 to 15 mg. intravenously, and relaxation occurs in three to four minutes, and lasts for 15 to 20 minutes. A second injection of 3 to 5 mg. may be given if necessary. The relaxant effects are reversed by neostigmine but care is necessary when halothane has been used, as severe bradycardia may occur unless the anaesthetic has been eliminated. *Brand name :* Alloferin.†

Gallamine Triethiodide †

Gallamine is a synthetic muscle relaxant that resembles tubocurarine in its general properties, but it has a less prolonged action, and larger doses are necessary to produce comparable effects. It may also cause tachycardia in some patients, due to an atropine-like action on the vagus nerve, and such tachycardia may persist longer than the relaxant action. The average adult dose of gallamine is 80 to 120 mg. by intravenous injection; relaxation of the muscle occurs within two minutes, and continues for about twenty minutes, and can be maintained by a second dose of 40 to 60 mg. Gallamine is used in a wide range of operative procedures requiring muscle relaxation, and is regarded as particularly useful in association with halothane (*q.v.*). The action of the drug, like that of tubocurarine, can be reversed by neostigmine, and atropine should also be given beforehand both to minimise the cardiac effects and to reduce bronchial secretions. Gallamine causes less histamine release than tubocurarine, so that the risk of bronchospasm is correspondingly reduced. *Brand name:* Flaxedil.†

Pancuronium bromide †

Pancuronium is related to the steroids, but has a muscle-relaxant action similar to tubocurarine. The onset of action is more rapid, but the duration rather less, and with few side-effects. No release of histamine and consequent bronchospasm follows the use of pancuronium, and the drug is of value in poor-risk patients. The dose is 4 to 6 mg. intravenously, followed by later doses of 2 mg. as required. The relaxant effect can be reversed by neostigmine, together with atropine. *Brand name :* Pavulon.†

Suxamethonium †

Suxamethonium, also known as succinylcholine, is a short-acting muscle relaxant, with an effect following intravenous injection that lasts from three to five minutes. It is therefore of value in procedures where a brief relaxation is adequate, as in manipulations, and the reduction of fractures, but a longer action can be obtained by repeated injections, or by the administration of a diluted solution by intravenous drip infusion. Suxamethonium causes an initial painful muscle fibrillation before relaxation occurs, and its use should therefore be preceded by an intravenous anaesthetic such as thiopentone sodium. An average adult dose of suxamethonium varies from 30 to 60 mg., and as it is rapidly destroyed in the body an antagonist is not required. The mode of action differs from that of tubocurarine, as suxamethonium blocks neuromuscular transmission by another mechanism. In consequence, neostigmine does not antagonise the action of suxamethonium, and may actually increase the relaxant action.

In a few patients, suxamethonium may have an unexpectedly long action, with marked apnea. *Brand names :* Anectine, Brevidil,† Scoline.†

Mephenesin † (dose, 0·5 to 1 G.)

Certain other drugs used as muscle relaxants exert their effects by a selective action on the spinal cord and not on the muscle endplate. Such drugs are not suitable as relaxants in surgery, but have therapeutic applications in acute muscle spasm, fibrositis, and other musculo-skeletal conditions.

Mephanesin was introduced as a muscle relaxant in surgery, but proved to be of limited value, and is now used orally for the symptomatic treatment of spastic conditions, the relief of anxiety and tension states, and by intramuscular injection in the treatment of tetanus. It may also be given by intravenous injection, but the standard 10 per cent. solution must be diluted before use to prevent haemolysis and local thrombosis. *Brand name :* Myanesin.†

A longer-acting oral form of the drug is mephenesin carbamate (Tolseram†), and other muscle relaxants of this type, used in the treatment of spondylitis, myositis, and related conditions are carisprodol † (Carisoma), methocarbamol † (Robaxin) and chlormezanone (Trancopal). Mixed products containing an analgesic are represented by Norgesic.

Some tranquillising drugs such as meprobamate (*q.v.*), diazepam (*q.v.*) and chlordiazepoxide (*q.v.*) also have mild muscle-relaxant properties, and are useful in various musculo-skeletal disorders, especially when an emotional component is present.

CHAPTER V

CARDIOVASCULAR DRUGS

THE heart, although only weighing about 10 oz., is a remarkably efficient and reliable pump. During a normal span of life it may beat about 2,000 million times, and in health it has enough reserve of power to cope with any physiological demands that may be made upon it. Reduction in the efficiency of the heart influences the whole body, and is a correspondingly serious matter. In the early stages of cardiac weakness the inability of the heart to cope with the demands made upon it may be apparent only after stress or exercise, but later, if the cardiac output continues to fall, blood begins to accumulate behind the weakened heart, leading to the congested lungs and liver, oedema of the tissues, and cyanosis that are characteristic of heart failure.

Apart from cardiac weakness or failure, the heart may also show disturbances of rhythm. Normally the auricles and ventricles beat in unison, but in auricular (atrial) fibrillation, the auricles contract independently at a very high rate. Some of these auricular impulses continue to reach the ventricles, which in turn contract rapidly but irregularly. Owing to these rapid but erratic impulses the ventricles do not fill regularly or completely with blood, in consequence the cardiac output suffers, and the pulse becomes weak and irregular.

In heart block some of the impulses from the auricles fail to reach the ventricles, which therefore beat independently, and the heart block may be complete or partial according to the degree of blockade. These variations in cardiac rhythm, though not directly or necessarily associated with cardiac failure, may precipitate such failure by adding to the burden of an already weakening heart.

CARDIAC THERAPEUTICS

In this field natural drugs still hold pride of place, as so far no synthetic drug has been produced which can rival the remarkable effects of digitalis on the failing heart. Digitalis is

4   87

the leaf of the common foxglove, and was introduced into medicine by William Withering in 1785 for the relief of dropsy. In spite of misuse by Withering's contemporaries and later physicians, digitalis eventually achieved an established place in cardiac therapeutics, although in recent years it has been supplanted to an increasing extent by digoxin (*q.v.*) the active principle of the Austrian foxglove.

Digitalis † (dose, 100 to 200 mg.)

Digitalis may be given as tablets of the dried leaf, and is absorbed fairly rapidly after oral administration, exerting its maximum effect in about six hours. Although it is of little value in heart failure associated with infection or anaemia, in congestive heart failure digitalis is the drug of choice. By its powerful and selective action on the myocardium or heart muscle, it produces more powerful and effective contractions so that the heart empties more completely. With this increase in cardiac output there is an improvement of the circulation, a lowering of the venous pressure, a slowing of the heart-rate, and a reduction in the size of the enlarged heart. This increase in efficiency occurs without any increase in the oxygen demand.

The improved blood supply to the kidneys leads to an increase in urinary output, and this increased elimination of fluid leads to a reduction in the oedema that accompanies heart failure. The blood pressure is not affected directly by digitalis, but as the cardiac output and circulation improve, the elevated blood pressure tends to return to normal.

The dose of digitalis and the product used depend to some extent on the rapidity of action desired. For rapid digitalisation a single large dose of 1 to 1·5 G. has been given, but for this purpose digoxin (*q.v.*) is usually preferred. In all cases when high-dosage digitalis therapy is to be started, care must be taken to check that the patient has not already taken digitalis during the previous 10 to 14 days in order to avoid overdosage. Alternatively, and preferably, digitalisation may be carried out more slowly by giving doses of 60 to 120 mg. of digitalis leaf three or four times a day, later reduced according to need and response. The maintenance dose, which is normally required indefinitely, should be adjusted so that the pulse-rate becomes steady at about sixty beats per minute.

Digoxin †

Preparations of digitalis leaf cannot be standardised chemically, as the active principles, sometimes referred to as cardiac glycosides, are not easily extracted. Digitalis products are therefore tested for activity by measuring the effects on the heart of a test animal (cat or frog), and such biological assays have certain disadvantages.

The Austrian foxglove, however, differs from the common foxglove in possessing a glycoside that can be extracted in pure form as digoxin, and being of constant composition, its action is more consistent and it is now the preferred product. Digoxin has the advantage of rapid and complete absorption when given orally, and it may also be given by injection when a very rapid action is required, or when oral treatment is not possible.

The standard tablet of digoxin contains 0·25 mg., equivalent to about 60 mg. of digitalis leaf, and for rapid digitalisation an initial dose of four to six tablets may be given followed by maintenance doses of one or two tablets daily. If a particularly rapid effect is required, the drug may be given by slow intravenous injection in doses of 0·5 to 1 mg., equivalent to 2 to 4 ml. of Injection of Digoxin B.P. The action then begins in a few minutes, and reaches a maximum in about one hour. Alternatively the injection can be made intramuscularly.

TOXIC EFFECTS.—In general, digitalis preparations are slowly excreted, and most toxic side-effects are due to the cumulative action of the drug. Nausea and vomiting are early signs of overdosage, as is the slowing of the pulse-rate below sixty. The drug should then be withdrawn for a few days. This nausea should be distinguished from any gastric disturbance which may occur early in treatment, and is a local irritant effect, and may be reduced by dividing the dose. Other toxic manifestations are confusion and disturbances of cardiac rhythm, such as extrasystoles and coupled beats. In severe cases these disturbances of cardiac rhythm, which indicate an increased excitability of the ventricles, may lead to a fatal ventricular fibrillation.

Toxic reactions may also occur if the potassium reserves of the body are depleted. This may happen during extended additional therapy with the chlorothiazide type of diuretic when appreciable amounts of potassium are excreted in the urine, and potassium chloride is often given in association with these diuretics to offset such potassium loss.

It should be remembered that elderly patients require smaller doses of digitalis preparations, possibly because of increased sensitivity of the myocardium and a less efficient renal function. Children tolerate relatively large doses, and to permit easy adjustment of dose for these two groups of patients, tablets of digoxin containing 0·0625 mg. are available as Lanoxin P.G. (paediatric-geriatric).

Other Products

Certain other digitalis products are available, such as lanatoside C or Cedilanid † (dose, 0·5 to 1 mg. orally or intravenously), and may be useful occasionally as alternatives. Cardiac properties are also found in plants such as strophanthus.† This drug, used as the active principles strophanthin and oubain, is excreted more rapidly than digitalis, and has no cumulative action, but although it has some reputation abroad, it is rarely prescribed in Britain.

CARDIAC ARRHYTHMIAS

Valuable as digitalis is in the treatment of heart failure, in disturbances of cardiac rhythm its action is less specific, and the main effect of the drug is to control such disturbances rather than that of restoring a normal rhythm. On the other hand, particularly in early auricular (atrial) fibrillation, it may be desirable to attempt to restore the normal rhythm, and the drugs used for this purpose include quinidine, procainamide, lignocaine, phenytoin, propranolol and related drugs.

Quinidine Sulphate (dose, 300 to 600 mg.)

This substance is closely related to quinine, and is extracted from the same source, the bark of cinchona trees. It has a specific action on the muscle of the auricle, and extends the 'refractory period,' *i.e.* the brief rest period between successive contractions of the muscle. In atrial fibrillation such an extension of the refractory period may break up the sequence of excessive impulses that results in fibrillation and allow a normal rhythm to be resumed and maintained.

Quinidine was once used extensively as a myocardial drug, but has been largely superseded by more active substances. If used, a test dose of 200 mg. should be given, as a few patients have an idiosyncrasy to quinidine. If the drug is tolerated, doses of 300 mg. gradually increasing, may be given up to five times a day for seven to ten days. Restoration of normal rhythm, if it occurs, may occur quite suddenly, and the dose of quinidine can then be reduced slowly to maintenance levels of 300 mg. or so twice daily. The drug should be withdrawn if no benefit is experienced within ten days.

Procainamide (dose, 0·5 to 1 G.)

Procaine, the well-known local anaesthetic, has a depressant action on the myocardium, similar to that of quinidine, but the drug is broken down so rapidly in the body that it is useless for routine treatment. The chemically related procainamide is more stable, and active orally. It is used principally for ventricular arrhythmias, and is given in doses of 0·5 to 1 G. every four to six hours. In full doses, which may be necessary for an adequate response, the drug may cause nausea and vomiting.

Procainamide is occasionally given by intramuscular or intravenous injection in doses of 250 to 500 mg., but its use requires care as it may cause cardiovascular collapse. *Brand name :* Pronestyl.

Lignocaine †

This local anaesthetic is chemically related to procainamide, and that similarity has led to the use of lignocaine in the treatment of acute cardiac arrhythmias. Initially a loading dose of 1 to 2 mg. per kg. is given intravenously, followed by a dose of 1 to 2 mg. per minute as a solution of 500 mg. of lignocaine hydrochloride in 500 ml. of 5 per cent. dextrose solution. The addition of 500 units of heparin is advisable to prevent thrombophlebitis. This solution is of particular value in acute ventricular fibrillation, particularly that occurring during cardiac surgery, or after acute myocardial infarction.

Phenytoin Sodium (dose, 250 mg.)

Phenytoin sodium, in addition to being a valuable anticonvulsant, is also useful in some cardiac arrhythmias. The drug is given by slow intravenous injection in doses of 250 mg., and may be successful, particularly in drug-induced arrhythmias, when other measures fail. Slow injection is essential.

Propranolol (dose, 10 to 80 mg.)

Noradrenaline and adrenaline, sometimes referred to as catecholamines, exert their effects on two types of receptor points, the alpha and beta receptors. Alpha-receptors are found mainly in the peripheral vessels, and when stimulated by noradrenaline, cause vasoconstriction and a rise in blood pressure. Beta-receptors are found mainly in the heart, and respond more to adrenaline, resulting in an increased cardiac output, and greater oxygen demands by the myocardium. Stimulation of an already damaged heart in this way may cause severe or even fatal arrhythmias, and substances that can block the beta-receptor sites, and so inhibit the cardiac effects of adrenaline, are of considerable therapeutic importance. Propranolol is a beta-receptor blocking agent of this type, and has been used in cardiac arrhythmias, arrhythmias occurring during anaesthesia or associated with digitalis therapy, and in angina pectoris. The drug is given orally in doses of 10 to 30 mg. up to four times a day, but in emergencies it is given by slow intravenous injection in doses of 5 mg. Propranolol in doses up to 80 mg. four times a day is also effective in hypertension. The drug is slow in action but continued therapy produces a slow but steady fall in blood pressure. With propranolol, the peripheral vessels are not constricted, and so can respond to sympathetic stimulation. The faintness, postural hypotension and pooling of blood in the vessels, which may occur with other antihypertensive drugs, is thus avoided.

Propranolol is also useful in the treatment of angina pectoris. That condition is usually an indication of ischaemic heart disease, where the supply of oxygenated blood passing through the heart is insufficient to meet the physiological demands. These demands may arise from physical exertion or from stress. In conditions of stress, the heart is stimulated by the sympathetic nervous system, there may be an increase in the amount of catecholamines in the blood, followed by a rise in heart rate and blood pressure. The oxygen demands of the heart rise accordingly, and when the supply is insufficient, it is experienced as the paroxysmal chest pain known as angina pectoris. This stress response can be inhibited by the use of beta-receptor blocking agents such as propranolol. These drugs modify the myocardial response to adrenergic stress, and the tachycardia and increased oxygen demands that result in angina, can be reduced or prevented. Propranolol in oral doses of

10 to 30 mg. gives a high degree of relief and protection in patients subject to angina, as well as improving exercise tolerance. Its introduction marked a new approach to angina, although the drug is not without disadvantages. It may cause bronchospasm in asthmatic patients, and may reduce myocardial efficiency to a less than desirable level, and alternative drugs are now available. *Brand name :* Inderal.

Practolol (dose, 100 to 300 mg. daily)

Practolol represents an extension of propranolol therapy, as although both compounds have basically similar properties, practolol has a more selective action on the cardiac beta-receptors. In standard doses of 100 mg. three times a day it gives adequate relief in angina without depressing the cardiac output. Practolol has virtually no broncho-constrictor action, and may be used in asthma and other conditions associated with bronchospasm. It may be used if required in association with isoprenaline.

Practolol is also valuable in the management of cardiac arrhythmias. Mild conditions may respond to oral doses of 100 mg., twice or more daily, but in severe conditions the drug should be given in doses of 5 mg. by slow intravenous injection. The dose may be repeated if necessary. *Brand name :* Eraldin.

Oxprenolol (dose, 50 to 200 mg. daily)

Oxprenolol is a beta-receptor blocking agent of the propranolol type. It protects the heart against excessive stimulation induced by physical or emotional stress, and by slowing down the heart rate it reduces the oxygen requirements of the myocardium. At the same time, oxprenolol has a mild stimulant action of its own, so that the cardiac output is largely unchanged. The drug reduces the frequency and severity of anginal attacks, and is given in initial doses of 40 mg. orally, increasing according to need and response. Oxprenolol is also useful in the control of cardiac arrhythmias, and in the tachycardia of hyperthyroidism. *Brand name :* Trasicor.

ANTIHYPERTENSIVE DRUGS

The blood pressure of the body is maintained by two forces, the pumping action of the heart and the elastic response of the muscle fibres of the blood vessel walls. The tone of these muscle fibres is largely controlled by the sympathetic nervous system, but is also subject to some extent to the influence of the central nervous system, as emotions such as fear and anger, which bring about a release of adrenaline, can also cause a temporary rise in blood pressure. In health, the vascular system is so adjusted that it can respond rapidly to all the physiological demands made upon it, yet permit a prompt return to the normal blood pressure when the immediate stress has passed. In later life, the blood pressure tends to rise to a permanently higher level, and is associated with progressive changes in the artery and arteriole walls. There is a thickening of the connective tissue of the intima in response to the higher pressure, and the arterial walls lose some of their former elasticity. But this thickening, initially a structural adaptation, leads eventually to irreversible vascular change, and if untreated the arteries and other vessels lose their ability to respond to physiological stress, and the peripheral resistance rises. As a consequence, the heart enlarges in an attempt to overcome the increased resistance, and the increase in arterial pressure leads to kidney damage and a reduction in renal blood flow, and the attempt at adaptation finally becomes a destructive process.

This process may be halted, and the condition relieved by the use of drugs which relax the muscle of the arterial walls, and the vasodilatation thus produced results in a lowering of the elevated blood pressure. Such antihypertensive therapy not only brings about a relaxation of the arterial walls and a reduction in peripheral resistance, but also reduces the size of the enlarged heart, improves the blood flow through the kidneys, and repairs retinal damage as the retinal oedema is relieved.

The drugs used may reduce the blood pressure by several mechanisms. Ganglion blocking agents (p. 69) inhibit the transmission of nerve impulses, so no stimulation of the post-ganglionic sympathetic nerves and consequent release of noradrenaline occurs, and the blood pressure falls as the vessels relax. These blocking agents are not very selective, and drugs that act on the sympathetic nerve endings and which prevent the release or formation of pressor amines are now preferred. Sedatives may also have some hypotensive properties by reducing the activity of those areas of the brain concerned with vascular tone, and so bring about a lowering of blood pressure by a less direct action. With any drug or combination of drugs, therapy in hypertension is aimed at lowering the blood pressure to a point consistent with age and the condition of the individual patient. Too rapid or too great a fall in blood pressure may lead to thrombosis, or a reduction in renal function that could have serious consequences. The ideal drug would lower the blood pressure without disturbing the controls which govern normal variations in response to exercise or movement. Such a drug is still unknown, and therapy remains a compromise.

Amyl Nitrite (dose, 0·12 to 0·3 ml. by inhalation)

Amyl nitrite is a clear yellow liquid with a characteristic odour, and is one of the few drugs given by inhalation. It is supplied in crushable glass capsules, which are broken at the time of use, and the vapour inhaled. Following such inhalation, a general vasodilatation occurs, and the blood pressure falls. The response is rapid, but evanescent, and as the drug has a marked odour, which draws attention to the patient, its use has declined. Amyl nitrite is used chiefly in angina pectoris but is occasionally of value in biliary colic and spasmodic asthma.

Glyceryl Trinitrate (dose, 0·5 to 1 mg.)

Glyceryl trinitrate is an oily liquid, and is of interest as the explosive constituent of dynamite. The action is much slower than that of amyl nitrite, but more prolonged, and doses may be repeated according to need. It is usually given as tablets containing 0·5 mg., which for maximum effect should be dissolved under the tongue. The vasodilator action begins within two minutes, and lasts for about twenty minutes. Side-effects such as headache may be experienced, and tolerance, necessitating larger doses, may develop.

Glyceryl trinitrate tablets are reasonably stable if kept in airtight containers, but should be used within a year of manufacture. Sustac is a long-acting form of the drug intended for prophylactic use. Tablets are available in two strengths (2·6 mg. and 6·4 mg.) and should be swallowed whole.

Pentaerythrityl Tetranitrate (dose, 10 to 30 mg.)

This drug is much slower in action than glyceryl trinitrate, and the effects may last as long as five hours. It is used mainly for prophylaxis, as side-effects are less troublesome, and tolerance less common. *Brand names:* Mycardol, Peritrate, Pentral.

Propatyl Nitrate

Propatyl nitrate has the general vasodilator action of glyceryl trinitrate, and is given in doses of 10 mg. sublingually at the first warning of an attack of angina. It may be useful prophylactically if taken regularly in doses of one to three tablets daily. *Brand name:* Gina.

Sorbide nitrate (Vascardin) and trolnitrate (Vasomed) are representative of other nitrate products used as vasodilators in the prophylaxis and treatment of angina pectoris.

Pentolinium (dose, 10 to 200 mg. orally; 2·5 to 20 mg. by subcutaneous injection)

Pentolinium tartrate is a ganglion-blocking agent and prevents the transmission of nerve impulses in both the sympathetic and parasympathetic nervous systems beyond the ganglion (see diagram on page 69. The blockade thus set up causes the arterial walls to relax, with a fall in blood pressure. It is now chiefly used in diagnosis to assess response after a subcutaneous dose of 2·5 mg. *Brand name :* Ansolysen.

Mecamylamine (dose, 5 to 60 mg. daily)

Mecamylamine is a ganglion-blocking agent of high potency, and is well absorbed when given orally. It has been widely used in the treatment of the more severe forms of hypertension, but following the introduction of drugs which inhibit the formation or release of noradrenaline at sympathetic nerve endings, the use of mecamylamine has declined. *Brand name :* Inversine.

Pempidine (dose, 10 to 80 mg. daily)

Pempidine tartrate is a ganglion-blocking agent similar in general properties to mecamylamine but it is absorbed more rapidly. *Brand name :* Perolysen.

Bretylium Tosylate (dose, 0·6 to 4 G. daily)

By virtue of their mode of action in blocking both sympathetic and parasympathetic nerve impulses, the ganglion-blocking agents produce a variety of unwanted side-effects, and more selective drugs are now preferred. Bretylium tosylate was one of the first of these compounds, and by acting on the post-ganglionic sympathetic nerve endings, transmission of nerve impulses was inhibited at a later stage. The drug is now little used, as tolerance soon developed, but its introduction led to the discovery of more reliable compounds. *Brand name :* Darenthin.

Guanethidine (dose, 10 to 300 mg. daily)

Guanethidine lowers the blood pressure by preventing the release of noradrenaline and adrenaline at the sympathetic nerve endings. The action is thus much more selective than that of the ganglion-blocking agents, the response is smoother and more predictable, and tolerance to the drug is uncommon. Treatment is commenced with a single daily dose of 10 to 20 mg., increased at weekly intervals by increments of 10 mg., until an optimum response has been obtained. Average maintenance doses vary from 30 to 60 mg. or more as a single daily dose. The drug is one of the most effective yet available, particularly in severe and malignant hypertension. Side-effects in doses adjusted to evoke the best response are few, but diarrhoea and some slowing of the pulse may occur with full doses. Thiazide diuretics potentiate the action of guanethidine, thus permitting a reduction in dose, and they also control the oedema which sometimes occurs during treatment. It is of interest to note that the drug has been used as eye-drops in the treatment of glaucoma (see page 264). *Brand name :* Ismelin.

Bethanidine Sulphate (dose, 10 to 200 mg.)

This compound has chemical relationships with bretylium and guanethidine, and has similar neurone-blocking properties. The initial dose is 10 mg. twice daily, increased by 5 to 10 mg. according to need. Side-effects, such as diarrhoea, are less common, and may often be avoided by a small reduction in dose. The rapid action of the drug is an advantage should it be necessary to suspend treatment, as in preparation for surgery, or where a more flexible control of blood pressure is required. *Brand names:* Bethanid, Esbatal.

Debrisoquine Sulphate (dose, 10 to 20 mg.)

Debrisoquine resembles bethanidine in its type and pattern of action, and following oral use, the maximum response occurs within two hours, and extends over twelve hours. The drug is well tolerated, and may be effective when the response to other hypotensive drugs is unsatisfactory. Overdose is indicated by

postural hypotension, weakness and diarrhoea. *Brand name :*
Declinax.

Methyldopa (dose, 0·5 to 2 G. daily)

This substance is related to one of the amino acids present in
the body, and functions in part as an enzyme inhibitor. It interferes with the production and availability of noradrenaline and so
has therapeutic applications in the treatment of hypertension.
The initial dose of methyldopa is 250 mg. three times a day, and
the maintenance dose varies from 0.5 to 2 G. daily. It is well
absorbed orally, and produces a smooth reduction in blood
pressure without significant side-effects or fluctuations in pressure
as the result of exercise. A sedative effect may occur early in
treatment, and water and salt retention is not uncommon. Combined administration of a thiazide diuretic increases the hypotensive action, thus permitting a reduction in dose and side-effects.
Brand name : Aldomet.

Other Synthetic Drugs

Several other anti-hypertensive drugs are available, and are
represented by Envacar (guanoxan ; tablets of 10 and 40 mg.),
Vatensol (guanoclor) and Eutonyl † (pargyline; tablets of 10 and
25 mg.). These drugs inhibit sympathetic activity by several
mechanisms, and provide useful alternative forms of treatment for
patients resistant to other drugs. Verapamil † (Cordilox) reduces
the cardiac response to sympathetic stimulation, and is used in the
treatment of angina pectoris (dose, 40 to 80 mg.). The use of
propranolol (Inderal) in hypertension is referred to on page 92.

Reserpine † (dose, 0·5 to 2 mg. daily)

The root of the Indian shrub, *Rauwolfia serpentina* contains
several alkaloids used in the treatment of the less severe forms of
hypertension. The main constituent is reserpine, and the hypotensive action is linked with a reduction in the stores of noradrenaline. The response to the drug is slow and variable and some days
may elapse before the full effects can be expected. The action
may be increased by the use of one of the thiazide diuretics, and
this potentiation permits the dose of reserpine to be reduced
without loss of hypotensive activity. Because of the slow onset of
effect, it is of no value in hypertensive crises. The drug has a

number of side-effects, and nasal congestion, lethargy and depression may occur even with standard doses. With higher doses, the central depression may be severe.

Reserpine is available as Serpasil †; Rauwiloid † is a mixture of reserpine and other alkaloids from Rauwolfia root, available as tablets of 2 mg., and Raudixin † is a preparation of the powdered whole root, issued as tablets containing 50 mg. Drugs related to reserpine include deserpidine † (Harmonyl) and methoserpidine † (Decaserpyl).

Hydrallazine (dose, 50 to 200 mg. daily)

Hydrallazine is a synthetic compound with a peripheral vasodilator action and some anti-adrenaline properties. In hypertension the response to treatment is slow and variable and side-effects, such as nausea and headache, limit its value. Hydrallazine is sometimes given by intramuscular injection or intravenous drip infusion in doses of 20 to 40 mg. in the treatment of the high blood pressure associated with the toxaemia of pregnancy. *Brand name :* Apresoline.

Supplementary Drugs

The thiazide group of diuretics (*q.v.*) also have some hypotensive properties, but from that point of view their chief value is their power of increasing the effects of other drugs used in the treatment of hypertension. This potentiation permits lower doses of the main drug with a consequent reduction in side-effects. Many proprietary products containing a thiazide diuretic and a hypotensive drug are available, but do not permit adjustment of dose of the main constituent to suit the individual patient. Some of these mixed products also contain potassium chloride, and are intended to offset the urinary loss of potassium caused by the thiazide diuretics. Such loss may cause muscle weakness, severe cardiac disturbances, and an increased sensitivity of the heart to digitalis.

PERIPHERAL VASODILATORS

Although these drugs are of no value in the treatment of hypertension, they are considered here for convenience. Reference has already been made (page 92) to the alpha-receptors in the peripheral vessels. When noradrenaline is released by stimulation of a sympathetic nerve, it acts upon these receptors and causes vasoconstriction. Alpha-receptor blocking agents can inhibit such vasoconstriction, and have therapeutic value in the treatment of vasospasm. Some compounds also have a direct vasodilator action.

Tolazoline (dose, 25 to 75 mg. orally; 10 to 20 mg. by intramuscular or intravenous injection)

Tolazoline is used in the treatment of Raynaud's disease and other conditions of peripheral vasospasm. Such vasospasm, by limiting the blood supply to the limbs and extremities, may cause pain, and in long-standing cases may lead to necrosis. Peripheral vasodilators such as tolazoline give relief by improving the local blood supply but the response may be brief and disappointing. Tolazoline is also useful in counteracting the arterial spasm that occurs when alkaline anaesthetic solutions, such as thiopentone sodium, are inadvertently injected into an artery instead of a vein. The prompt injection of tolazoline may reduce the severe arterial spasm, and so limit damage and prevent necrosis. *Brand name :* Priscol.

Phenoxybenzamine (dose, 10 to 20 mg.)

This compound has the peripheral vasodilator and alpha-receptor blocking action of tolazoline, but a much longer duration of effect. It is useful in the treatment of peripheral vascular disorders, and to control the hypertension associated with adrenaline-liberating tumours. *Brand name :* Dibenyline.

Phentolamine (dose, 40 to 100 mg. orally; 5 to 10 mg. by injection)

Phentolamine is effective orally in the treatment of arteriospasm and vasospasm, and in diabetic arteriosclerosis and related conditions, but its main therapeutic value is in the diagnosis of chromaffin tumour (phaeochromocytoma). These tumours liberate large amounts of adrenaline, and bring about a rise in blood pressure that could be mistaken for essential hypertension. The high blood pressure associated with such tumours can be differentiated from that of hypertension by an injection of phentolamine which temporarily neutralises the vasoconstrictor effects of the adrenaline. If the high blood pressure is due to the adrenaline liberated from the tumour, it will fall very soon after an intravenous injection of phentolamine, but will return to the previous level within a few minutes, whereas in essential hypertension no significant change in blood pressure will occur. *Brand name :* Rogitine.

Thymoxamine (dose, 40 mg.)

Thymoxamine is an alpha-receptor blocking agent with a more specific action than related compounds, and so has fewer side-effects. It is used in a variety of conditions, characterised by peripheral ischaemia, and is well tolerated. *Brand name:* Opilon.

Other synthetic drugs used for their peripheral vasodilator action are represented by buphenine (Perdilatal), inositol nicotinate (Hexopal), isoxsuprine (Duvadilan), cyclandelate (Cyclospasmol), nicotinyl tartrate (Ronicol).

Kallikrein is a vasodilator substance extracted from the pancreas and has been used in the treatment of severe vascular disease and circulatory disturbance, mainly by injection as Depot-Glumorin.

CHAPTER VI

DRUGS ACTING ON THE URINARY SYSTEM

DIURETICS

DIURETICS are substances that increase the excretion of urine by the kidneys, and the drugs used for this purpose show a great diversity of character, as they range from simple organic salts to complex synthetic chemicals. The kidneys are the organs of excretion of unwanted soluble substances, and anatomically each kidney is made up of several million nephrons, each consisting of a glomerulus and two tubules. Each nephron functions as a filtering unit and can be represented diagrammatically thus :—

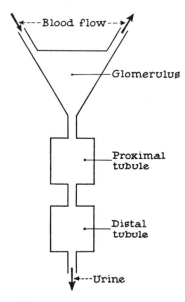

The glomerulus consists of a group of fine blood vessels, and functions as a filter, for at this point a large amount of water and dissolved salts is separated from the protein constituents of the blood passing through the glomerulus. This protein-free filtrate passes on to the tubules, where much of the water, dextrose, sodium chloride, sodium bicarbonate, the potassium chloride and other substances are selectively reabsorbed and pass back into the circulation, leaving the excess water, urea and other unwanted substances to be excreted as urine. Thus the kidney is an organ of considerable complexity, and in health it is capable of maintaining the composition of the blood within narrow limits in spite of varying fluid intake or extremes of climatic conditions. The antidiuretic hormone of the pituitary gland present in vasopressin (q.v.) plays an important part in this control of the electrolyte balance of the body, but disease can upset this delicate balance, and heart failure and liver disease are among the most important causes of kidney dysfunction.

In heart failure the blood supply to the glomerulus is reduced as a consequence of the impaired circulation, and the filtration rate is slowed down. Yet tubular reabsorption continues unchecked, so that water and salts soon begin to accumulate in the body tissues. In such conditions diuretics can afford relief by checking tubular reabsorption, and so increasing the elimination of water and the dissolved salts. Owing to the complex nature of the kidney, different diuretics may produce the same final effect by different modes of action. Thus diuresis may be achieved by drugs which dilate the renal blood vessels and so increase the glomerular filtration rate, or by the use of substances which prevent the reabsorption of salts and water by the proximal or distal tubules.

Osmotic Diuretics

Soluble salts, such as potassium citrate (dose, 1 to 2 G.) and ammonium chloride (dose, 1 to 2 G.) are rapidly absorbed and excreted, and by their osmotic action prevent the reabsorption of water by the tubules. The diuretic effect of potassium citrate is not very great, and as citrates are metabolised in the body to bicarbonates, potassium citrate is mainly used to make the urine alkaline. Ammonium chloride has a similar but reversed action, as it makes the urine acid.

Certain sugars also function as osmotic diuretics, especially when given by intravenous injection. Thus mannitol, injected as a 20 per cent. solution, prevents the reabsorption of water by the tubules, and is useful in renal insufficiency, and in the forced diuresis treatment of barbiturate poisoning. Urea by injection has a similar action, but is used mainly to reduce cerebral oedema.

Xanthine Diuretics

These include caffeine (dose, 250 to 500 mg.), theobromine (dose, 300 to 600 mg.) and theophylline. The latter is the most powerful, but it is used mainly as the more soluble derivative aminophylline (dose, 100 to 500 mg. orally; 500 mg. intramuscularly or 250 mg. by intravenous injection. The xanthine diuretics act by reducing the reabsorption of water and salts by the tubules, and by increasing the renal blood flow and glomerular filtration rate. As diuretics these drugs are not very potent, and aminophylline is employed mainly for its bronchodilator action in bronchospasm, asthma and Cheyne-Stokes respiration.

Mercurial Diuretics

Mersalyl and Neptal are organic mercurial compounds that have diuretic properties, and produce diuresis by inhibiting the enzymes concerned with the reabsorption of chloride and sodium by the tubules. This inhibition indirectly reduces the reabsorption of water, and the final result is an increased excretion of sodium chloride and water. Injection of Mersalyl † is the official preparation, and is given by intramuscular injection in doses of 1 to 2 ml.

In severe oedema the excretion of fluid may be considerable, but the response to subsequent injections becomes less as the oedema is relieved. The action is increased if the urine is acidified by the previous administration of ammonium chloride. The mercurial diuretics were once widely employed in the treatment of cardiac oedema, in some forms of nephritis, and in ascites, but with the introduction of the powerful oral diuretics of the thiazide type, the use of the mercurial diuretics has declined.

Thiazide Diuretics

The ideal diuretic would cause the increased excretion of salts in physiological proportions, whereas the mercurials mainly increase the loss of sodium of chloride, and during the search for alternative drugs some diuretic action was found in compounds related to the sulphonamides. Acetazolamide (Diamox) was used for a time as an oral diuretic as it inhibits the enzyme system responsible for the reabsorption of bicarbonate by the tubules, and results in the elimination of an alkaline urine. The action is self-limiting, and the effects are not sustained and acetazolamide is now mainly used in the treatment of glaucoma, where it reduces the formation of the aqueous humour.

Other and more effective oral diuretics have since been synthesised, and the thiazide group of diuretics is now of outstanding importance. In addition to their diuretic properties, the thiazides bring about a slight reduction in blood pressure, but they also potentiate the action of more powerful hypotensive drugs, and combined therapy may evoke the best response.

Chlorothiazide † (dose, ½ to 2 G. daily, or on alternate days)

Chlorothiazide was the first of the thiazide diuretics, and the oral use of this drug is characterised by an increased excretion of

TABLE OF DIURETICS

Approved Name	Brand Name	Products
Bendrofluazide	Aprinox	Tablets, 2·5 mg.; 5 mg.
	Berkozide	Tablets, 2·5 mg.; 5 mg.
	Centyl	Tablets, 2·5 mg.; 5 mg. and Vials, 5 mg./c.c.
	Neo-Naclex	Tablets, 2·5 mg.; 5 mg.
Chlorthalidone	Hygroton	Tablets, 50 mg.; 100 mg.
Chlorothiazide	Saluric	Tablets, 0·5 G.
	Lyovac Saluric	Vials, 0·5 G.
Clopamide	Brinaldix	Tablets, 20 mg.
Clorexolone	Nefrolan	Tablets, 10 mg.; 25 mg.
Cyclopenthiazide	Navidrex	Tablets, 0·5 mg.
Ethacrynic Acid	Edecrin	Tablets, 50 mg.
Frusemide	Lasix	Tablets, 40 mg. Ampoules, 20 mg.
Hydrochlorothiazide	Direma	Tablets, 25 mg.; 50 mg.
	Esidrex	Tablets, 25 mg.; 50 mg.
	Hydrosaluric	Tablets, 25 mg.; 50 mg.
Hydroflumethiazide	Hydrenox	Tablets, 50 mg.
	Naclex	Tablets, 50 mg.
Methyclothiazide	Enduron	Tablets, 5 mg.
Polythiazide	Nephril	Tablets, 1 mg.
Quinethazone	Aquamox	Tablets, 50 mg.
Triamterene	Dytac	Capsules, 50 mg.

The suffix ' K ' is added to the brand name of several of the above products when a compound tablet containing both potassium chloride and diuretic is available. It should not be assumed that these products contain the same amount of diuretic as the plain tablet, as in some cases they contain less. In some mixed tablets potassium chloride is contained in an enteric coated core of the tablet, and the release of the potassium chloride in the small intestine may cause small-bowel ulceration and obstruction. Patients taking such tablets should be advised to report any gastro-intestinal disturbances.

water, chlorides, sodium and some potassium. It is given daily in severe conditions, and it produces a diuresis comparable with that of an injection of mersalyl. This effect is achieved by limiting the reabsorption of salts and water by the proximal tubule, so that more fluid is available to be excreted as urine. There is also an increased potassium excretion during thiazide therapy, and if treatment is prolonged potassium loss in the urine may be excessive. Such loss of potassium may cause severe cardiac irregularities and muscle weakness, and the supplementary administration of potassium is necessary. That may be done by giving potassium chloride as an enteric coated tablet, or a delayed release product such as Slow-K. Effervescent tablets of potassium are also available and are well tolerated. Newer compounds such as hydrochlorothiazide (dose, 25 to 100 mg. daily) are more powerful and cause less potassium loss, but for prolonged treatment some additional potassium is still advisable. The table on page 105 indicates the wide range of thiazide and other potent diuretics now available.

It is of interest to note that in diabetes insipidus, a disease characterised by an excessive excretion of urine, the thiazide diuretics may have an antidiuretic action. That paradoxical effect is difficult to explain, but salt retention occurs in some cases of diabetes insipidus, and the use of a thiazide diuretic, by increasing the elimination of sodium, could bring about an indirect antidiuretic response.

Frusemide † (dose, 40 to 120 mg. daily)

Frusemide is a powerful diuretic of unusual chemical structure, and appears to act by inhibiting reabsorption in both the proximal and distal tubules. It is frequently effective when response to thiazide diuretics or mersalyl is inadequate. Frusemide may be given orally in doses of 40 mg. or more, and the onset of diuresis is rapid and may extend over four hours. If oral therapy is inadequate owing to malabsorption, the drug may be given by intramuscular or intravenous injection in doses of 20 mg. and the response may be dramatic both in the rapidity of action and magnitude of the diuresis. Nausea and weakness may follow the copious diuresis, and dehydration may cause a temporary hypotension. The potassium loss following frusemide therapy may be less than that induced by some thiazide diuretics, but potassium supplements may still be necessary if treatment is prolonged. Frusemide is indicated in oedema generally, but is of particular value in severe pulmonary oedema and water-retention. It is also useful in ascites and in the treatment of hypertension. *Brand name :* Lasix.†

Ethacrynic Acid † (dose, 50 to 150 mg. daily)

Ethacrynic acid is a powerful diuretic which is chemically distinct from other diuretic drugs. In doses of 50 mg. initially, subsequently increased according to response, the drug evokes a prompt and copious diuresis, which is greater than that produced by hydrochlorothiazide, and is associated with a reduced potassium excretion. Ethacrynic acid inhibits the reabsorption of salts and water in both the proximal and distal tubules and the loop of Henle, and may produce a diuresis in patients with a high blood urea who have failed to respond to other drugs. A test dose of 50 mg. is advisable, as hepatic coma may occur in cases of severe liver damage, and occasionally an excessive response may result in water and salt depletion. With continued treatment, potassium supplements are usually required, as the loss of potassium, although reduced, is not completely suppressed. *Brand name:* Edecrin.†

Spironolactone (dose, 50 to 200 mg. daily)

Spironolactone is a synthetic steroid which blocks the action of aldosterone on the kidney. Aldosterone is one of the steroid hormones of the adrenal cortex, and is concerned with the electrolyte balance of the body by its influence on the reabsorption of sodium and excretion of potassium by the distal tubules. Some patients with cardiac oedema and ascites do not always respond to diuretics, and such resistance to treatment appears to be linked with the fact that many oedematous patients excrete excessive amounts of aldosterone. When that occurs, the effects of a diuretic on the proximal tubules are largely nullified by the increased reabsorption in the distal tubules under the influence of aldosterone. In such cases spironolactone may permit a diuresis by its aldosterone blocking action, and the drug is of value in many conditions associated with water-retention, such as resistant cardiac oedema, ascites, and nephrotic syndrome. It is given in doses of 25 mg. four times a day, together with a thiazide diuretic. The initial response is slow in onset, and if the diuresis is still inadequate after five days, the higher dose of 200 mg. daily should be given. These high doses may cause headache and drowsiness, and the drug should be used with care in hepatic disease. *Brand name:* Aldactone-A.

Triamterene (dose, 50 to 100 mg.)

Triamterene represents a type of diuretic that functions by inhibiting the reabsorption of salts and water by the distal tubules of the kidney. Although the final effect of triamterene is similar to that of spironolactone, the mechanism of action is different, and in severe conditions both drugs can be given together. Triamterene is given in initial doses of 50 mg. twice daily, adjusted later to a single dose, or given on alternate days, according to response. It is usually given with a thiazide diuretic, so that a proximal and distal blockade can be achieved, but the combined action is a powerful one, and laboratory control of blood electrolytes during treatment is necessary. *Brand name:* Dytac.

Metyrapone (dose, 3 G. daily in divided doses)

Metyrapone inhibits the formation of aldosterone by the adrenal cortex, and so has an indirect diuretic action. It is sometimes of value in resistant conditions and is usually given in association with spironolactone or a thiazide drug. Metyrapone is also used as a test for pituitary function. *Brand name:* Metopirone.

Urea (dose, 5 to 15 G.)

Urea is a normal constituent of urine, as it is one of the end products of protein metabolism but it also has useful diuretic properties. Urea has in fact been described as the ' forgotten diuretic ' as, although it is now little used, it has the advantages of low toxicity, ready solubility and effectiveness. Urea may also be given by intravenous drip infusion in doses of 30 to 90 G. to reduce intracranial tension. In renal damage the ability of the kidneys to excrete urea is reduced, and the drug is given in oral doses of 15 G. as a renal clearance test.

URINARY ANTISEPTICS

The organisms associated with urinary infections are those commonly found in the intestines, such as *E. coli*, but *Proteus* and *Pseudomonas pyocyanea* may also be present. Urinary infections are often very difficult to treat as an initial response may be followed by a relapse, and some clinicians prefer a course of four or more different drugs, taken successively, in order to obtain the maximum response.

Certain antibiotics and sulphonamides have some value as urinary antiseptics, and are considered in more detail in the sections dealing with those drugs. The other drugs used as urinary antiseptics vary widely in their nature and activity. Many compounds with antiseptic properties lose their activity during their passage through the body, but a urinary antiseptic must be excreted in the urine in an active form and should retain its activity in spite of changes in the acidity or alkalinity of the urine. The range of effective substances is regrettably limited.

Methylene Blue (dose, 60 to 300 mg.)

This drug has a mild antiseptic action and has been used in cystitis, often in association with hexamine (q.v.). Another dyestuff, phenazopyridine (Pyridium), is used mainly for analgesia of the urinary tract (dose, 100 mg.).

Hexamine (dose, 0·6 to 2 G.)

Hexamine is a compound of formaldehyde and ammonia. The drug is rapidly absorbed and if excreted in an acid urine the hexamine is slowly decomposed to liberate formaldehyde, to which the antiseptic action is due. To achieve the necessary degree of urinary acidity, sodium acid phosphate or ammonium chloride should be given with each dose of hexamine. Alternatively hexamine may be given in combination with mandelic acid (q.v.), as Mandelamine or Mandurin. Although far less effective than the sulphonamides, hexamine is virtually non-toxic, and may be given even when some renal damage is present.

Nitrofurantoin (dose, 50 to 150 mg.)

This compound is an antiseptic substance with a wide range of activity against gram-negative and gram-positive bacteria, including many associated with urinary infections, although most strains of Pseudomonas pyocyanea are resistant. Following oral administration, much of the drug is excreted unchanged in the urine, and the compound is of value in urinary tract infections such as cystitis and pyelonephritis, particularly those that have not responded to other forms of treatment.

Dosage is based on a scale of 5 to 10 mg. per kg. body-weight daily, and an average adult dose is 100 mg. four times a day. Recent infections often respond within a week but treatment is normally continued up to a maximum of fourteen days, and in resistant or recurrent infections may be repeated after a rest period. Care is necessary in renal damage. Nausea is a not uncommon side-effect of treatment, and the drug is best taken after meals. Part of the absorbed drug is excreted as breakdown products which colour the urine brown, but is of no significance.

Peripheral neuropathy and haemolytic anaemia have followed the use of nitrofurantoin, and the drug is mainly used in the treatment of urinary infections resistant to other compounds. *Brand name:* Furadantin.

Nalidixic Acid (dose, 1 G.)

Nalidixic acid represents a different type of chemotherapeutic agent, and is active against a wide range of gram-negative organisms. The drug is rapidly absorbed when given orally and a large proportion is excreted in the urine in an active form. Nalidixic acid is effective against many organisms responsible for urinary tract infections, particularly *Proteus*, and there is some evidence that the drug may be concentrated in renal tissues. The standard dose is 1 G. four times a day for at least seven days, but prolonged treatment may be necessary in chronic conditions. Bacterial resistance to nalidixic acid may develop, and sensitivity tests should be carried out if the infection persists. The drug may cause nausea and visual disturbances in some patients. *Brand name:* Negram.

Mandelic Acid (dose, 2 to 4 G.)

Mandelic acid is occasionally employed in the treatment of urinary infections as an alternative to the sulphonamides when the latter are ineffective or poorly tolerated. It is usually given as calcium or ammonium mandelate, and for optimum results the urine must be kept acid, if necessary by the administration of ammonium chloride. Mandelic acid may also be given in combination with hexamine as Mandelamine or Mandurin. The degree of acidity of the urine is important and should be not less than *p*H 5·3 (*p*H *q.v.*). With urine of higher *p*H the drug is much less effective. *Brand names:* Mandecal (calcium mandelate), Mandelamine (hexamine mandelate).

pH

This symbol refers to the hydrogen-ion concentration (acidity or alkalinity of aqueous solutions). This is of considerable importance when the efficacy of urinary antiseptics is concerned, as some substances, such as streptomycin and the sulphonamides, are more effective in alkaline urine, but hexamine and mandelic acid are inactive unless the urine is acid. Nurses are familiar with the use of litmus paper to detect whether a solution is acid or alkaline, but such papers give no indication of the *degree* of acidity. Thus blue litmus will change to red in both weak and strong acids, but for many purposes greater accuracy is required, and here the pH scale is useful. On this scale the neutral point is pH 7, and all acid solutions have a lower pH, and the lower the figure the greater the degree of acidity. Conversely, all alkaline solutions have a pH higher than 7, and solutions of pH 13 are very much more alkaline than solutions of pH 8.

The degree of pH can be determined by the changes in colour of certain dyes produced by the solution under test, or by special meters. Thus methyl red, used to test the pH of the urine during mandelic acid therapy, changes from red at pH 4 to yellow at pH 6·5 and bromocresol green is yellow in strongly acid solutions up to about pH 3·5, green from pH 3·5 to 5·5, and blue from pH 5·5 to 13.

By a suitable combination of dyes, a ' universal indicator solution ' can be prepared, and the changes in colour of this indicator from red to blue correspond to changes in pH from strongly acid (pH 3) to strongly alkaline (pH 13).

CHAPTER VII

CHEMOTHERAPY AND ANTIBIOTICS

CHEMOTHERAPY

CHEMOTHERAPY can be defined as the treatment of bacterial or related diseases by drugs which can attack the invading organisms without being toxic to the patient. The ease with which bacteria can be killed by antiseptics led to the search over a long period of years for a non-toxic antiseptic that could be given systemically, although to many the expression ' non-toxic antiseptic ' was a contradiction of terms, as any substance that could kill bacteria would seem to be automatically toxic to other cells.

The problem was eventually solved when the unusual antibacterial properties of certain dyes were discovered, as in 1932 it was found that a red dye, later known as Prontosil, could protect laboratory animals against streptococcal infections, and by 1935 Prontosil was being used clinically with great success.

It is difficult now to appreciate the importance and excitement of this discovery, which for the first time enabled the physician to treat systemic bacterial diseases with active but relatively non-toxic drugs. A puzzling feature of Prontosil was that it had little direct antibacterial action outside the body, but was undoubtedly effective systemically. It was soon found that after administration Prontosil was metabolised and released a simpler substance, sulphanilamide, to which the antibacterial action is ultimately due. The discovery led to the synthesis of thousands of related substances known as the sulphonamides, of which only a few have won and retained an established place in therapeutics.

Mode of Action

The sulphonamides have an unusual mode of action, as they are bacteriostatic rather than bactericidal, *i.e.* they inhibit the growth of bacteria and do not kill them directly. This effect is achieved by preventing the take-up of para-aminobenzoic acid (Fig. 1) and subsequent formation of folic acid by the organisms. That substance is an essential growth factor for many bacteria, and sulphonamides, which are chemically related to para-aminobenzoic acid, can inhibit the formation of folic acid, and thus indirectly prevent further bacterial growth. The organisms, in effect, are unable to distinguish between para-aminobenzoic acid and the sulphonamides, represented here by sulphanilamide (Fig. 2). Figures 1 and 2 show the close chemical relationship between the two compounds.

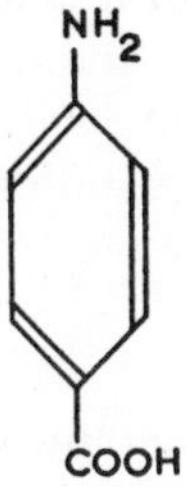

FIG. 1 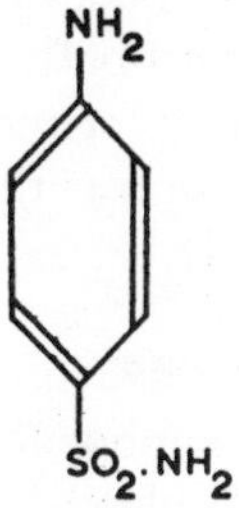   FIG. 2

It follows that bacteria which do not require para-aminobenzoic acid for their metabolic processes are not sensitive to the action of the sulphonamides. In practice, the sulphonamides are active against a wide range of organisms, including the streptococci, meningococci, *Escherichia coli*, Shigella and pneumococci. They therefore have applications in the treatment of tonsillitis, septicaemia, pneumonia, meningococcal meningitis, bacillary dysentery and a number of infections of the urinary tract. The staphylococci are less sensitive to the sulphonamides, and as the action of the drugs is inhibited by pus, they are of no value in suppurating lesions caused by staphylococcal infection.

Absorption, Excretion and Toxic Effects

With few exceptions, which will be referred to later, the sulphonamides are rapidly absorbed after oral administration, and are well distributed in the body fluids. In the liver the drugs are partly acetylated, or combined with acetic acid, and are excreted in the urine as such, together with any unchanged sulphonamide. With some of the older sulphonamides these acetylated forms are less soluble than the parent drug, and an adequate fluid intake was maintained during treatment to prevent any crystal formation in the urinary tract. With the sulphonamides in current use the acetylated forms are more soluble, and urinary complications such as haematuria are less common.

The toxic side-effects of the sulphonamides vary considerably, and may have little relationship to the dose. Nausea and vomiting, once common with the older sulphonamides, are now less frequent, but allergic reactions, skin sensitisation and drug fever may occur. Cyanosis, drowsiness and haemolytic anaemia are among the less frequent reactions. The most serious toxic reaction to the sulphonamides is agranulocytosis, but it is fortunately uncommon if treatment is standard both in dose and duration. Administration is rarely necessary for more than seven to ten days, but any jaundice, haematuria or sore throat are indications for withdrawing the drug immediately.

Sulphonamide Dosage

In all systemic sulphonamide therapy it is essential rapidly to reach an optimum blood level and maintain it for seven to ten days. Treatment with low doses may not only be ineffectual but is potentially dangerous, as although the sulphonamides are active against a wide range of bacteria, resistant strains of normally susceptible organisms are not uncommon, and resistance may even be acquired during treatment. An initial or ' loading ' dose of 2 to 3 G. (or double the maintenance dose) is usually given, followed by 1 to 1·5 G. every four or six hours. This dose should give a sulphonamide blood level of 5 to 10 mg. per 100 ml. An adequate fluid intake during treatment is important. In general, children tolerate the sulphonamides well, and the daily dose may be calculated on the basis of 0·1 G. per kg. body-weight for administration in divided doses four or six times a day. The numerous sulphonamide compounds now on the market are basically similar in action, and differ mainly in their absorption, degree of binding to plasma protein, excretion rates and degree of alteration in the body. The following are representative compounds :

Sulphadimidine †

One of the most widely used and least toxic of the sulphonamides, and adequate blood levels can be maintained by six-hourly doses. It is well tolerated, and the nausea and vomiting so characteristic of early sulphonamide therapy seldom occur. Sulphadimidine and its metabolic derivatives are fairly soluble, even in an acid urine, so that renal complications and other toxic effects are uncommon.

In systemic infections sulphadimidine is given orally in doses of 3 G. initially, followed by maintenance doses of 1 G. four-hourly or 1·5 G. six-hourly. In urinary infections, a lower initial dose of 2 G., followed by maintenance doses of 1 G. six-hourly are commonly given. Oral administration is usually adequate, but solutions of the sodium salt may be given by injection when oral use is impossible, or absorption is not satisfactory. Such injection solutions are very alkaline, and are mainly intended for slow intravenous injection, but may be given by deep intramuscular injection if adequate care is taken. No sulphonamide solution should ever be given by intrathecal injection, as serious injury to the spinal cord may result. *Brand name:* Sulphamezathine.†

Sulphadiazine †

Sulphadiazine resembles sulphadimidine in general properties, but diffuses more readily into the cerebrospinal fluid. It is therefore often preferred for the treatment of meningococcal meningitis. An initial dose of 3 G. is followed by maintenance doses of 1 G. six-hourly. In acute infections, large initial doses (2 G. or occasionally more) of the sodium salt may be given by slow intravenous injection or by intravenous drip infusion. The solution is not suitable for intramuscular injection.

Solutions of sulphadiazine sodium, like those of sulphadimidine sodium, are very alkaline, and great care is necessary during intravenous injection to avoid any leakage into the surrounding tissues.

Sulphafurazole †

Sulphafurazole is a well-absorbed sulphonamide with a wide range of activity, associated with a reduced risk of toxic side-effects. Like sulphadimidine, it is effective in many systemic infections, and as it is excreted in an active state in the urine it is often used in urinary infections. The standard dose in systemic infections is 3 G. initially, followed by 1·5 G. every four hours, but slightly smaller doses may be adequate in urinary infections. A soluble form of the drug is available for intramuscular or intravenous use when oral treatment is not possible. *Brand name :* Gantrisin.†

Sulphamethizole †

Sulphamethizole is an exceptional sulphonamide, as in urinary infections it is effective in doses of 100 mg. to 200 mg. five or six times a day. With these low doses the fluid intake should be limited, in order to prevent excessive dilution of the excreted drug by the urine. *Brand name:* Urolucosil.†

Sulphamethoxazole

Sulphamethoxazole is one of the longer-acting sulphonamides, and in common with related drugs, acts by blocking the formation of folic acid by bacterial cells. This synthesis of folic acid is but one stage in a complex metabolic process, as folic acid is finally converted into folinic acid. A compound that could inhibit this final stage, if given with a sulphonamide, would permit a sequential double metabolic blockade, and the combination would have a greatly increased antibacterial action. Septrin and Bactrim are mixed products with this double action, and contain trimethoprim 40 mg. as the second stage antibacterial, together with sulphamethoxazole 400 mg. Sulphamethoxazole is preferred to other sulphonamides as the pattern of excretion is basically similar to that of trimethoprim. The combination marks a valuable extension of sulphonamide therapy, as it has a wide range of activity that includes *Haemophilus influenzae*, *E. coli*, *Proteus* and many penicillinase-producing organisms. The standard dose of the mixed product is two tablets twice a day. A loading dose of four tablets may be given in severe infections, but in cases of renal damage reduced doses are necessary to avoid toxic effects. It is not suitable for use in pregnancy.

Sulphacetamide †

Sulphacetamide is a survivor from the early days of sulphonamide therapy. It is active orally, and useful in urinary infections, but it has now been replaced to a great extent by more potent compounds. Sulphacetamide sodium is very soluble in water, and is widely used in ophthalmology, as unlike the sodium salt of other sulphonamides, it is not irritant to the tissues. Eye drops of 10 to 30 per cent. are available, and eye ointments containing 6 to 10 per cent. of sulphacetamide are also used. *Brand names :* Albucid,† Ocusol.†

Other Sulphonamides

Other systemically acting sulphonamides are sulphapyridine, sulphathiazole and sulphamerazine. Sulphapyridine, † one of the early sulphonamides, is now used solely for the treatment of dermatitis herpetiformis. Sulphathiazole,† one of the most active but also most rapidly excreted sulphonamides, is now rarely used for systemic infections, but is occasionally applied locally. Sulpha-merazine † is also an active drug but is more toxic as it is excreted more slowly than many other sulphonamides. Sulphatriad,† a mixture of sulphathiazole, sulphamerazine and sulphadimidine, represents an attempt to minimise reactions by the use of mixed sulphonamides in lower individual doses.

Long-acting Sulphonamides

The frequency of dose of a drug is closely related to the rate of breakdown in the body or the rate of excretion. The sulphon-amides generally are rapidly excreted, necessitating four-hourly or six-hourly doses, but in recent years a number of sulphonamides have been introduced which become bound to plasma protein, and are excreted so slowly that doses of 500 mg. daily may be sufficient to maintain an adequate blood level. Such compounds are of value in the treatment of chronic infections, especially those of the urinary tract, but the slow excretion of these drugs may increase the risk of side-effects which in the occasional very susceptible patient may be severe. As excretion is slow, elimination of the drug and control of side-effects is correspondingly difficult. Representative products include sulphamethoxypyridazine † (Lederkyn, Midicel), sulphamethoxydiazine † (Durenate), sulpha-phenazole † (Orisulf), sulphamethoxazole † (Gantanol) and sulphadimethoxine † (Madribon).

Poorly-absorbed Sulphonamides

Certain sulphonamide derivatives are not absorbed to any significant extent when given orally, and so are useless for the treatment of systemic infections. In the intestines these deriva-tives break down slowly and release the active sulphonamide, but the released drug is not absorbed by the colon, so a high concen-tration can be obtained by local release, without risk of systemic effects. These poorly-absorbed compounds are of considerable value in the treatment of bacillary dysentery, and are sometimes given in association with streptomycin and kaolin to increase their effects. They are also used for the pre-operative preparation or patients before bowel surgery.

These sulphonamides also suppress the non-pathogenic intestinal organisms which synthesise vitamin K and the vitamins of the B group, so vitamin supplements are necessary during long treatment.

Phthalylsulphathiazole †

One of the most effective compounds for the treatment of bacillary dysentery, and is also of value in ulcerative colitis. It reduces the bacterial flora of the intestines by the slow release of sulphathiazole and is used in the pre-operative preparation and post-operative care of patients requiring bowel surgery, in order to reduce the risk of peritonitis. The average dose is 2 G. four times a day, and as only a small amount of the drug is absorbed it may be given for long periods in the treatment of ulcerative colitis. *Brand names :* Sulfathalidine,† Thalazole.†

Succinylsulphathiazole †

Succinylsulphathiazole is similar to phthalylsulphathiazole in general properties, but it is less effective in watery diarrhoea and dysentery. An initial dose of 6 G. four-hourly for one day is often given, followed by doses of 4 G. four times a day for seven days. Although absorption is normally slight, it may be increased in ulcerative colitis, and as prolonged treatment in that condition may be necessary, phthalylsulphathiazole is often preferred. The drug is occasionally used as a retention enema in doses of 7 to 10 G. in 100 to 200 ml. of water. *Brand name :* Sulfasuxidine.†

Sulphaguanidine †

Sulphaguanidine was one of the first of the poorly absorbed sulphonamides to be used for intestinal therapy. Average doses are 3 G. up to four times a day, but as a large proportion of an oral dose may be absorbed, especially in ulcerative colitis, sulphaguanidine has now been replaced to a great extent by more active and less potentially toxic drugs.

Sulphasalazine †

Also known as salicylazosulphapyridine, this drug appears to be taken up selectively by the connective tissues of the intestines, where it is slowly broken down to release sulphapyridine. Sulphasalazine is used in the treatment of ulcerative colitis, but the response is variable. The drug is given in doses of 1 G. four or more times a day, and treatment may be continued with half doses as improvement occurs. *Brand name :* Salazopyrin.†

ANTIBIOTICS

Antibiotics can be defined broadly as antibacterial substances produced by fungi and other organisms. They owe their introduction into therapeutics to an observation by Professor Fleming, in 1928, that the growth of some cultures of staphylococci had been inhibited by a mould which had appeared in the culture as a chance contaminant. Experiments showed that some substance excreted by the mould into the culture medium could

TABLE OF ANTIBIOTICS

INDICATING MAIN TYPE OF ACTIVITY

Against Gram-positive Organisms	Against Gram-negative Organisms	Against Gram-positive and Gram-negative Organisms	Antitubercular Antibiotics

Penicillin
Penicillin V
Cloxacillin
Erythromycin
Flucloxacillin
Lincomycin
Methicillin
Novobiocin
Sodium fusidate
Spiramycin
Triacetyl-
    oleandomycin
Vancomycin
	Colistin
	Polymyxin
		Ampicillin
		Carbenicillin
		Cephalexin
		Cephaloridine
		Chloramphenicol
		Gentamicin
		Kanamycin
		Neomycin
		Tetracycline and
		    modified
		    tetracyclines
			Capreomycin
			Cycloserine
			Rifamycin
			Streptomycin
			Viomycin

prevent the growth of bacteria, and this substance, when extracted, was named penicillin (derived from the name of the mould *Penicillium*).

Since that time thousands of different moulds have been cultured, and examined for antibacterial properties, and many therapeutically active antibiotics are now available.

Penicillin †

Also known as penicillin G, soluble penicillin, or benzyl-penicillin. It is a metabolic by-product of the mould *Penicillium*

5

notatum, and although in normal circumstances the yield of penicillin is low, large-scale culture methods have resulted in greatly
increased yields at low cost.

Penicillin is chiefly effective against gram-positive bacteria, but
a few gram-negative and other organisms are also susceptible.
It is thus of great value in a wide range of infections, including
the following :—

Organism	*Disease*
β-haemolytic streptococcus	Septicaemia, tonsillitis
Staphylococcus	Septicaemia, boils
Pneumococcus	Pneumonia
Meningococcus	Meningococcal meningitis
Streptococcus viridans	Subacute bacterial endocarditis
Clostridium tetani	Tetanus
Clostridium welchii	Gas gangrene
Corynebacterium diphtheriae	Diphtheria
Treponema pallidum	Syphilis
Actinomyces	Actinomycosis

Although the antibacterial range of penicillin is wide, the
degree of activity may vary very considerably, as bacteria differ
markedly in their sensitivity to the drug, even amongst those
groups which are normally susceptible. This variation is particularly common amongst the staphylococci, where the sensitivity
to penicillin may range from a high degree of sensitivity to the
point of complete resistance.

Many of these resistant organisms owe their immunity to the
fact that they produce an enzyme, penicillinase, which inactivates
penicillin, and at one time the treatment of penicillin-resistant
infections was a therapeutic problem. The difficulties have
largely been overcome by the discovery of a method of producing
chemically modified penicillins which are not inactivated by
penicillinase, and thus have an extended range of activity. These
modified penicillins are referred to on page 125.

Penicillin is most active against young organisms, and the
antibacterial action appears to be due to an interference with
enzyme systems concerned with growth and development of
the bacterial cell wall.

It should be noted that although penicillin is active against the
organisms causing gas-gangrene and diphtheria, it does not

neutralise the toxins produced by these organisms, and early treatment of these diseases with antitoxin is still essential.

Penicillin is a stable substance in the dry state, but aqueous solutions soon decompose and lose their activity. Injection solutions are therefore best prepared as required, but may retain their activity for a few days if stored in a refrigerator.

ADMINISTRATION AND DOSE.—Penicillin G is not very effective orally unless given in very large doses, as it is rapidly broken down by the gastric acid, and the drug is best given by intramuscular injection. Absorption is rapid and the drug diffuses into most of the body tissues, but it does not pass into the cerebrospinal fluid or brain unless the meninges are inflamed or damaged, neither does it penetrate well into the pleural cavity, or into the synovial or ocular fluids. Penicillin is rapidly excreted by the kidneys, and as much as 95 per cent. of an injected dose may be lost within four hours. Frequent injections are therefore necessary to maintain an adequate blood level of the drug, and initial doses of one million units of penicillin are often given, followed by three-to-four-hourly maintenance doses of 250,000 to 500,000 units.

This clumsy method of expressing doses of penicillin in units is a legacy of the past when penicillin was very impure, and of low potency. With the highly purified products now available, there is no good reason why the doses should not be expressed as milligrams. One million units is equivalent to 600 mg. of penicillin. When the organism is susceptible to penicillin, response to treatment is usually prompt, but failure to respond may be due to an inadequate dose, and is not necessarily due to resistant organisms. In mixed infections, penicillin and streptomycin are sometimes given together to extend the range of antibacterial activity, and Crystamycin and Soluvone represent products containing both antibiotics.

Although the action of penicillin is not inhibited by pus or the products of tissue breakdown, penetration of the drug into pus-laden and sloughing areas is slow and the use of penicillin does not remove the need for surgical drainage.

In bacterial endocarditis very large doses are necessary. In this disease the valves of the heart are infected by *Streptococcus viridans* (although other organisms may also be involved) and become inflamed, and the so-called ' vegetations ' are formed. These are growths or excrescences of inflamed tissue in which large numbers of bacteria are found, and in order to achieve an adequate level of penicillin in such vegetations, daily doses of two to five million units are required. This high dose must be continued for at least six weeks to avoid a relapse.

In meningitis, penicillin penetrates through the normally resistant blood-brain barrier, but supplementary intrathecal injections of penicillin are also necessary. The maximum adult dose by the intrathecal route is 20,000 units, and special ampoules for the purpose are available.

Although penicillin G and its modifications are virtually nontoxic, allergic reactions to the drug may occur. These are usually due to hypersensitivity, and resemble serum sickness in general character. The reaction is usually that of an urticarial rash, but like serum sickness may be accompanied by shock and bronchospasm, and cardiac arrest has occurred. In severe reactions adrenaline or corticosteroids may be necessary. Occasionally injections of penicillinase have proved useful. As indicated earlier, some bacteria, such as *E. coli*, owe their resistance to penicillin to an enzyme, penicillinase, which rapidly inactivates the antibiotic. This enzyme is now available in a pure form as Neutrapen, and in a penicillin reaction may be given by injection to destroy any penicillin in the tissues. This allergic reaction is considered to be due to the presence in penicillin G of traces of a highly allergenic fraction formed during the manufacture of penicillin. Means of removing this fraction have been devised, and a highly purified penicillin is available as Puropen. The product is intended for routine use to avoid the development of sensitivity, and not for administration to patients known to be penicillin-sensitive, as the risk of a reaction, although markedly reduced, has not been eliminated.

LONG-ACTING FORMS.—The rapid elimination of soluble penicillin from the body, and the consequent need for frequent injections, has led to the introduction of a number of long-acting products. One of the most useful of these products is Procaine Penicillin Suspension. Penicillin reacts with procaine to form an insoluble derivative, and following injection, the compound is slowly broken down in the body and the penicillin is released over a period of twelve to twenty-four hours. The onset of action of procaine-penicillin is therefore slow, and to overcome this disadvantage, Fortified Procaine Penicillin containing 100,000 units of soluble penicillin and 300,000 units of procaine penicillin per dose is available. With this product a high initial blood level is obtained from the soluble constituent, which is followed by the sustained action of the procaine penicillin.

Other penicillin derivatives with a still longer action include benethamine penicillin and benzathine penicillin, and mixed preparations are also available containing one of the above with both soluble and procaine penicillin. A single injection may give antibacterial cover for several days.

Apart from the products containing soluble penicillin, which must be reconstituted by the addition of sterile water before use, these ' delayed release ' or depot forms of penicillin are supplied as suspensions ready for use. The solid constituents of all suspensions tend to settle on standing, so before a dose of long-acting penicillin is drawn into a syringe it is *essential* to shake the vial *thoroughly*. If merely a perfunctory shake is given, the penicillin will not become remixed and the patient will receive little more than an injection of sterile water. This matter is very much a nurse's responsibility, and its importance should be recognised and acted upon.

Some Brand Names

Procaine Penicillin—

> Distaquaine G. †   Lenticillin †

Fortified Procaine Penicillin—
> Distaquaine Fortified †

Preparations of Fortified Procaine Penicillin with other Depot Forms—
> Penidural All-Purpose †   Triplopen †

Penicillin V † (dose, 125 to 250 mg.)

Soluble penicillin is rapidly broken down by the gastric acid, and very large doses must be given orally to produce an adequate blood level. In patients with hypoacidity or achlorhydria, and in infants, who also have a gastric secretion low in acid, absorption of penicillin is almost complete, but for routine oral use soluble penicillin is unsatisfactory.

That disadvantage has been overcome by the introduction of

acid-stable forms of penicillin, such as penicillin V, and oral penicillin treatment now has an established place in therapeutics.

Penicillin V, also known as phenoxymethylpenicillin, is rapidly absorbed after oral administration, and effective blood levels are obtained in half an hour.

Like soluble penicillin, this oral derivative is indicated in the treatment of infections due to penicillin-sensitive organisms. The standard dose of penicillin V is 250 mg. every four hours, and although the highest blood levels are obtained when it is given on an empty stomach, absorption is not greatly reduced if the drug is given after food. In acute conditions, treatment should be initiated by an injection of soluble penicillin, followed by full oral doses of penicillin V. Oral penicillin is also useful in the treatment of rheumatic fever. Although it does not influence the acute course of the disease, penicillin reduces the risks of associated staphylococcal infection. Recurrence of rheumatic fever in susceptible patients can also be prevented by prophylactic penicillin treatment, and penicillin V may be given for such prophylaxis in doses of 125 mg. twice daily.

Phenoxymethylpenicillin, in common with other oral penicillins, is not considered suitable for the treatment of subacute bacterial endocarditis and other conditions where exceptionally high blood levels of penicillin are required, or for deep-seated and chronic infections.

Penicillin V is an organic acid, and available products may contain the free acid, or the potassium or calcium salt, or other form of the drug. *Brand names include:* Compocillin V-K,† Crystapen V,† Distaquaine V-K,† Icipen V,† Stabilin-V-K.†

Phenethicillin † (dose, 125 to 250 mg.)

Phenethicillin is also known as phenoxyethyl penicillin, and has chemical relationships with other acid-stable, orally active penicillins. In its general activity it resembles both penicillin V and penicillin G, but is better absorbed, and the blood level reaches a peak within a half to one hour. The standard dose is 125 to 250 mg. three or four times a day before food according to the severity of the infection. Response is usual within four days of treatment, but haemolytic streptococcal infections should be treated for longer periods to reduce the risk of relapse. It is not suitable for deep infections such as endocarditis. *Brand name :* Broxil.†

Propicillin † (dose, 250 to 500 mg.)

Propicillin is the phenoxypropyl derivative of penicillin. It is thus chemically related to penicillin V and phenethicillin, and has similar antibacterial properties. The average dose is 250 mg. every four to six hours, increased to 500 mg. in severe infections. *Brand names :* Brocillin,† Ultrapen.†

Methicillin †

Reference has already been made (p. 120) to the fact that penicillin is broken down and inactivated by penicillinase, and in consequence penicillin is ineffective against penicillinase-producing organisms. Chemical modification of the penicillin nucleus has resulted in the introduction of new penicillin derivatives which differ from ordinary penicillin. The first of these new compounds was methicillin, which although less potent than other forms of penicillin, had the outstanding advantage of being resistant to the action of penicillinase. It was thus effective in staphylococcal infections hitherto resistant to penicillin. The standard dose is 1 G. four-hourly by intramuscular injection. Methicillin is easily decomposed by acids, and is therefore unsuitable for oral administration, and it has been replaced to a great extent by cloxacillin. Occasionally, however, methicillin may be more effective than cloxacillin when the invading organisms produce very large amounts of penicillinase. It should be noted that methicillin is less effective than soluble penicillin in the treatment of infections due to non-resistant organisms, and in such infections the older drug is still the antibiotic of choice. *Brand name :* Celbenin.†

Cloxacillin †

Cloxacillin is a semi-synthetic penicillin and like methicillin (*q.v.*) is active against penicillinase-producing organisms, but it is more potent, and effective in lower doses. It is also active against other organisms, and so is of value in mixed infections due to gram-positive bacteria. Cloxacillin is given by intramuscular injection in doses of 250 mg. four-to-six hourly, but as it is also acid-resistant, it may be given orally before food in doses of 500 mg. It is less active than soluble penicillin against penicillin-sensitive organisms, and for the treatment of infections due to such organisms the older form of penicillin is still the preferred drug. Cloxacillin has very little action against gram-negative bacteria.

It should be remembered that both cloxacillin and methicillin are penicillin derivatives, and are not suitable for patients who have become sensitised to any form of penicillin. *Brand name :* Orbenin.†

Ampicillin † (dose, 250 to 750 mg.)

Ampicillin represents an interesting extension of the range of activity of penicillin. Like penicillin V and associated derivatives, ampicillin is active orally, but it possesses a much wider range of antibacterial activity. This range includes many of the gram-negative organisms such as *E. coli*, Salmonella and Shigella, *Haemophilus influenzae* and some species of Proteus, but *Pseudomonas* and *Proteus mirabilis* are not affected. Absorption is variable after oral administration, and the drug should be given before meals, but in severe infections it should be given by intramuscular injection or intravenous drip infusion. It is useful in a wide range of infections, particularly those due to gram-negative organisms, or where the infection is a mixed one. It is also valuable in the prophylaxis as well as the treatment of respiratory infections especially those due to *Haemophilus influenzae*. Ampicillin is not effective against penicillinase-producing staphylococci as it is destroyed by penicillinase, but may be given in association with cloxacillin as Ampiclox. It is less active than soluble penicillin against some gram-positive cocci, but the general pattern of activity is similar to that of the tetracyclines. The dose varies according to the nature of the infecting organism ; 250 mg. six-hourly are given in urinary tract infections and those due to gram-positive organisms, but larger doses of 500 to 750 mg. are required for infections due to the gram-negative group. Allergic reactions of the urticarial type are more common with ampicillin than other penicillin derivatives. *Brand name :* Penbritin.†

Carbenicillin †

Carbenicillin is a semi-synthetic derivative of penicillin which resembles ampicillin in being active against many gram-positive and gram-negative organisms. This activity is exceptional as it extends to *Pseudomonas pyocyanea* and some species of *Proteus*, and the drug has considerable therapeutic value in the treatment of infections due to those organisms. The drug is not very potent, so that large doses are necessary, but that disadvantage is offset by the low toxicity of the drug, which is characteristic of penicillin derivatives. Carbenicillin is given in doses of 1 G. six-hourly by intramuscular injection for urinary tract infections, but for severe systemic infections much larger doses, ranging from 12 to 30 G. daily, or even more, may be necessary. Such large doses are given by intravenous drip infusion. Probenecid (q.v.) may also be given orally to delay excretion of the carbenicillin, and so increase the blood level.

Carbenicillin may be given in association with other drugs active against gram-negative organisms, i.e., colistin and gentamicin, and such combined treatment may have an increased antibacterial action. It should be noted that carbenicillin is inactivated by penicillinase, and is not suitable for the treatment of resistant staphylococcal infections. *Brand name :* Pyopen.†

Cephalexin † (dose, 1 to 4 G. daily)

Cephalexin is an orally active derivative of cephalosporin, and has a pattern of activity similar to that of cephaloridine (q.v.). It attacks *E. coli* and other gram-negative organisms more rapidly than the gram-positives, and as it is excreted unchanged in the urine, it is of value in cystitis and other infections of the urinary tract. It is also effective in respiratory tract infections, and may be given to patients sensitive to penicillin. *Brand names :* Ceporex, Keflex.

Cephaloridine † (dose, 500 mg. to 1 G.)

The extensive use of wide-range antibiotics and of penicillin-streptomycin mixtures reflects the frequency with which mixed infections are encountered, and the problems of drug-resistance. Chemical modification of known antibiotics may increase the range of activity, as exemplified by the penicillin derivatives cloxacillin (q.v.), ampicillin (q.v.) and carbenicillin (q.v.), and cephaloridine, derived from cephalosporin, represents a similar development.

Cephalosporin was the name applied to a mixture of antibiotics produced by a mould obtained from a sewage outflow in Sardinia in 1948. Investigation showed that cephalosporin had some interesting properties, but was of little clinical interest. Further research resulted in the discovery of a new derivative, cephaloridine, characterised by a wide range of activity, and a marked bactericidal action. Cephaloridine is active against penicillin-resistant *Staphylococci* and *Streptococci*, and many gram-negative organisms such as *E. coli* and *Salmonella*, but it is not effective against *Pseudomonas pyocyanea* or *Proteus*. It is of value in endocarditis and septicaemia, in respiratory and bone infections, and as it is excreted unchanged in the urine, it is effective in urinary tract infections.

Cephaloridine may be given by intramuscular injection in doses of 1 G. two or three times a day in mixed or gram-negative infections, and in 500 mg. doses twice daily in gram-positive infections. It is usually but not invariably tolerated by patients who are sensitive to penicillin. Cephaloridine may also be given by intravenous injection, and in meningitis the intramuscular injections may be supplemented by intrathecal doses of 50 mg. Most systemic and urinary tract infections respond well to cephaloridine therapy within two to five days, and treatment beyond ten days is rarely necessary. Side-effects are uncommon but care should be taken in renal dysfunction to reduce the dose, and so avoid the accumulation of the drug to possibly toxic levels. Cephalothin (Keflin) is a related drug with a similar action. *Brand name* : Ceporin.†

Chloramphenicol † (dose, 1·5 to 3 G. daily)

Chloramphenicol is a broad spectrum antibiotic originally obtained from cultures of *Streptomyces venezuelae*, but it is now prepared synthetically. Like the tetracyclines, it is active against a wide range of organisms, which includes *Proteus, E. coli, Brucella, Salmonella, Haemophilus influenzae* and others. The therapeutic value is limited to some extent by its toxicity, as although in general it is well tolerated, in some patients it brings about a severe depression of the bone marrow, which may lead to aplastic anaemia and agranulocytosis. Intestinal overgrowth with *Candida* may occur as with other wide-range antibiotics, and because of the toxic side-effects, the therapeutic applications of chloramphenicol are limited, but within those limits the drug is of outstanding value.

In practice the chief therapeutic application of chloramphenicol is in the treatment of typhoid and paratyphoid fever, as in these conditions it is superior to other antibiotics. It is also of value in meningitis due to *Haemophilus influenzae* and other susceptible organisms, as it penetrates easily into the cerebrospinal fluid. Chloramphenicol is effective in urinary, viral and rickettsial infections, but it should be reserved for use in conditions not responding to other forms of treatment. Chloramphenicol is also useful for local application, particularly for eye infections.

The standard dose of chloramphenicol is 500 mg. orally four times a day, but larger doses are sometimes given. In very severe infections, or when oral administration is not practicable, chloramphenicol succinate, a water-soluble form of the drug, may be given by intravenous, intramuscular or subcutaneous injection. As soon as the infection is under control the dose should be reduced, and the course should be terminated within ten days or so. The risk of toxic effects increases with higher doses and longer administration, but such effects can also occur with standard doses, and frequent blood counts should be made during treatment. The drug has a bitter taste, and for children a flavoured suspension of chloramphenicol palmitate is available. Care should be taken with new-born infants, as they may react badly to chloramphenicol, exhibiting the so-called ' grey syndrome ' of vomiting, depressed respiration and cyanosis. This reaction may be due to the inability of the infant to metabolise and excrete the drug. *Brand name:* Chloromycetin.†

Colistin † (dose, 3 to 9 mega units daily by intramuscular injection, 9 to 18 mega units daily orally)

This antibiotic, also known as polymyxin E, has the general properties of polymyxin B (*q.v.*), but is less toxic and less irritating. It is effective against *Ps. pyocyanea* and most other gram-negative organisms, with the exception of *Proteus*, *Brucella* and *Neisseria*. It is not absorbed orally, and for the treatment of systemic infections due to gram-negative organisms, colistin is given by intramuscular injection as colistin sulphomethate in doses of 1,000,000 units four times a day. As much of the drug is excreted by the kidneys, it is also useful in infections of the urinary tract. Colistin may be given by mouth for the treatment of gastro-enteritis, especially in children with *E. coli* infections. A syrup is available containing 250,000 units in 5 ml. *Brand name :* Colomycin.†

Erythromycin † (dose, 250 to 500 mg.)

Erythromycin resembles penicillin in being active mainly against gram-positive organisms, but it has the advantage of being effective orally. The activity extends to many penicillin-resistant organisms, and haemolytic streptococci are usually very sensitive to erythromycin.   Other organisms may develop a resistance to erythromycin, but this occurs mainly when treatment is prolonged.   It is best used for intensive short-term treatment, or where the patient is sensitive to penicillin.   Erythromycin is also of particular value in staphylococcal enteritis due to organisms resistant to other antibiotics.

It penetrates rapidly into the body tissues and much is excreted in the bile.   The standard adult dose is 0·5 G. four times a day, and following such administration, a peak blood level is reached in one to two hours, and effective levels persist for about six hours. Erythromycin is best given as coated tablets, as some inactivation might otherwise occur, particularly if absorption of the drug is delayed by food in the stomach.   In severe infections it may be given by intramuscular injection (dose, 100 mg.) or by slow intravenous drip infusion (dose, 300 mg.).   Some oral preparations contain erythromycin estolate, and jaundice has followed the use of this form of the antibiotic.   *Brand names :* Erythrocin,† Erythrocin I.M.,† Erythrocin Lactobionate † (intravenous injection), Erythroped,† Ilosone,† Ilotycin.†

Flucloxacillin

Flucloxacillin is closely related chemically to cloxacillin (*q.v.*), and has the penicillinase-resisting properties of the older drug. In addition, flucloxacillin is absorbed more completely after oral administration, and adequate blood-levels of the drug may be obtained from doses of 250 mg. every six hours.   Such doses are best given one hour before meals.   In severe infections, flucloxacillin may be given in standard doses of 250 mg. by intramuscular injection, or by slow intravenous infusion.   Flucloxacillin has the low toxicity characteristic of the penicillin derivatives, and larger doses may be given if required.   Conversely, it should not be given to penicillin-sensitive patients.

Flucloxacillin is mainly indicated in infections due to penicillinase-producing staphylococci, but it is also active against other gram-positive organisms such as the streptococci and pneumococci. It is also of value in mixed infections, and in patients who have failed to respond to other drugs. *Brand name :* Floxapen.

Gentamicin sulphate † (dose, 0·4 to 0·8 mg. per kg. body weight)

Gentamicin is an antibiotic obtained from cultures of *Micromonospora*.   It has a wide range of activity against many gram-negative organisms and also against some gram-positive cocci, including those resistant to other antibiotics. Gentamicin is not absorbed to any great extent when given orally, and for systemic infections the drug is given by intramuscular injection. It is more stable than most antibiotics, and that stability permits the injection to be supplied as a solution ready for use.

Gentamicin is used mainly for the treatment of infections of the urinary tract, but it is also useful in chest infections, in septicaemia, and infections due to penicillin-resistant staphylococci and haemolytic streptococci. In general, gentamicin is well tolerated, but as it has chemical links with kanamycin and neomycin, it should be used with care in renal or vestibular dysfunction. In any case treatment should not be given for more than seven consecutive days in order to reduce the risk of auditory or kidney damage. The average adult dose is up to 80 mg. daily divided into two or three doses, with lower doses where renal dysfunction would lead to unnecessarily high blood levels. Gentamicin is also useful for topical application in skin infections associated with *Ps. pyocyanea* or *Proteus*, and a cream and ointment are available. *Brand names:* Cidomycin,† Genticin.†

Kanamycin † (dose, 1 G.)

Kanamycin is related to neomycin (*q.v.*) and is active against a wide range of gram-positive and gram-negative organisms, including many resistant to other antibiotics. It is less toxic than neomycin, and it is used for the treatment of staphylococcal infections, and in urinary infections due to *Proteus*. Kanamycin is not absorbed orally, and for systemic use must be given by intramuscular or intravenous injection. The standard adult dose is 1 G. daily in divided doses. Treatment should not be continued for more than six days, as the drug, like streptomycin, may cause tinnitus and deafness in full and prolonged doses. A good fluid intake during kanamycin treatment is important and reduced doses of the drug are necessary if renal function is impaired. *Brand names :* Kannasyn,† Kantrex.†

Lincomycin † (dose, 500 mg. to 1 G.)

This antibiotic differs chemically from others presently available, and is effective against most of the gram-positive pathogens. It is useful in infections of the respiratory tract, soft tissue infections and osteomyelitis, and may be given orally in doses of 500 mg. eight-hourly, in mild infections, or by intra-muscular injection in doses of 600 mg. once or twice daily in severe infections. Lincomycin may also be given by slow intra-venous drip infusion in very severe infections. It is also useful in patients sensitive to penicillin or other antibiotics. Clindamycin (Dalacin C) is a more powerful derivative, given in doses of 150 to 300 mg. *Brand names :* Lincocin,† Mycivin.†

Neomycin †

Neomycin is related chemically to streptomycin, and has a basically similar range of activity against gram-positive and gram-negative organisms. It is too toxic for systemic use, but is widely employed in the treatment of topical infections, particularly those of the eye and ear. Together with one of the topically effective corticosteroids, neomycin is present in a wide range of products used for the local treatment of inflamed and infected conditions. Although sensitivity to neomycin is not common, it is by no means unknown, and contact dermatitis and allergic reactions have followed topical application of neomycin-containing products. Neomycin is not absorbed orally, and in doses of 1 G. every four or six hours it has been used for intestinal infections and in preparation for bowel surgery.

Brand names: Nivemycin,† Mycifradin.†

Novobiocin † (dose, 250 to 500 mg.)

Novobiocin is an orally active antibiotic effective against many gram-positive organisms, and a few gram-negative organisms, including some strains of *Proteus*. Novobiocin has been used in the treatment of staphylococcal infections resistant to penicillin and other antibiotics, or in patients sensitive to penicillin and the tetracyclines. Its use has declined as new and more effective antibiotics have become available.

The standard dose is 250 mg. six-hourly, or 500 mg. twelve-hourly. Fever is not uncommon during treatment and nausea and skin reactions may also occur. *Brand names :* Albamycin,† Cathomycin.†

Paromomycin † (dose, 1 to 1·5 G. daily)

Paromomycin is an antibiotic effective against gram-positive and gram-negative organisms, and it is also active against *Enta-moeba*. The drug is not absorbed when given orally, so its use is largely restricted to the treatment of gastro-intestinal disorders due to *Salmonella* and *Shigella*, both in the acute and carrier states. Paromomycin is sometimes used pre-operatively before bowel surgery to reduce the bacterial flora of the intestines, and it is also of value in the treatment of intestinal amoebiasis.

It is given in doses of 1 to 1·5 G. daily in divided doses according to body weight, but sometimes much larger doses are required. A five-day course of treatment is usually adequate, as longer use may result in the overgrowth of non-susceptible organisms. Paromomycin is sometimes used in hepatic coma on the basis that such coma may be associated with the absorption of toxic nitrogenous products produced by bacteria in the intestines. By inhibiting the growth of intestinal organisms, the formation and absorption of these toxic products is prevented. *Brand name :* Humatin.†

Polymyxin B †

A mixture of related substances, referred to as polymyxins, is produced in cultures of *Bacillus polymyxa*, and the most important are polymyxin B and polymyxin E (colistin *q.v.*). Polymyxin B is characterised by its activity against many pathogenic gram-negative organisms such as *E. coli, Haemophilus influenzae, K. aerogenes* and *Ps. pyocyanea*, but it is much less active against *Proteus* and is inactive against gram-positive organisms. The systemic use of polymyxin B is restricted to the treatment of infections due to gram-negative organisms which have not responded to other forms of therapy. It is given in doses of 250,000 units by intramuscular injection every four to six hours. The injection may cause pain and a local reaction, but the most serious toxic effect is kidney damage. Alternatively, polymyxin methanesulphonate, (Thiosporin †) may be used, as this derivative, although less active, is less toxic and causes less tissue irritation.

Polymyxin B is also used topically as drops, creams and ointments in *Ps. pyocyanea* and related infections.

Brand name : Aeroporin.†

Cortisporin,† Otosporin,† Polybactrin † and Polyfax † represent products for local use containing polymyxin and other substances.

Sodium Fusidate (dose, 1·5 G. daily)

Sodium fusidate is active against a wide range of gram-positive and gram-negative organisms, and is used mainly in the treatment of staphylococcal infections that are resistant to penicillin. The standard dose is 0·5 G. eight-hourly, and is best given with food to reduce possible gastro-intestinal disturbance. In severe infections, sodium fusidate may be given by intravenous drip infusion. *Brand name :* Fucidin.†

Spiramycin † (dose, 2 to 5 G. daily)

Spiramycin is a mixture of closely related antibiotics, and has a pattern of antimicrobial action very similar to that of erythromycin. Its chief use is in the treatment of infections due to gram-positive organisms in patients sensitised to penicillin and other antibiotics. Spiramycin is also of value in the treatment of staphylococcal enteritis following the use of the wide-range antibiotics. It is active orally, and standard doses are 0·5 to 1 G. six-hourly and treatment should be continued for 48 hours after the signs of infection have disappeared. Much of the drug is excreted in the bile. A syrup is available for paediatric use. *Brand name:* Rovamycin.†

Triacetyloleandomycin † (dose, 250 to 500 mg.)

Triacetyloleandomycin resembles erythromycin in its range of activity, but its therapeutic value is limited. It is sometimes used in the treatment of penicillin-resistant staphylococcal infections, or in patients sensitised to other antibiotics. Liver damage has been reported after extended treatment. *Brand name :* Evramycin.†

Vancomycin † (dose, 0·5 G.)

Vancomycin is effective against many gram-positive organisms, including those resistant to other antibiotics. The introduction of newer drugs has limited its value, and it is used mainly for the treatment of staphylococcal infections which do not respond to other drugs or in fulminating conditions when rapid control of the infection is essential. Vancomycin is given by slow intravenous drip infusion in doses of 0·5 G. six-hourly. It may cause pain and phlebitis at the injection site, and tinnitus and deafness may occur with full doses. *Brand name :* Vancocin.†

The Tetracyclines and other Broad-spectrum Antibiotics

The early antibiotics such as penicillin, erythromycin and streptomycin are somewhat restricted in their range of activity, but following a world-wide investigation of products of fungal metabolism, substances active against both gram-positive and gram-negative organisms, as well as against spirochaetes, rickettsias and some viruses were discovered. One large group consists of substances that are closely related chemically, and are referred to in general terms as the tetracyclines. They include chlor-tetracycline (Aureomycin †), oxytetracycline (Terramycin,† Imperacin †), tetracycline (Achromycin,† Steclin,† Totomycin,† Tetracyn †), demethylchlortetracycline (Ledermycin †), metha-cycline (Rondomycin †), clomocycline (Megaclor †), doxycycline (Vibramycin†) and lymecycline (Tetralysal†). Because of their wide range of activity, the tetracyclines are referred to as broad-spectrum antibiotics, and although there are certain differences between them, they are so closely linked that they will be considered together.

The following table indicates the wide range of conditions in which the tetracyclines are effective.

Organism	*Disease*
Brucella abortis	Abortus fever
Clostridia spp	Gas gangrene
Escherichia coli	Urinary infections
Gonococcus	Gonorrhoea
Haemophilus pertussis	Whooping-cough
Haemophilus influenzae	Pneumonia, meningitis
Staphylococcus spp	Boils, etc.
Streptococcus haemolytica	Septicaemia, tonsillitis, etc.
Pneumococcus spp	Pneumonia
Treponema pallida	Syphilis
Viruses	Virus pneumonia
Rickettsias	Q fever, scrub typhus

The tetracyclines are less effective in infections caused by *Proteus*, *Pseudomonas*, *Salmonella* and other gram-negative organisms, and in such infections other drugs, such as colistin (*q.v.*), and carbenicillin (*q.v.*), are preferred. The chief therapeutic applications of the tetracyclines include the treatment of infections which do not normally respond to penicillin or the sulphonamides, mixed infections and infections which are due to bacteria that have acquired a resistance to the older drugs. The tetracyclines are also useful in pulmonary infections that do not respond to penicillin.

These infections may be viral in origin, or due to mycoplasma, and the associated bacterial invaders, such as *H. influenzae*, may also be more sensitive to the action of the tetracyclines. Oral therapy is usually effective, and although in severe infections treatment may be commenced with parenteral doses, the change to oral administration should be made as soon as possible. Treatment should be continued for at least forty-eight hours after the temperature has become normal. This group of drugs is also used in the prophylactic treatment of chronic bronchitis, and irreversible lung damage may be prevented by tetracycline treatment during the winter months.

The wide range of activity of the tetracyclines has led to their use in many conditions that might be expected to respond to other forms of treatment. When in doubt concerning the nature of the infecting organisms there is a temptation to use a wide-range drug, but indiscriminate use has its dangers, and may increase the incidence of tetracycline-resistant infections.

ADMINISTRATION AND DOSE.—Following oral use initial absorption is fairly rapid, and effective blood levels of tetracycline can be maintained with six-hourly doses of 250 mg. The tetracyclines may be given by slow intravenous drip infusion, but the solutions are potential irritants, and oral treatment should be instituted as soon as possible. Absorption after intramuscular injection is less regular, the injection is painful, and only small doses of 100 mg. may be tolerated.

However administered, the tetracyclines penetrate into all body fluids, with the exception of the cerebrospinal fluid, unless the meninges are inflamed. Part of an oral dose of a tetracycline is excreted unabsorbed in the faeces (and absorption is further reduced if aluminium hydroxide is also given). Of the absorbed or injected drug much is excreted in the urine, but significant amounts also appear in the bile.

The average dose of the tetracyclines is 250 to 500 mg. four times a day, but larger doses are given in very severe infections. In the prophylactic treatment of bronchitis, the lowest dose necessary to keep the sputum free from pus should be used, and 0·5 G. daily may be adequate.

SIDE-EFFECTS.—In general, the tetracyclines are well tolerated, but some nausea and vomiting may occur. The gastric irritant effects may be minimised by taking the drug with food or milk, but aluminium hydroxide gel should not be given as it hinders absorption. The tetracyclines are deposited in teeth and calcifying tissues and the yellow staining of the teeth may be permanent if the drugs are given to children. Clomocycline (*q.v.*) is largely free from that disadvantage. Because of this take-up of tetracycline by bone, the drugs are best avoided during pregnancy. The most important side-effects are directly related to their wide range of activity, as by reason of this activity the normal bacterial flora of the intestines is changed, the faeces become more fluid, and pruritus may occur. Further, the bacteria in the oral cavities may be affected, resulting in stomatitis and glossitis. This change may be related in part to the suppression of vitamin B synthesis, the lack of which is easily remedied, but much more serious is a ' supra infection ' or staphylococcal enteritis.

It will be appreciated that many non-pathogenic organisms are normally found in the intestinal tract, and some of these are beneficial, as they are concerned with the formation of vitamin K and vitamins of the B group. If wide-range antibiotics are given in full doses for extended periods, growth of all susceptible organisms in the intestines will be inhibited and the balance which normally prevents the excessive growth of any one organism will be disturbed. A severe staphylococcal enteritis due to the overgrowth of a tetracycline-resistant organism can occur very suddenly, with the development of a shock-like state with dehydration, low blood pressure and high temperature. Immediate change of antibiotic to cloxacillin or methicillin is essential, together with intravenous fluids and other supportive measures, if a fatal outcome is to be avoided. Fungal overgrowth with *Candida* may also occur in the same way.

Clomocycline † (dose, 170 mg.)

Clomocycline is a derivative of chlortetracycline, but is more soluble, and is absorbed more rapidly. The standard adult dose is 170 mg. four times a day, children's doses are 12 mg. per kg. body weight daily. Unlike the more slowly absorbed derivatives, clomocycline is not deposited in calcifying areas, is less likely to cause staining of the teeth and may be safer in the later stages of pregnancy. *Brand name:* Megaclor.†

Demethylchlortetracycline † (dose, 150 mg.)

A derivative of chlortetracycline, with a similar range of activity, but an increased potency. That increase is reflected in the lower dose of the drug, which is 150 mg. four times a day. *Brand name:* Ledermycin.†

Doxycycline † (dose, 100 mg.)

Doxycycline has the wide range of activity of the tetracyclines, but is characterised by an exceptionally high degree of absorption, and a slow rate of excretion. After an initial dose of 200 mg., therapeutic blood levels can be maintained with a dose of 100 mg. daily. *Brand name :* Vibramycin.

Lymecycline † (dose, 150 mg.)

Lymecycline is a combination of tetracycline with the amino-acid lysine. The compound is much more soluble than tetracycline, and adequate blood levels are obtained with oral doses equivalent to 150 mg. of tetracycline. A preparation of lymecycline for intramuscular injection is also available, and has the advantages of increased solubility and stability. *Brand name:* Tetralysal.†

STREPTOMYCIN AND OTHER TUBERCULOSTATIC DRUGS

Streptomycin † (dose, 0·5 to 1 G. daily)

Streptomycin was one of the first antibiotics to be introduced after the discovery of penicillin. It is effective against many gram-negative organisms, a group against which penicillin is of no value, although its range includes a few gram-positive organisms, notably *Mycobacterium tuberculosis*, as indicated in the following table.

Organism	*Disease*
M. tuberculosis	Tuberculosis
Escherichia coli	Cystitis, pyelitis and related conditions; meningitis
Haemophilus influenzae	Pneumonia, meningitis
Pseudomonas pyocyanea	Urinary infections
Pasteurella pestis	Plague
Streptococcus faecalis	Bacterial endocarditis

Streptomycin is soluble in water, and stabilised solutions retain their activity for several weeks, or even longer if stored in a refrigerator ; slight discoloration may occur, but this does not necessarily indicate any reduction in potency.

ADMINISTRATION AND DOSE.—Streptomycin is not absorbed orally, and for systemic use it must be given by intramuscular injection. It becomes widely distributed throughout the body, but it does not normally penetrate into the cerebrospinal fluid unless the meninges are inflamed. Special ampoules containing 50 mg. and 100 mg. of the drug are available for the preparation of intrathecal injections for the treatment of meningeal infections.

The standard dose of streptomycin in urinary and other non-tuberculous infections is 0·5 to 1 G. twice daily for four to five days, but the usefulness of the drug is limited by the rapidity with which bacterial resistance appears, so unless response to the drug is prompt, longer treatment is useless.

Streptomycin is not broken down in the body to any great extent, and is excreted by the kidneys in an active form. It is therefore useful in the short-term treatment of urinary infections due to *Pseudomonas pyocyanea*, *E. coli* and associated organisms, particularly when resistant to other forms of treatment. The effectiveness of streptomycin in such infections is increased if the urine is made alkaline by giving potassium citrate. In renal dysfunction exceptionally high blood levels may occur owing to delayed excretion, and the risk of toxic side-effects is thereby increased.

Although streptomycin is freely soluble in water it is not absorbed when given orally, but is used in oral doses of 0·5 to 1 G. three or four times a day for intestinal infections, and for pre-operative and post-operative use in abdominal surgery.

The chief use of streptomycin is in the treatment of tuberculosis, but it should never be given alone, both because of its toxic effects and the development of drug resistance. The drugs usually employed with streptomycin are isoniazid (*q.v.*) and aminosalicylic acid (*q.v.*). A standard initial course of treatment is streptomycin 1 G. daily with isoniazid 200 mg. daily, with aminosalicyclic acid 15 G. daily. For patients over 40, and when less intensive treatment is adequate, streptomycin is given two or three times a week. Other combinations of drugs or doses may be used according to response. The best results are obtained in the early inflammatory stage of pulmonary tuberculosis, and in tubercular meningitis. The less impressive results in some other forms of tuberculosis may be due to poor penetration of the drugs into the caseous areas,

TOXIC EFFECTS.—Streptomycin has neurotoxic properties and may cause tinnitus, vertigo and other disturbances of hearing and balance by a toxic effect on the eighth cranial nerve. These effects are slow in onset, and permanent deafness has followed prolonged treatment with full doses. Hepatic and renal damage has also been associated with streptomycin therapy. The drug may also cause a sensitisation dermatitis, and nurses should take care that streptomycin solutions do not come into contact with the skin.

Aminosalicyclic Acid (dose, 10 to 15 G. daily)

Often referred to as PAS, it is more accurately described as para-aminosalicylic acid, and is used mainly as the sodium salt. It is chiefly of interest because of its powerful antitubercular properties, and in association with isoniazid and streptomycin it is now part of the standard treatment of tuberculosis. Resistance to the drug occurs, as with streptomycin, but the resistance is slower in onset, and can be delayed still further by combined treatment with other antitubercular drugs such as isoniazid (*q.v.*). This question of combined treatment is of great importance, and several products containing both aminosalicylic acid and isoniazid are available to simplify and ensure combined administration. Aminosalicylic acid is effective orally, but as excretion is rapid, frequent administration is necessary to maintain an adequate blood level. Doses of 3 G. four or five times a day may be given but as the drug has a very unpleasant taste, which is difficult to disguise, it is usually given in cachets. The calcium salt is also available, and is given in similar doses. *Brand names :* Aminacyl, Dantyl, Paramisan Sodium, Pasade.

An alternative preparation is calcium benzamidosalicylate. This compound is broken down in the body to release the aminosalicylate, and as it is better tolerated than sodium aminosalicylate and excreted more slowly, it has some advantages. *Brand names:* Calcium B-PAS, Therapas.

Isoniazid † (dose, 300 to 600 mg. daily)

Isoniazid is an example of a highly selective antibacterial drug, as although it has a remarkable inhibitory effect on *M. tuberculosis* it has virtually no action against other organisms. Following oral administration, isoniazid is rapidly absorbed and penetrates easily into the body tissues and fluids, including the cerebrospinal fluid, and also into caseous areas. This rapid penetration is of great value in the treatment of tubercular meningitis. As with streptomycin and aminosalicylates, drug resistance may occur if the compound is used alone, and combined therapy is essential.

Isoniazid is well tolerated and side-effects are not usually serious. Skin rashes and urticaria may occur, and peripheral neuropathy is an occasional serious hazard with higher doses. Pyridoxine in doses of 50 to 100 mg. daily has been given as a prophylactic, as isoniazid may interfere with normal pyridoxine metabolism. Some patients experience mild euphoria whilst taking isoniazid, and it is of interest to note that a study of that effect led to the introduction of the monoamine oxidase inhibitor type of antidepressant drug. *Brand names :* Nicetal,† Pycazide,† Rimifon.† *Brand names* of products containing both isoniazid and aminosalicylate : B-Pasinah,† Inapasade,† Pasinah,† Pycamisan,† Pycasix,† Therazid.†

Other synthetic antituberculous drugs include salinazid (Nupasal †), ethionamide (Trescatyl †), ethambutol (Myambutol †), prothionamide (Trevintix †), pyrazinamide (Zinamide †) thiacetazone and thiocarlide (Isoxyl †). Salinazid is a derivative of isoniazid which has the antitubercular properties of the parent drug, but has reduced toxic effects. It is sometimes useful when isoniazid is badly tolerated. Ethionamide and prothionamide (dose, 0·5 to 1 G. daily) have some chemical relationships with isoniazid, and are sometimes effective when the tubercular organisms have become resistant to the older drug. Their value is limited by the side-effects, which include vomiting, jaundice and depression, although prothionamide is less likely to cause gastric disturbance. Combined treatment with other antitubercular drugs remains essential. Pyrazinamide has similar tuberculostatic properties, and in combination with streptomycin and isoniazid has proved of value in patients resistant to other drugs. Resistance to pyrazinamide may develop during long-term treatment, and the drug may also cause liver damage.

Thiazetazone is also used occasionally when the response to other drugs is inadequate. Doses of 10 to 25 mg. have been given, in association with other antitubercular drugs, but toxic effects, such as agranulocytosis and hepatic dysfunction, limit the use of the drug to the treatment of resistant conditions.

Viomycin † (dose, 1 G.)

Viomycin is an antibiotic with properties similar to those of streptomycin but it is used only when the causative organism has become resistant to other forms of treatment or when the patient is streptomycin-sensitive. Viomycin is given by deep intramuscular injection in doses of 1 G. twice daily every third day, in association with aminosalicylic acid and isoniazid. It is of little value when caseation or fibrosis has occurred, as diffusion into such areas is poor. Like streptomycin, viomycin may cause partial deafness, but the principal toxic effect is on the kidneys, and the drug should be used with care in patients with renal disease. *Brand names :* Viocin,† Viomycin P,† Vionactane.†

Cycloserine † (dose, 250 to 750 mg. daily)

Although cycloserine is an antibiotic active against many organisms, it is of limited therapeutic value owing to its low potency. The main use of the drug is in the treatment of severe pulmonary tuberculosis where the organism is resistant to other tuberculostatic drugs. It is not considered suitable for long-term treatment. Like streptomycin, the drug must be used together with other antitubercular compounds. It is occasionally used for the treatment of non-tuberculous infections of the urinary tract. Cycloserine is excreted slowly, and if doses of more than 1 G. daily are given, it may accumulate in the body, causing side-effects such as drowsiness, twitching and other symptoms involving the central nervous system. Epilepsy is a contra-indication.

Capreomycin † (dose, 1 G. daily)

Capreomycin is an antibiotic of occasional value in tuberculosis when other drugs fail to evoke an adequate response. It is given by intramuscular injection in doses of 1 G. daily, always in association with isoniazid or alternative drugs. It is of no value when the condition is resistant to viomycin or kanamycin.

Rifampicin † (dose, 450 to 600 mg. daily)

Rifampicin is one of the rifamycin group of antibiotics, and is highly effective against *Mycobacterium tuberculosis* and related organisms. It is of low toxicity and well tolerated, and is of particular value when resistance to other drugs has developed.

Rifampicin is given as a single daily dose of 450 to 600 mg., preferably on an empty stomach to obtain maximum absorption. Combined therapy with other tuberculostatic drugs remains essential, and in pulmonary tuberculosis the change to a negative sputum may occur rapidly. The drug is excreted mainly in the bile, so care is necessary in cases of liver dysfunction. It is contra-indicated in pregnancy. Rifampicin has a red colour, and may discolour the urine, sputum and tears, but is of no significance, and the discoloration may be used as a test of continuity of treatment. *Brand names :* Rifadin,† Rimactane.†

Mould against Mould

It is remarkable that whilst various fungal organisms produce antibacterial substances, a few also produce antifungal compounds, and these have no significant antibacterial properties. These antifungal products are mainly used in superficial fungal infections, as systemic fungal infections are fortunately uncommon.

Nystatin †

Nystatin is used mainly for oral and intestinal fungal disorders such as thrush and moniliasis. Such conditions may occur during extended therapy with broad-spectrum antibiotics, and the administration of nystatin is valuable both for prophylaxis and treatment.

It is given orally for intestinal moniliasis in doses of 500,000 units or more three times a day; for local application to the mouth the drug is used as a suspension. Pessaries are available for the treatment of vaginal moniliasis. Nystatin is not well absorbed orally, and it is of no value in systemic moniliasis. *Brand name :* Nystan.†

Amphotericin B †

Amphotericin is active against many yeast-like and filamentous fungi, and is the most effective drug for the treatment of deep fungal infections such as cryptococcosis, histoplasmosis and systemic moniliasis. It is given in doses of 0·25 mg. per kg. body weight daily by slow intravenous drip infusion in dextrose solution. Such solutions should be freshly prepared, and protected from light during administration. The dose is slowly increased to

1 mg. per kg. body weight, but long treatment is necessary, as the response to treatment in deep mycotic infections is slow. Febrile reactions, which can be severe, and headache may necessitate a temporary reduction in dose.

Amphotericin B is not absorbed orally, but is of value in the treatment of oral and intestinal moniliasis, and lozenges and tablets containing 10 mg. are available. The drug is also effective when applied locally. *Brand names :* Fungizone intravenous,† Fungilin.†

Candicidin †

Candicidin is an antifungal antibiotic, particularly effective against candida. It is used in the treatment of vaginal candidiasis by the application of a vaginal ointment or vaginal tablet, daily for fourteen days. Relief of symptoms is rapid, but the full course of treatment is necessary to eradicate the infection. *Brand name :* Candeptin.

Griseofulvin †

Griseofulvin has no antibacterial properties but is effective in ringworm and other fungal infections of the hair, skin and nails, *i.e.* those tissues containing keratin. Griseofulvin appears to be taken up selectively by such tissues, and prevents further penetration by the fungus. The new tissues formed are therefore free from infection, but response to treatment is correspondingly slow, and complete elimination of the fungus awaits the natural shedding of infected hair or nails, and replacement by healthy tissues. The drug is not effective in moniliasis or systemic fungal infections.

Griseofulvin is given orally in doses of 125 to 250 mg. four times a day for some weeks. In general it is well tolerated, but headache, allergic reactions and gastro-intestinal disturbances may occur. *Brand names :* Fulcin,† Grisovin.†

Antiviral Drugs

The advance made in the treatment of bacterial disease by chemotherapeutic agents has not yet been paralleled by comparable achievements in the control of virus diseases. Certain antibiotics such as the tetracyclines are effective against some of the larger viruses, and so are used in the treatment of atypical pneumonia, but specific antiviral drugs await discovery. One advance that may be a forerunner of others is the introduction of idoxuridine (I.D.U.), for the treatment of ocular herpetic keratitis. The drug is related to thymidine, one of the constituents of nuclear protein, and was originally synthesised as a possible cytostatic drug.

Subsequent research showed that it had antiviral properties, and it has since proved of value in viral infections of the eye. Even severe keratitic conditions respond to the local application of idoxuridine as a 0·1 per cent solution, and the compound may be useful in dermatology for the treatment of herpes simplex. Idoxuridine is also used occasionally by intravenous injection in lethal conditions such as viral encephalitis. Hitherto, that condition has been fatal, but some remarkable recoveries have followed early diagnosis and prompt treatment with idoxuridine. *Brand names :* Dendrid, Kerecid.

Another development is the discovery of methisazone (Marboran). This compound prevents the development of the virus of smallpox, and is useful for the temporary protection of smallpox contacts, and in the treatment of eczema asssociated with smallpox vaccination. It is given in doses of 3 G. twice daily.

Interferon

Interferon is a substance of considerable potential value in the treatment of virus diseases. It is a protein produced in mammalian cells following exposure to viruses, and has the power of inhibiting the growth of many viruses in the affected cells, and of protecting surrounding cells from attack. Such a substance has great potentialities as a therapeutic weapon against viral attack, and as all mammals produce interferon, attempts have been made to extract interferon from animal cells for clinical use. So far these attempts have not been very successful, as interferon is difficult to extract, is mainly effective in the species from which it was obtained, and is inactive in other animals. The problem may be solved by finding substances that stimulate the production of interferon, in which case as great a control of virus diseases might be achieved as is now possible with bacterial infections.

CHAPTER VIII

ANTICOAGULANTS AND HAEMOSTATICS

THE clotting of blood is such a complex process that a final explanation has still to be devised. The main factors concerned are fibrinogen, thrombin, thromboplastin and calcium. Fibrinogen is the soluble protein of the blood plasma, and is changed into insoluble fibrin by the action of thrombin. Thrombin is present in the blood in an inactive state as prothrombin, and is converted to active thrombin by the action of thromboplastin in the presence of calcium. A number of auxiliary factors are also concerned, but for practical purposes the process may be summarised thus :—

$$Prothrombin + thromboplastin + calcium \rightarrow thrombin$$
$$Thrombin + fibrinogen \rightarrow fibrin$$

The fibrin forms a matrix upon which the blood clot is built up. Thromboplastin is normally present in blood platelets and tissue cells, and is released when cells are injured. Normally the clotting of blood in undamaged blood vessels is prevented by heparin and other anticoagulant factors in the plasma, but occasionally, for reasons that are not yet clear, intravascular clotting or thrombosis may occur. One explanation is that some change in the vascular epithelium leads to a deposit of blood platelets, which release thromboplastin, which in turn releases thrombin, so that a clot is eventually formed. If this process takes place in one of the coronary arteries the supply of blood to the heart is restricted, the local concentration of thrombin may rise again and the dangerous condition of coronary thrombosis may result.

Thrombosis may also occur in the deep veins of the legs, expecially during prolonged bed rest, and there is the added danger that the clot may become detached at a later stage, and may eventually cause a pulmonary embolism.

Heparin

Thrombosis can be treated both actively and prophylactically by various anticoagulant drugs, of which one of the most important is heparin. This substance is a natural anticoagulant, and is present, as the name implies, in the liver and also in the lungs and intestinal mucosa. The mode of action of heparin is very complex, but following combination with some fractions of the plasma proteins, it inhibits the conversion of prothrombin to thrombin and the interaction of thrombin and fibrinogen. It is inactive orally, and is best given by intravenous injection, when the effect is prompt and reliable.

Heparin is used extensively in the treatment of arterial and venous thrombosis, and prophylactically after surgery to reduce the risks of thrombo-embolic complications. Initial doses of 10,000 units or more are often given, followed by maintenance doses every four to eight hours. The maintenance doses should be based on the clotting time of the blood, and consequently heparin should be used only when adequate laboratory facilities for determining clotting times are available. The aim of heparin treatment is to extend the clotting time to double or treble that of normal blood, thus preventing further clotting, and the risk of embolism.

Excessive doses of heparin cause haematuria and bleeding, but such overdosage can be neutralised by the infusion of fresh blood or by the intravenous injection of a solution of protamine sulphate. Protamine is a simple protein obtained from fish sperm, and has a specific effect in neutralising the action of heparin, as well as having some intrinsic anticoagulant properties. It is given in doses of 1 mg. for each 100 units of heparin, but not more than 50 mg. should be given as a single dose.

Heparin is also used to prevent the thrombophlebitis that occurs during and after prolonged drip infusion of intravenous fluids, and amounts of 1000 units or so may be added to each bottle of the transfusion solution. The rapid action of heparin when injected intravenously complicates the treatment of thrombosis, and a number of attempts have been made to prepare intramuscular products. Such intramuscular injections are less satisfactory than the intravenous solutions, as the injection is more painful, absorption is less regular and reliable, and a haematoma may occur at the injection site. *Brand name:* Pularin.

ORAL ANTICOAGULANTS

It has been known for many years that cattle fed with badly prepared sweet clover hay may develop a haemorrhagic disorder.

Research showed that an antiprothrombin substance was present in the hay, later identified as dicoumarol, and the therapeutic value of the compound was soon realised.

Dicoumarol differs sharply from heparin in several ways, as it is active orally but response is slow. Following oral administration there is a time-lag of twenty-four to forty-eight hours before any response can be detected, and as this delay is virtually independent of the dose given, the drug is thought to act by inhibiting the formation of prothrombin by the liver. Prothrombin already circulating in the blood is unaffected. Dicoumarol is not used therapeutically, as more reliable and effective compounds are now available.

Ethyl Biscoumacetate (dose, 150 mg. to 1·2 G. daily)

This anticoagulant is chemically related to dicoumarol, but absorption and excretion are more rapid, and treatment is more easily controlled. The initial dose is 1·2 G., given as a single dose, or as 300 mg. six-hourly. Subsequent doses vary from 150 to 900 mg. daily, based on estimations of the blood prothrombin levels. *Brand name :* Tromexan.

Phenindione (dose, 25 to 100 mg. daily)

Phenindione is one of the most widely used of the oral anti-coagulants. In common with related drugs, it inhibits the formation of prothrombin and other factors, and the onset of action is correspondingly slow. The rate of excretion is less rapid than that of ethyl biscoumacetate, and the general response to phenindione is more consistent and reliable.

The standard dose is 200 to 300 mg. initially, repeated after twelve hours. Subsequent daily doses vary from 25 to 100 mg. according to response. With a suitable maintenance dose the prothrombin time is double or treble that normally found.

Phenindione is of great value in the treatment and prophylaxis of coronary thrombosis, and it can prevent further clotting when thrombosis has already occurred.

When rapid treatment is required it is necessary to give heparin intravenously for the first twenty-four to thirty hours, and to commence oral therapy with phenindione at the same time. This affords anticoagulant cover immediately and also over the interim period before the phenindione (or other oral anticoagulant) begins to exert its effects. Treatment may have to be continued for some weeks. Phenindione has been employed extensively as a reliable anticoagulant with few side-effects but these side-effects, although uncommon, may be severe, and both liver and kidney damage may occur. There is now a tendency to use warfarin (*q.v.*) as the standard anticoagulant. *Brand name :* Dindevan.

Warfarin

Warfarin is a synthetic anticoagulant, resembling phenindione in its general pattern of activity. It is given in initial doses of 30 to 50 mg., with subsequent daily doses of 3 to 10 mg., based on laboratory reports of the blood-clotting times. With elderly and frail patients, the smaller doses should be used. The drug appears to have fewer side-effects than other oral anticoagulants, and is regarded by many haematologists as the drug of choice. *Brand name :* Marevan.

Related Drugs

Several other oral anticoagulants are available, and phenprocoumon (Marcoumar) and nicoumalone (Sinthrome) are representative products.

Toxic effects.—The chief danger of oral anticoagulant therapy is overdosage, which may cause bleeding from the gums and other mucous areas, the skin or internal organs. This side-effect occasionally occurs even with therapeutic doses, and immediate withdrawal of the drug is essential if the haemorrhage is severe.

At the same time an antidote should be given, and the compound most effective against the orally active anticoagulants is phytomenadione or vitamin K_1, which is given in doses of 10 to 50 mg. by intravenous injection. Alternatively, a transfusion of fresh whole blood may be given. (NOTE : Vitamin K_1 is a modification of vitamin K. Standard forms of vitamin K (such as Synkavit) are much less effective than K_1 in the treatment of overdosage with oral anticoagulants.) The treatment of overdosage with heparin is referred to on page 147. It should be noted that anticoagulant treatment is contra-indicated in severe hypertension, liver or renal disease, ulcerative lesions of the alimentary tract, in pregnancy, or soon after injury or operation.

HAEMOSTATICS

The factors concerned in the formation of a blood clot have been referred to on page 146, and certain blood fractions containing some of these factors have a limited therapeutic use as haemostatics when applied to bleeding areas. They are mainly of use in controlling capillary oozing, and are of little value when bleeding occurs from a vein or artery. Oxidised cellulose and other products are also used to control excessive bleeding.

Thrombin

Thrombin is the enzyme which converts fibrinogen into fibrin. It is usually obtained from bovine plasma and is supplied as a powder, to be dissolved in normal saline at the time of use. It is intended for local application, to control capillary bleeding, and must not be used by injection. Thrombin is also used in association with fibrinogen to form fibrin foam which has specialised haemostatic applications.

Fibrinogen

Fibrinogen is the soluble protein constituent of plasma. When mixed with thrombin it forms fibrin, which is an insoluble protein, and acts as a framework or scaffolding on which a blood clot can be built up. When supplied for haemostatic purposes fibrinogen is issued as a dry powder, to be dissolved in water and mixed with thrombin immediately before use. It is used in skin grafts and in the fixing of nerve sutures.

Fibrin Foam

The fibrin formed by the mixing of fibrinogen and thrombin can, by suitable manipulation, be prepared as a dry, spongy material. In this form it is used as a haemostatic in brain and lung surgery and may be left in place when the wound is closed as the foam is eventually absorbed.

Gelatin Sponge

Gelatin sponge is prepared by whipping highly purified gelatin solution into a foam. This foam is freeze-dried and sterilised, and the spongy product has valuable haemostatic properties. It is used in all branches of surgery and for packing cavities, and may be used alone, or in association with thrombin. When implanted into tissues as a haemostatic the wound may be closed, as the sponge is slowly absorbed over a period of four to six weeks. *Brand name :* Sterispon.

Oxidised Cellulose

Surgical gauze can be modified by chemical means so as to acquire haemostatic properties, although its physical appearance remains virtually unchanged. When applied to a bleeding surface the gauze swells and forms a soft mass, and it is used as temporary packing in abdominal and other forms of surgery. Small amounts of the material are slowly absorbed within a few days, but larger amounts may take several weeks, and care should be taken if the wound is to be closed. *Brand names:* Oxycel, Surgicel.

Calcium Alginate

Calcium alginate, derived from certain seaweeds, can be formed into products resembling gauze and cotton wool, and these products have useful haemostatic properties. The material is used to pack sinuses, bleeding tooth sockets and in surgery, and is slowly absorbed if left *in situ*. Alternatively, it may be removed by irrigation with water or sodium citrate solution. *Brand name :* Calgitex.

Ethamsylate

Ethamsylate is a synthetic compound which has haemostatic properties that are useful in the prevention and treatment of haemorrhage associated with damage to the capillary vessels. The mode of action is not clear, but the stimulation of the clotting process may be linked with an increase in the number of circulating platelets. Ethamsylate may be given orally in doses of 500 to 750 mg., or by intravenous or intramuscular injection in doses of 250 to 500 mg. *Brand name:* Dicynene.

Aminocaproic Acid

In health, fibrinogen is converted into fibrin in the blood as part of a repair process to maintain the vascular system, and excessive deposits of fibrin are prevented by a fibrinolytic enzyme system. The main component of this system is plasminogen, which is normally inert, but is converted into plasmin by activator

6

substances present in various tissues, notably the lungs. Plasmin has marked fibrinolytic properties, and normally there is a dynamic balance according to physiological needs between the activity of plasmin and the formation of fibrin. Some haemorrhagic conditions, however, appear to be associated with an increased fibrinolytic activity, and excessive bleeding may occur in prostatic diseases, and following surgical shock. This excessive breakdown of fibrin can be inhibited by various substances, particularly by aminocaproic acid, sometimes referred to as epsilon-aminocaproic acid. This compound inhibits the action of plasmin and so has an indirect haemostatic action, by preventing the breakdown of fibrin. It is used to control the haemorrhage associated with prostatic disease and after prostatectomy, in carcinoma of the pancreas, in leukaemia, and after surgery generally. It may be given orally in doses of 6 G. four-hourly, as a syrup or effervescent powder, or by intravenous drip infusion in doses of 1·5 G. hourly, after dilution with normal saline. Aminocaproic acid is well tolerated, and side-effects, apart from occasional nausea and diarrhoea, are slight. *Brand name :* Epsikapron.

Russel's Viper Venom

This snake venom contains a substance with the properties of thromboplastin and has powerful haemostatic properties when applied locally. It is supplied as a dry powder, to be dissolved in water to make a 1 : 10,000 solution and is occasionally of value in controlling excessive bleeding after extraction of teeth, especially in haemophiliacs. *Brand name :* Stypven.

CHAPTER IX

ANTI-ANAEMIC DRUGS

ANAEMIA can be broadly defined as an insufficiency of mature red cells in the blood. The most frequent and important cause is impaired blood formation, but excessive blood loss or destruction of red cells may also lead to anaemia. The blood cells or erythrocytes begin in the bone marrow as large cells, termed megaloblasts, which gradually diminish in size as they mature, and are then referred to as normoblasts. At a later stage these normoblasts acquire haemoglobin (the red iron-containing protein of the blood cells), and then enter the circulation as fully developed and mature erythrocytes. Haemoglobin is concerned with the transport of oxygen from the lungs to all the body tissues, and iron is an essential element of its constitution. Anaemia can therefore arise simply from a deficiency of iron, and in such iron-deficiency anaemias an adequate number of normoblasts may develop, but they lack the oxygen-carrying capacity of the mature red cells. Other and more serious forms of anaemia are due to a true deficiency of fully developed and mature erythrocytes owing to impaired cell formation by the bone marrow.

IRON-DEFICIENCY ANAEMIA

In health the loss of iron from the body is only about 2 mg. daily, and as this small amount is easily compensated for by the absorption of iron in the diet, the body has few reserves of iron.

A deficiency of iron, with consequent anaemia, therefore arises mainly from excessive blood loss, and may be due to the haemorrhage associated with peptic ulcer, profuse menstruation, and many other conditions. Deficiency may also occur during pregnancy and lactation, and in tropical countries hookworm infestation may cause anaemia.

The treatment of this type of anaemia is directed to a replacement of the deficiency of iron, and the history of the medicinal use of iron is interesting and instructive. From the earliest times iron has been regarded as the symbol of strength, and water in which swords had been allowed to rust was used as a tonic by the early physicians. The true therapeutic importance of iron was first realised early in the nineteenth century by the Frenchman Blaud, who introduced the once famous Blaud's pill. His pill contained ferrous sulphate and potassium carbonate, and was given in large doses. High-dose treatment is a fundamental principle of the therapy of iron-deficiency anaemia, and this principle was successfully applied for over a century.

Later, the use of large doses was considered unnecessary on the grounds that only small amounts of iron were required to balance even a severe blood loss, and that theoretical view prevailed until it was shown that to ensure the absorption of even small amounts of iron, doses much greater than those theoretically sufficient are essential.

The process by which iron is absorbed is a very complex one, and is influenced by a number of factors. Briefly, absorption of a soluble ferrous salt occurs in the duodenum, and the mucosal cells lining the small intestine appear to play an important part in regulating the absorption to balance a deficiency. Thus there is an increased absorption of iron in deficiency states, or when nutritional requirements are increased as in pregnancy. The absorbed iron combines with a protein to form ferritin, and as ferritin the iron is carried to the bone marrow for ultimate use in the formation of haemoglobin. Small amounts of iron are also deposited in the liver, spleen and other tissues. Many compounds of iron have been used as haematinics, and the following are in current use :

Ferrous Sulphate (prophylactic dose, 200 mg. daily; therapeutic dose, 0·6 to 1·2 G. daily)

Ferrous sulphate is one of the most widely used therapeutic forms of iron, as it is soluble, effective and inexpensive. It is usually given as tablets containing 200 mg. The drug is astringent and may cause occasional gastric disturbance, but this can be reduced by taking the tablets after food. The standard compound tablets of ferrous sulphate contain small amounts of copper and manganese, on the basis that traces of these metals play some part in the haemopoietic process (copper, for example, is essential for the synthesis of haemoglobin). As the diet contains adequate amounts of these metals, their inclusion in the standard tablet is hardly necessary. Ferrous sulphate may also be given in solution as Mixture of Ferrous Sulphate, and in small doses is a very suitable product for the administration of iron to small children. Tablets of ferrous sulphate are usually coated to prevent oxidation, and have been taken by children in mistake for sweets. The gastric irritation thus set up may be severe, leading to haematemesis, shock and cardiovascular collapse. Many deaths have occurred in small children from this cause. Immediate treatment includes emetics, gastric lavage with weak solutions of sodium bicarbonate, and injections of desferrioxamine (Desferal).

This substance is a chelating agent that binds the iron as a water-soluble non-toxic complex. It is given as soon as possible by intramuscular injection of 2 G., followed by doses of 20 mg. per kg. body-weight by intravenous drip infusion, to eliminate any absorbed iron. The further absorption of any iron remaining in the stomach may be prevented by giving an oral dose of 5 G. of desferrioxamine dissolved in 50 to 100 ml. of water.

Ferrous Gluconate (prophylactic dose, 300 mg. daily; therapeutic dose, 1·2 to 2·4 G. daily)

Ferrous gluconate has the same action as ferrous sulphate, but is much less astringent and less irritant, and is often acceptable when ferrous sulphate is not tolerated. Weight for weight it contains less iron than the sulphate, so that larger doses are required. Ferrous gluconate is present in a number of proprietary iron preparations, many of which contain vitamins to supplement any dietary deficiencies that may be associated with the anaemia. Such vitamin supplements, with the exception of vitamin C, do not increase the absorption of the associated iron compound.

Ferric Ammonium Citrate (dose, 1 to 3 G.)

This preparation is one of the older preparations of iron, and was once widely used as Ferric Ammonium Citrate Mixture B.N.F. It has little astringent or gastric irritant action, and is well tolerated, but it must be given in large doses. Although effective, and much less expensive than other liquid preparations of iron, it is now less popular, perhaps because it may blacken the teeth.

Other Iron Salts

Ferrous fumarate, ferric hydroxide and ferrous succinate are other iron salts with reduced side-effects, and are present in a number of proprietary anti-anaemic preparations. They are useful for patients who cannot tolerate other forms of iron, but have few other advantages. Some are available as special slow-release forms of iron salts, designed to delay absorption until the product has passed into the intestine, and thus reduce the risk of gastric disturbance still further.

Colliron, Sytron and Neo-Ferrum represent liquid preparations. The iron in Sytron is combined with an organic complex, which is broken down in the body to release the iron in an absorbable form. It is useful when gastric intolerance to other oral iron preparations is severe.

Some iron deficiency is common in pregnancy, and such deficiency may be associated with a folic acid deficiency, which manifests itself in late pregnancy as a megaloblastic anaemia. Several preparations of iron and folic acid are now available for prophylactic use throughout pregnancy, and representative products include Folaemin, Folvron, Fefol and Pregamal.

IRON BY INJECTION

In very severe iron deficiency, or when oral iron is not tolerated, it may be necessary to give iron by injection. Solutions of ordinary iron salts are too irritant and toxic for this purpose, but injectable products are available in which the iron is bound up in a complex with various carbohydrates. Preparations of this type are tolerated fairly well, and are of value in the rapid treatment of severe iron deficiency. As such iron injections by-pass the mechanism that normally controls the degree of iron absorption, the dose must be based on the actual iron deficiency as shown by laboratory tests, otherwise an overdose may be given.

Dextriferron

Dextriferron is a stabilised complex of ferric hydroxide and dextrin (a soluble derivative of starch), prepared for intravenous use, and is largely free from the toxic side-effects associated with earlier intravenous products. It is used when oral iron is unsuitable, or when the iron deficiency is severe and a rapid restoration is necessary. A test dose of 2 ml. is first given to detect any exceptional sensitivity, and if tolerated, daily doses of 5 ml. (100 mg. iron) may be given by slow intravenous injection. The total dose is based upon the degree of haemoglobin deficiency.

Extravascular injection may cause an inflammatory local reaction. *Brand name :* Astrafer I.V.

Iron-Dextran

Dextran is a carbohydrate used as a blood-plasma substitute in the treatment of shock, but it is also employed as an iron-dextran complex to make a solution suitable for intramuscular injection. The total dose, like that of the intravenous iron injections, is based on the degree of iron deficiency. The solution is given in doses of 5 ml., equivalent to 250 mg. of iron, at daily or longer intervals until the full calculated dose has been injected. It must be given by deep intramuscular injection, as more superficial injections are absorbed less completely and may discolour the skin. An alternative scheme of treatment is referred to as T.D.I. (total dose infusion). By this method the total dose of iron required (calculated from the haemoglobin level and the weight of the patient), is added aseptically to 500 to 1000 ml. of 5 per cent. dextrose or normal saline, and given by slow intravenous drip infusion over a period of four to six hours. This method has advantages, but the patient should be kept under constant observation, as occasional general reactions have occurred. *Brand name :* Imferon.

A related product also suitable for intramuscular use is Iron Sorbitol Injection. Sorbitol is a sugar-like substance, and the injection contains a stabilised solution of an iron-sorbitol-critic acid complex. The product contains the equivalent of 50 mg. of iron per ml., and is absorbed much more rapidly than the iron-dextran complex. *Brand name :* Jectofer.

ANAEMIAS NOT DUE TO IRON DEFICIENCY

Anaemia may occur in some people on a full diet even in the absence of any significant blood loss, and the lack of response to iron or other forms of treatment led to the term ' pernicious anaemia.' In this condition the number of erythrocytes is reduced, and they are of abnormal size and shape. In 1926 it was discovered that raw liver could alleviate the symptoms of pernicious anaemia, later a liquid extract of liver was developed, and eventually refined extracts suitable for injection were introduced.

The discovery of the value of liver extract was a great advance at the time, but it is now known that a number of factors are concerned with the production of mature red cells by the bone marrow. One of these factors is cyanocobalamin, or vitamin B_{12}, which is present in milk, eggs and meat, and is also formed by some of the intestinal bacteria. Pernicious anaemia can be relieved by injections of cyanocobalamin, so that basically the disease is due to an inability to absorb dietary vitamin B_{12}. The vitamin is also referred to as the extrinsic factor, as another substance, produced by the stomach, and termed the intrinsic factor, is necessary for its absorption. The nature of this intrinsic factor is not known, but it appears to be a mucoprotein. When both the intrinsic and extrinsic factors are present the vitamin is absorbed, stored in the liver, and released as required for blood formation. The process can be summarised thus :

Dietary vitamin B_{12} + stomach factor
$\downarrow$
vitamin absorbed from intestines
$\downarrow$
stored in the liver
$\downarrow$
released to enter bone marrow
$\downarrow$
erythrocytes formed
$\downarrow$
released into circulation.

A deficiency of cyanocobalamin not only causes a megaloblastic anaemia, but may also bring about a degeneration of the spinal cord and peripheral nerves (combined subacute degeneration). This neurological involvement can also be relieved by vitamin B_{12}.

Cyanocobalamin (dose, 250 to 2000 micrograms)

Cyanocobalamin was originally extracted from liver, but is now obtained as a by-product of the fermentation process used for aureomycin and streptomycin extraction. It has a specific effect in the treatment of pernicious anaemia. Initial doses of 1 to 2 mg., followed by doses of 250 micrograms once or twice weekly by intramuscular injection, bring about a rapid improvement in the blood picture, but long treatment is required if the disease has caused any damage to the spinal cord. Oral treatment is unreliable as absorption is poor and erratic.

Much larger initial doses are sometimes given in order to build up the reserves in the liver, and very large doses have been used in neuroblastoma in children.

Cyanocobalamin is also given in large doses in the treatment of trigeminal neuralgia, polyneuritis and related conditions. The drug is occasionally used as a dietary supplement in malabsorption conditions such as coeliac disease. Hydroxocobalamin (Neo-Cytamen) is a closely related compound that is excreted more slowly, and has a correspondingly longer action. *Brand names :* Cobalin, Cytamen, Cytacon.

Stomach Extracts

Desiccated stomach tissue contains the intrinsic factor already referred to, as well as some vitamin B_{12} and has been used in pernicious anaemia as an oral product. Concentrates of stomach extracts are also available, but the response to these products may be variable. *Brand names :* Bifacton, Biopar.

Liver Extracts

Extracts of liver suitable for injection are survivors from the early days of liver therapy, but they are still used occasionally in the treatment of pernicious anaemia although they are now standardised on the amount of cyanocobalamin that they contain.

These extracts are given by intramuscular injection in doses of 1 to 5 ml., in amounts and at intervals determined by need and response. They occasionally cause allergic reactions in sensitive patients, and as a rule injections of cyanocobalamin are preferred. *Brand names :* Anahaemin, Hepacon.

Folic Acid (dose, 5 to 20 mg. daily)

Folic acid is regarded as a member of the vitamin B complex, and is one of the many factors concerned in blood formation. Deficiency of folic acid may lead to a megaloblastic anaemia, and the administration of folic acid is of value in dietary deficiency anaemias, and is exceptionally useful in some disturbances of fat metabolism such as tropical sprue.

The prophylactic use of folic acid in the megaloblastic anaemia that may occur in pregnancy is referred to on page 156. Folic acid was used at one time in the treatment of pernicious anaemia, as it can restore the blood picture to normal, but unfortunately it does not prevent or reverse associated neurological damage. The use of folic acid alone in pernicious anaemia is therefore dangerous, and has now been abandoned.

CHAPTER X

DRUGS ACTING ON THE GASTRO-INTESTINAL TRACT

GASTRO-INTESTINAL disturbance of some kind afflicts most people at times from the cradle to the grave, and the variety of these disturbances is matched by the variety of preparations available. These preparations vary widely in nature and pharmacological properties, and will be considered under the headings of antacids, spasmolytics, carminatives, bitters, anti-emetics, sedatives, adsorbents and laxatives.

ANTACIDS

Antacids are widely employed to partially neutralise gastric acid in the treatment of peptic ulcer. Both hydrochloric acid and pepsin are formed and liberated in the stomach to aid the breakdown and digestion of food, and in health the protective mucosa of the stomach effectually prevents any autodigestion. Sometimes this protective mechanism breaks down, and an erosion occurs which may develop into an ulcer. The reason for this breakdown is unknown, but both acid and pepsin are concerned, as ulcers occur only in those areas in contact with the gastric juices.

Ulcer patients may secrete more than the normal amount of pepsin, but in the absence of hydrochloric acid, as in achlorhydria, ulcers do not occur. Experimental evidence suggests that a decrease in the resistance to the action of hydrochloric acid is the main cause of peptic ulcer, but many other factors, such as sex, age, diet, occupation and smoking also play a significant part in ulcer formation.

When an ulcer is formed the acid normally present in the stomach causes pain and spasm, and such spasm inhibits healing. Many substances have been used to neutralise the gastric acid in such conditions and thus promote the repair of damaged tissues and the wide choice available indicates that the ideal antacid still awaits discovery. A compound is required that will reduce the level of gastric acid without neutralising it completely, will have a prolonged action, but will not have any significant systemic or local side-effects.

A drug that neutralises gastric acid completely may lead to a compensatory oversecretion of more acid, with a consequent increase in pain and spasm. Absorption of the antacid may disturb the acid-base balance of the body and cause alkalosis, and local effects may cause constipation or diarrhoea. For these reasons mixtures of antacids are often used, and the proportions of each constituent can be adjusted to suit the individual patient. The following products are in general use as antacids :—

Aluminium Hydroxide Mixture (dose, 4 to 8 ml.)

This product, also known as aluminium hydroxide gel, has valuable antacid properties. Like magnesium trisilicate (*q.v.*) it reduces the degree of acidity to a point at which attack on the inflamed stomach wall is minimal, and as it is slow acting it affords a considerable degree of protection.

It is not absorbed and so cannot cause alkalosis, and frequent administration in the acute stages of peptic ulcer is possible without many side-effects. The gel, after dilution with water, is sometimes given by intragastric drip and the extended action thus obtained may give prolonged relief. Several tablet products with a long action are also available. Thus Gastrils contain an aluminium hydroxide-magnesium carbonate complex incorporated in a slow-dissolving pastille base. Neutrolactis and Nulacin tablets contain antacids and milk solids, and are intended to be sucked slowly at frequent intervals and thus provide the equivalent of a prolonged and continuous effect.

A large number of proprietary products are available containing standard or newer antacids, but all have a basically similar pharmacological action. In some, the antacid action is augmented by the use of auxiliary drugs to reduce spasm and inhibit the secretion of gastric acid and the value of these products depends largely on individual need and response.

Calcium Carbonate (dose, 1 to 5 G.)

Chalk is natural calcium carbonate, and has a useful and extended antacid action. It is often used in association with magnesium carbonate as in Magnesium Carbonate Compound Powder B.P.C., for its antacid effects, but unlike most other antacids, it has a constipating effect. That action makes chalk a useful drug for diarrhoea, especially in association with opium as in Chalk and Opium Mixture B.P.C.

Magnesium Carbonate (dose, 250 to 500 mg.)

Magnesium carbonate is insoluble in water, and therefore has a much longer action than sodium bicarbonate.   It is not absorbed and so does not cause alkalosis, but like other magnesium compounds, *i.e.* Epsom salts (*q.v.*), it may have laxative effects if large doses are given.   This can be minimised by formulation with other antacids, as in Calcium Carbonate Compound Powder B.P.C.   Magnesium hydroxide (cream of magnesia) has similar antacid properties, but does not cause any release of carbon dioxide, but it also has a laxative action that may be undesirable.

Magnesium Trisilicate (dose, 0·5 to 2 G.)

Magnesium trisilicate is an insoluble powder with a slow and prolonged antacid action.   It is widely used in the treatment of peptic ulcer, as the interaction with gastric acid results in the formation of a hydrated silica gel, which has a valuable protective action.   The neutralisation of acid is not complete, so there is no danger of alkalosis or rebound formation of acid, and magnesium trisilicate is one of the most useful antacids available. During the neutralisation of acid some magnesium chloride is formed, which has a laxative action, and in large doses magnesium trisilicate alone may cause some diarrhoea.   Magnesium Trisilicate Compound Powder B.P.C. is a useful alternative.

Sodium Bicarbonate (dose, 1 to 4 G.)

Sodium bicarbonate is soluble in water and neutralises gastric acid very quickly, with the evolution of carbon dioxide.   Continued use may lead to alkalosis and rebound acid formation, and it is therefore seldom given alone except for the immediate relief of gastric pain.   For such occasional use sodium bicarbonate is invaluable.   The carbon dioxide liberated in the stomach by the reaction of gastric acid with the sodium bicarbonate may also relieve distension as the gas is eructed, and such eructation is useful as a proof to the patient of the efficacy of the antacid.

Carbenoxolone (dose, 50 to 100 mg.)

Carbenoxolone represents a quite different approach to the treatment of peptic ulcer.   It is a derivative of an acid present in liquorice root, and has anti-inflammatory properties similar in some respects to those of the corticosteroids.   When given orally in doses of 50 to 100 mg. three times a day, carbenoxolone appears to have a stimulating action on the ulcer, and healing, associated with an increased protection by mucus, normally occurs in about four weeks. Salt and water retention may occur in a few patients. The drug is also used in the treatment of duodenal ulcer, and is then given in a special capsule, designed to release the contents in the duodenum at the site of the ulcer. *Brand names :* Biogastrone, Duogastrone.

SPASMOLYTICS

The pain of peptic ulcer is due not only to the action of the gastric acid on the ulcerated areas but also to spasm and hypermotility of the stomach. Atropine or belladonna, or synthetic equivalents, are often added to antacid preparations to reduce such spasm, and the reduction of gastric motility thus brought about not only relieves pain but extends the action of the antacid by delaying the emptying of the stomach. The side-effects of atropine, such as dryness of the mouth, limit its value, and many synthetic compounds, claimed to have a more selective action on the gastric mucosa and fewer side-effects, are available. Brief reference to these synthetic atropine-like compounds with a spasmolytic action is on page 79.

CARMINATIVES

Carminatives are examples of older therapy, and are drugs which relieve gastric distension by promoting the elimination of gas by belching. They also produce a feeling of warmth in the stomach. The drugs used for this purpose include oil of peppermint, tincture of ginger and compound tincture of cardamom. They may be given together with small doses of sodium bicarbonate as a mixture, and although now prescribed less often, they have a useful if limited place in the treatment of flatulence and dyspepsia.

BITTERS

Bitters are substances which by virtue of their taste produce a reflex secretion of gastric juice, and thus stimulate the appetite. They therefore have some value in debility and convalescence. The most commonly used bitter is gentian root, used as Gentian and Alkali Mixture B.P.C., B.N.F. Nux vomica, from which strychnine is obtained, also has an intensely bitter taste and is sometimes given with gentian as Nux Vomica and Alkali Mixture B.P.C., B.N.F.

All bitters should be given a short time before meals to obtain the maximum response.

ANTI-EMETICS

The function of vomiting is that of removing unwanted contents from the stomach, but the act is governed by a complex nervous system associated with the vomiting centre of the reticular formation of the brain. Stimulation of this centre causes vomiting, but the process may be initiated reflexly by impulses arising from almost any part of the gastro-intestinal tract, or from the urinary system, or may arise from shock or injury. Thus vomiting does not necessarily serve a useful purpose. Post-operative recovery may be hindered by vomiting, and the consequent loss of electrolytes may bring about serious metabolic disturbances. In view of the complex nature of the vomiting process, it is not surprising that an anti-emetic action is found in a wide variety of substances, many of which have some degree of central depressant activity. Hyoscine (q.v.) is a constituent of many travel-sickness remedies, but the ideal drug has yet to be found, as no substance is known that has a specific effect on the vomiting centre. Reliance has to be placed on drugs which act at some other point of the system, and many of the phenothiazine-derived tranquillisers have a powerful anti-emetic action. Chlorpromazine (Largactil), thiethylperazine (Torecan) and trifluoperazine (Stelazine) are representative compounds, and are of value in the nausea and vomiting due to surgery, X-ray therapy, and vomiting induced by drugs such as mustine (q.v.) Certain antihistamines such as cyclizine (Valoid) and dimenhydrinate (Dramamine) are also useful as anti-emetics. Pyridoxine, one of the vitamins of the B group, also has anti-emetic properties, and is present in several proprietary anti-nauseants.

Metoclopramide (Maxolon) differs from other anti-emetics by its multiple action. It not only has a central effect by depressing the vomiting centre (or raising the threshold of activity), but it also reduces the sensitivity of nerves linking that centre with sensitive areas in the pylorus and duodenum. Metoclopramide

also has a marked effect in increasing the motility of the hypo-
motile stomach, and the full anti-emetic response is the result of
the operation of several factors. The drug is given in doses of
10 mg., and is useful in a wide range of conditions associated with
nausea and vomiting, including gastritis, alcoholism, heart failure,
uraemia and malignancy. The stimulating effects of metoclopramide on the gastro-intestinal tract are also useful in facilitating
barium meal examinations.

A number of anti-emetic compounds have been used in the
treatment of vomiting in pregnancy, but some apparently safe
drugs are not without danger, and ideally, no drug should be
given during the first months of pregnancy unless such treatment
is essential, and due regard is paid to the possible effects on the
feotus.

ADSORBENTS

Certain substances have the power of adsorbing gases and toxic
substances, and a few have medicinal applications.

Kaolin (dose, 15 to 60 G.)

Kaolin, or china clay, is a purified silicate of aluminium. It
is used in the treatment of food poisoning, enteritis, dysentery
and diarrhoea. Mixture of Kaolin and Morphine B.P.C., B.N.F.
is widely employed in the treatment of mild gastro-intestinal
disturbances as the kaolin absorbs any toxins, and the morphine
constituent reduces gastro-intestinal motility.

Charcoal (dose, 4 to 8 G.)

Activated charcoal has adsorbent properties similar to those of
kaolin, and is sometimes used in the treatment of flatulence and
distension, and in poisoning by alkaloids and related drugs.

INTESTINAL SEDATIVES

Intestinal sedatives can be described as drugs which reduce
peristalsis and relieve diarrhoea and spasm. These include
astringents containing tannin, exemplified by the vegetable
substance catechu, and adsorbents such as chalk and kaolin.
Peristaltic movements are also reduced by morphine and opium,

and Chalk and Opium Mixture B.P.C., B.N.F. and Kaolin and Morphine Mixture B.P.C., B.N.F. are typical preparations for the symptomatic treatment of diarrhoea. Any associated spasm can be relieved by the addition of a suitable dose of atropine or tincture of belladonna, or by one of the synthetic spasmolytics referred to on page 79. Lomotil contains diphenoxylate with a small dose of atropine, and is useful in both acute and chronic diarrhoea.

LAXATIVES

Sometimes termed aperients, laxatives are substances which stimulate peristalsis, promote evacuation and relieve constipation. At one time they were used extensively regardless of real need, but their use has declined, presumably because they are now employed on a more rational basis. The more powerful laxatives are known as purgatives, and drastic purgatives are termed cathartics. The following groups may be distinguished :

SALINE LAXATIVES

Substances such as the well-known magnesium sulphate (Epsom salts) and sodium sulphate (Glauber's salt) are not absorbed when given orally, and in the intestines they prevent the absorption of water, thus increasing the bulk and fluidity of the faeces. They are given in doses of 2 to 16 G., well diluted, on an empty stomach, when the action is rapid and effective. Magnesium Sulphate Mixture B.P.C., B.N.F., or ' white mixture ', is a once-popular preparation containing magnesium sulphate and carbonate. Seidlitz powder is another saline laxative that once enjoyed considerable popularity. A dose is supplied in two packets, a blue packet containing sodium potassium tartrate and sodium bicarbonate, and a white packet containing tartaric acid. The contents of the blue packet are first dissolved in water, the contents of the white packet are added, and the mixture is taken whilst it is effervescing.

VEGETABLE LAXATIVES

These drugs cause a mild irritation of the intestines and increase the rate of peristalsis. They are slow in action and are best taken at night. They are used less extensively than in the past, but still have a limited place in therapeutics.

Cascara

Cascara bark is a useful purgative that has a mild slow action that results in the passage of a soft stool. It is available as a liquid extract (dose, 2 to 5 ml.), but owing to the bitter taste, elixir of cascara (dose, 2 to 5 ml.), or tablets of the dry extract (125 mg.) are now preferred.

Senna (dose, 0·5 to 2 G.)

Both the leaves and the seed pods of senna have laxative properties, and have long been used domestically as ' senna tea.' Senna is very effective but may cause some griping, and the once widely used black draught (Compound Senna Mixture) contained carminatives as well as magnesium sulphate.

Senokot and Pursennid are proprietary products containing senna extracts, which are more consistent in action and better tolerated.

Rhubarb (dose, 0·2 to 1 G.)

Chinese rhubarb root was once widely used as a purgative, and is occasionally prescribed as Rhubarb Compound Mixture B.P.C., B.N.F.

Castor Oil (dose, 4 to 16 ml.)

The oil expressed from castor seeds contains a derivative of ricinoleic acid, and following oral administration it is split up in the intestine like other fats, by the enzyme lipase. The liberated ricinoleic acid has a stimulant action on the small intestine, and castor oil is a useful purgative in diarrhoea and food poisoning. The action, though powerful, is self-limiting, as evacuation is followed by a quiescent period and subsequent constipation.

Cathartics

The drastic purgatives are represented by vegetable drugs such as aloes, colocynth and jalap, but are now rarely used. Pill of Colocynth and Hyoscaymus is one of the few surviving preparations.

SYNTHETIC LAXATIVES

Phenolphthalein (dose, 50 to 300 mg.)

A white insoluble powder with a mild irritant action on the intestines, and of value in habitual constipation. Some of the drug is absorbed, and excreted later in the bile, so that the action may extend over two or three days. Phenolphthalein is well tolerated, but may cause a rash in a few susceptible patients. It is often given in association with emulsion of liquid paraffin, and is the active constituent of various chocolate laxatives.

Bisacodyl (dose, 5 to 10 mg.)

Bisacodyl is not absorbed when given orally but has a stimulant action on the walls of the colon. It is sometimes described as a contact laxative, and is useful not only as a general laxative, but also to secure evacuation of the colon before X-ray examination. Tablets containing 5 mg. and suppositories of 10 mg. are available. *Brand name:* Dulcolax.

Dorbanex

This product is representative of those preparations containing a laxative and a faecal softening agent. It contains danthron and poloxalkol. The former is a systemic laxative, but appears to promote peristalsis by a selective stimulant action on the large intestine. Poloxalkol is a surface-active agent, increasing the penetration of water, thus promoting faecal softening.

Lactulose (dose, 50 per cent. solution, 15 to 50 ml.)

Lactulose is an artificial sugar based on a combination of fructose and galactose. Sugars are normally metabolised by specific enzymes, but as there is no enzyme in the gut capable of metabolising lactulose, it reaches the colon unchanged. It is then rapidly broken down by sugar-splitting bacteria in the colon to lactic and other organic acids, and this change promotes the formation of a softer stool. Lactulose thus relieves constipation and assists in a return to a normal bowel action. The drug may also be of value in hepatic coma by limiting the formation of nitrogenous breakdown products in the intestinal tract by proteolytic bacteria. These breakdown products such as ammonia are normally converted in the liver to urea, a process that may be impaired when liver damage has occurred. *Brand name :* Duphalac.

BULK AND LUBRICANT LAXATIVES

Bulk laxatives are vegetable substances of a mucilaginous nature that are not digested, but excreted unchanged. During this process they absorb water and increase the bulk of the faeces, and so act as mechanical laxatives. They are therefore useful in the treatment of constipation where the faeces are dry and hard.

Typical products are ispaghula and psyllium seeds (dose, 4 to 16 G.) and mucilaginous products from various plants form the basis of proprietary bulk laxatives such as Isogel and Normacol.

Liquid Paraffin (dose, 8 to 30 ml.)

A mineral oil that passes through the alimentary tract unchanged, and therefore acts as a simple lubricant laxative. It is particularly valuable in producing a soft stool after intestinal and rectal operations or in cases of haemorrhoids. Liquid paraffin may be given as such, or as emulsion of liquid paraffin, to which phenolphthalein (*q.v.*) is sometimes added. The oil-soluble vitamins of the diet may dissolve in liquid paraffin, and its extended use as a laxative may cause some vitamin deficiency. Some absorption of the oil may occur after prolonged use, and paraffinomas may develop, and extensive self-medication should be discouraged.

CHAPTER XI

EXPECTORANTS AND EMETICS

EXPECTORANTS

EXPECTORANTS are drugs which increase the amount and reduce the viscosity of bronchial secretion. This increase in the amount of sputum stimulates the cough centre by a reflex action, and thus helps to clear the bronchial tract by the act of coughing. A reduction in the viscosity of tenacious sputum is also a considerable help in the treatment of the symptoms of respiratory disease. Expectorants represent one of the older aspects of therapeutics, but in recent years their effectiveness and value have been questioned. In spite of this, expectorants are still widely prescribed, and the following drugs are in use :—

Ipecacuanha (dose, 25 to 125 mg.)

The root of a South American plant, introduced into European medicine as a constituent of Dover's powder (*q.v.*).

The principal active constituent is the alkaloid emetine, which in small doses is thought to increase bronchial secretion and preparations of ipecacuanha are widely used in the treatment of bronchitis, and for cough where the sputum is tough and scanty. Larger doses of ipecacuanha have an irritant effect on the gastric mucosa, and cause vomiting. Ipecacuanha is often used in association with alkalis such as ammonium bicarbonate, which are also said to liquefy bronchial secretions and Ammonia and Ipecacuanha Mixture (B.P.C., B.N.F.) is a familiar expectorant cough mixture containing these traditional drugs.

Potassium Iodide (dose, 0·3 to 2 G.)

Iodides such as potassium iodide are rapidly absorbed when given orally, and are partially excreted in the saliva and bronchial secretions. The amount and fluidity of the secretions is increased, and iodides are therefore given for that purpose with other expectorants in cough mixtures and in preparations for the treatment of bronchitis and asthma.

Bromhexine (dose, 8 to 16 mg.)

One of the symptoms of bronchitis is the increased production of thick sputum, and some of the older expectorants are not very effective in loosening and liquefying such sputum. The viscosity of sputum is associated with the formation of polysaccharide fibres, and bromhexine inhibits the formation of these fibres, and thus has an indirect action of liquefying sputum. The volume of sputum may increase during bromhexine treatment, but the more liquid and frothy nature of the sputum makes expectoration correspondingly easier. When the sputum is purulent, combined use of an antibiotic to control the infection may be necessary to obtain the full response. *Brand name :* Bisolvon.

Benzoin

Gum benzoin is a natural balsamic resin and is the main constituent of that time-honoured remedy known as Friars' Balsam which is still widely used as an inhalation for the treatment of bronchitis. The standard method of use is to add one teaspoonful of the tincture to a pint of hot water, and inhale the vapour that is given off, which contains the volatile ingredients of the balsam. Menthol is occasionally added to increase the effect.

Other natural expectorant drugs are senega and squills, but are now used less frequently.

Substances which reduce cough by a sedative action on the cough centre such as codeine and pholcodine, are not expectorants, and are discussed briefly on page 56.

A more recent development in expectorant therapy is the administration of certain drugs as aerosols. Aerosols are sprays of exceptionally fine drops, and the particle size is so small that the drug or solution is carried deeply into the lungs when inhaled, and not trapped in the upper respiratory tract.

Drugs used in this way to reduce the viscosity of sputum include acetylcysteine (Airbron) and Ascoxal. Airbron both increases the volume and decreases the viscosity of bronchial mucus, and is useful during anaesthesia and in broncho-pulmonary conditions. Ascoxal contains copper sulphate, sodium percarbonate and ascorbic acid, and also has mucolytic properties. It should be noted that some bronchodilator drugs such as isoprenaline (*q.v.*) can also be given as aerosols.

EMETICS

Most expectorants have an irritant effect on the gastric mucosa, and in full doses have an emetic action. They are therefore used occasionally in the treatment of poisoning. Tincture of ipecacuanha (emetic dose, 5 to 20 ml.) is a suitable preparation. A solution of common salt is also a useful and readily available emetic for emergency use. Emetics should not be used in poisoning by caustic substances, as if the stomach has been damaged by the caustic, the action of vomiting may increase the injury.

Apomorphine † is a centrally acting emetic, and following the subcutaneous injection of 2 to 8 mg., emesis occurs within a few minutes. Solutions of apomorphine do not keep well, and any injection solution that develops a green or yellow colour should be discarded. The drug, as its name implies, is derived from morphine, and although it has a stimulant action on the vomiting centre, it also has the depressant properties of the parent drug. Care is necessary when considering the use of apomorphine in poisoning from barbiturates or other sedative drugs.

CHAPTER XII

HORMONES AND THE ENDOCRINE SYSTEM

HORMONES are chemical substances released into the blood stream by the endocrine glands. These glands, sometimes referred to as ductless glands, are small pockets of highly specialised tissues situated in various parts of the body, and they play a fundamental part in growth and development and in the maintenance of the health of the body.

The hormones of the endocrine system are released according to physiological needs, but the hormones of one gland may influence the activity of another, others may be affected by impulses from the central nervous system, and the whole mechanism of production and release of hormones is so complex that the final response is due to the interaction of many factors. A number of these hormones have now been extracted from the glands concerned and much of their chemistry is known. Adrenaline and insulin are familiar examples of hormones used therapeutically, and in some cases it has been possible to make hormones synthetically, and even to devise compounds more powerful and selective in action than the natural hormones. These advances in biological chemistry have led to a wider understanding of the action and importance of hormones, and their value, and limitations, as therapeutic agents.

THE PITUITARY GLAND

The pituitary is a small gland about the size of a pea, situated in the base of the skull. It consists of two parts, the anterior and posterior lobes, and exerts an influence on the body out of all proportion to its size. It secretes a number of hormones which affect other endocrine glands as well as various physiological processes, and the relationship between the pituitary gland and the hormones which it ultimately controls is indicated in the following diagram.

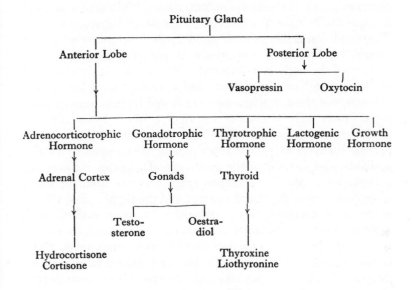

Posterior Lobe

This part of the pituitary gland secretes two hormones, vasopressin and oxytocin. An extract containing both hormones was once used therapeutically for its action on the blood pressure and to initiate uterine contractions. Posterior lobe preparations are still occasionally used, mainly by insufflation, in the control of polyuria of diabetes insipidus. *Brand names :* Di-sipidin,† Piton,† Pituitrin.†

Vasopressin Injection † (dose, 0·25 to 0·75 ml.)

Vasopressin has both pressor and antidiuretic properties, and following subcutaneous or intramuscular injection it causes a rise in blood pressure by a constrictor action on the smaller blood vessels. Although once used as a pressor agent it has now been replaced for that purpose by more reliable drugs. Vasopressin is of considerable physiological importance because of its powerful influence on the water balance of the body. It increases the reabsorption of water by the kidneys when the intake of water is low, and thus conserves the balance by reducing the amount of urine, whereas with a high intake the absorption of water is decreased, and the urinary output rises. This action is used therapeutically in the treatment and diagnosis of diabetes insipidus. That condition is due to some pituitary dysfunction by which the normal production of vasopressin is reduced, and the water-balance of the body is distributed. The disease is characterised by thirst, a high output of urine, and a corresponding high intake of water, but the symptoms can be relieved by injections of vaso-pressin twice daily in doses of 0·25 to 0·75 ml., or by injections of the longer-acting vasopressin tannate. A synthetic form of vaso-pressin referred to as lysinevasopressin (Syntopressin) is also available, and is used in the treatment of diabetes insipidus as a nasal spray. As it is a synthetic drug, it is free from the traces of protein present in natural extracts, and the slight risk of allergic reactions is correspondingly reduced. In some patients with diabetes insipidus, adequate control may be obtained by inhala-tions of dried extracts of the posterior lobe as pituitary snuff. Side-effects are unlikely to occur with the small doses used in diabetes insipidus, but larger doses may cause coronary artery constriction. *Brand names :* Pitressin,† Pitressin Tannate.†

Oxytocin Injection (dose, 2 to 5 units)

Oxytocin has a selective stimulating action on uterine muscle, but it has no pressor or antidiuretic properties. The degree of activity is related to the physiological state of the uterus, and is greatest during the later stages of pregnancy. In practice oxytocin is used mainly in uterine inertia and for the induction of labour, but its use in that way is not without risk unless the cervix is already fully dilated. If given by intravenous drip infusion in dextrose solution, the rapid response permits a more exact control of dose, and reduces the risk of uterine rupture or foetal asphyxia. Oxytocin is also used to control post-partum haemorrhage, often in association with the longer-acting ergometrine (*q.v.*) as Synto-metrine.†

Oxytocin may also be given orally as specially prepared buccal tablets. If these tablets are placed in the buccal space adjacent to the upper molar teeth, absorption of the oxytocin is rapid but controllable, as the effect on the uterus wanes quickly if the tablet is removed. Oxytocin also influences the mammary gland, and is used as Syntocinon spray to facilitate breast-feeding by stimulating

the so-called milk ' let-down ' response. *Brand names :* Pitocin,†
Pitocin Buccal,† Syntocinon.†

Ergot

Ergot is not a hormone, and is considered here solely because
it has a powerful action on the uterus similar to that of oxytocin.
Ergot is a fungus that develops in the ear of rye and occasionally
other cereals. Instead of the normal grains, dark-coloured
tapering cylindrical bodies about ½ to 1 in. long are produced,
which contain the toxic substances ergometrine and ergotamine.
Flour made from infected rye can cause severe ergot poisoning,
and epidemics due to such flour frequently occurred in the past
and are not unknown even to-day. Such ergot poisoning, or
ergotism, once known as ' St Anthony's fire,' is characterised by
agonising pain in the extremities, followed by gangrene, or less
commonly by epileptiform convulsions.

The therapeutic use of ergot is due to its powerful action on
the smooth muscle of the uterus, and it is widely employed as
ergometrine in the treatment of post-partum haemorrhage.

Ergometrine Maleate (dose, 0·5 to 1 mg. orally, 0·1 to 1 mg. by injection)

Ergometrine is the principal alkaloid of ergot, and is the
substance to which the oxytocic effects of ergot are due. It has
a specific and powerful action on the uterus, and uterine contractions commence a few minutes after the oral administration
of the drug. For a more rapid effect ergometrine may be given in
doses of 0·2 to 1 mg. by intramuscular injection, or 0·1 to 0·5 mg.
by intravenous injection. The main use of ergometrine is in the
control of post-partum haemorrhage, which is achieved by the
action of the drug in contracting the venous sinuses from which
the haemorrhage occurs. Owing to its powerful contractile
effects, ergometrine is usually given after the expulsion of the
placenta. It should not be given any earlier, as the uterine
contractions then produced may reduce placental circulation, and
cause foetal distress or may cause rupture of the uterus. Oxytocin
has a more rapid but less sustained action than ergometrine, but
the two drugs may be given together when a prompt but sustained
response is required. Syntometrine is formulated on that basis,
and contains synthetic oxytocin and ergometrine.

Anterior Lobe

The anterior lobe of the pituitary gland is one of the most important glands of the body. It secretes at least six hormones, including the adrenocorticotrophic (*q.v.*), the gonadotrophic (*q.v.*), the thyrotrophic (*q.v.*), the lactogenic (*q.v.*) and the growth hormone (*q.v.*). Some are used therapeutically, others in diagnosis, but as they are protein in nature they are not effective orally, and must be given by injection. With a few exceptions their therapeutic use is disappointing. Their action is basically that of stimulating the related endocrine gland, *i.e.* the thyrotrophic hormone controls the activity of the thyroid gland, and in therapy the use of the hormones of the glands concerned is preferred, the exception being the adrenocorticotrophic hormone.

Corticotrophin †

Also known as adrenocorticotrophic hormone and ACTH, this hormone is obtained from the pituitary glands of sheep and other animals. It has a direct action on the cortex of the adrenal gland, and stimulates the production of hydrocortisone and cortisone. The final action of the hormone is therefore that of hydrocortisone, and direct treatment with that drug or related steroids is usually preferred. In severe asthma, however, corticotrophin is often more effective than cortisone, and occasionally better results are obtained in other conditions. It will be appreciated that corticotrophin exerts its effects through the medium of the adrenal gland, and in health there is a balance between the activity of the gland and the level of corticosteroids in circulation. When the adrenal cortex is damaged, as in Addison's disease, or when the gland has been removed surgically, corticotrophin is of no value.

The drug is inactive orally as it is destroyed in the stomach and so must be given by injection. The method that evokes the maximal response is the slow intravenous infusion of doses of 15 to 20 units over six to twenty-four hours, although doses of 45 to 90 units are sometimes given. In practice, intramuscular injections, though less effective, are more convenient and standard doses range from 10 to 80 units. The intramuscular injection has an action lasting four to six hours, but longer acting preparations are also available. In these products the hormone is combined with zinc, or carboxymethylcellulose, or mixed with gelatin, and after injection the hormone is slowly released to give a pro-longed action. In some cases a single daily dose may be sufficient.

Corticotrophin is of chief value in status asthmaticus, when it may be effective, and indeed life-saving, when all other measures have failed. Large initial doses may be necessary, and subsequently decreased slowly over a period of some days. As the drug is palliative, and not curative, the symptoms may recur as the drug is withdrawn. Corticotrophin is also effective in a number of other conditions such as Bell's palsy. It is also used occasionally, as a diagnostic agent in suspected Addison's disease or Cushing's syndrome. *Brand names :* Acthar,† Acthar Gel,† Cortico-gel,† Corticotrophin-cmc,† Cortrophin,† Cortrophin-ZN.†

Tetracosactrin †

The corticotrophic hormone contains many amino acids, not all of which take part in ACTH-activity. Some of these unwanted amino acids cause the occasional allergic reactions to corticotro-phin, but the biologically active fragment of ACTH (tetracosac-trin), has been synthesised, and is free from the disadvantages of natural hormone. Tetracosactrin is used when a prompt and reliable ACTH-action is required, as in status asthmaticus and anaphylactic shock, and for such purposes is best given intra-venously in doses of 0·25 mg., equivalent to about 25 units. When a slower but more prolonged action is required, the drug may be given by intramuscular injection as a tetracosactrin-zinc phos-phate complex, 1 mg. producing an effect comparable to that of 80 units ACTH gel, but of longer duration. *Brand names :* Synacthen,† Synacthen Depot.†

Adrenal Cortex

Following stimulation by corticotrophin, the cortex of the adrenal gland produces a number of hormones of very great physiological importance. Chemically they have a complex four-ring or steroid structure (which is also found in cholesterol, calciferol, the sex hormones and the glycosides of digitalis). These corticosteroid hormones can be divided into two main groups, the glucocorticoid hormones exemplified by hydrocortisone and cortisone, which control carbohydrate and protein metabolism, and the mineraloid hormones, represented by aldosterone, which influence the salt and water balance of the body. This distinction is not a sharp one, as the glucocorticoid hormones also influence the electrolyte balance to some extent.

Glucocorticosteroids

Hydrocortisone and cortisone are well-known examples of glucocorticoid hormones, and are closely related as cortisone is converted in the liver to hydrocortisone. These steroids have a number of important actions, and are closely concerned with the metabolism of fats, proteins and carbohydrates. They promote the formation of glycogen by the liver, affect the excretion of salts and water, reduce capillary permeability, have a marked anti-allergic action, increase the resistance of the body to stress and shock, and have the power of suppressing inflammatory processes generally.

They are therefore used in the treatment of a wide range of conditions (apart from those due to adrenal cortical deficiency, *i.e.* Addison's disease) including rheumatoid arthritis, rheumatic fever, allergic reactions, shock and stress, skin and eye inflammatory conditions, and for the treatment of blood disorders such as auto-immune haemolytic anaemia and the various forms of leukaemia.

In inflamed conditions the action of the corticosteroids is both valuable and potentially dangerous, as the symptoms, and not their cause, are suppressed. If the suppressed inflammation is due to bacterial invasion, bacterial growth may continue unchecked during corticosteroid treatment, and is therefore essential to treat any infection at the same time. In other inflammatory conditions the relief of pain and inflammation permits a greater degree of movement, and in rheumatoid conditions their use not only gives relief but aids physiotherapy and rehabilitation.

The glucocorticosteroids influence many other activities of the body to a greater or lesser degree. Thus they inhibit the development of lymphocytes, and are of value in leukaemia and other blood disorders. In leukaemia large doses are given, especially in children, and a high degree of remission of symptoms may result. The corticosteroids cannot prevent an ultimate relapse, but as well as initiating a remission they may restore a sensitivity to other forms of treatment. Cortisone and its analogues are specific in Addison's disease, where treatment is replacement and not stimulant therapy, as in this disease the damaged suprarenal glands are no longer able to produce their own cortisone.

SIDE-EFFECTS.—The mode of action of these drugs is still not clear, and their profound influence on the physiological activities of the body are reflected in the side-effects of treatment. They increase gastric acidity, and may cause or exacerbate peptic ulcer, and the symptoms may be disguised by the anti-inflammatory action of the drugs, leading to delayed diagnosis of the real condition. The salt and water balance of the body is disturbed and muscle wasting, loss of calcium and osteoporosis may occur, especially after long treatment. The retention of normally excreted fluid may lead to oedema and hypertension. Moon-face and other signs of Cushing's syndrome may also occur, due to changes in the deposition of fat.

Potassium loss, causing muscle weakness and cardiac irregularities are other side-effects, and potassium supplements should be given if treatment with corticosteroids is prolonged. Psychotic disturbances may also be noted. With the newer synthetic steroids some of these side-effects have been reduced.

It will be appreciated that the administration of these glucocorticosteroids will depress their normal production by the adrenal cortex. Following treatment it is therefore usual to reduce the dose gradually, thus permitting the natural production of the hormones to rise again to the normal level. The potency of the corticosteroids is such that they should be used with great care, and patients should be warned of the potential dangers. They should carry a card stating that they are receiving the drugs, so that in cases of emergency, treatment can be adapted to the patient concerned.

Cortisone (dose, 10 to 400 mg. daily)

It had been known for some years that a remission of the symptoms of rheumatoid arthritis could occur during pregnancy, and when this effect was traced to an increased production of steroid hormones, cortisone was developed as a new and powerful therapeutic agent. It has been used extensively in the treatment of rheumatoid conditions, and in leukaemia, but wider experience revealed the limitations as well as the value of steroid therapy. In rheumatoid conditions the action is merely suppressive, and relapse may occur when treatment is stopped. The marked electrolyte and metabolic disturbances that follow cortisone treatment also limit its prolonged use. Except in Addison's disease, where the salt-retaining action of cortisone is an advantage, other corticosteroids with fewer side-effects are now preferred. Very large doses have been used to induce a remission in leukaemia. *Brand names :* Adreson,† Cortelan,† Cortisyl.†

Hydrocortisone † (dose, 12·5 to 400 mg. daily)

Hydrocortisone is considered to be the main glucocorticosteroid hormone of the adrenal gland. It differs from cortisone mainly in being effective when applied locally, and is widely used in creams, ointments and lotions in many inflamed and itching skin conditions such as pruritus, eczematous dermatitis and otitis externa. Many of these local preparations contain an antibiotic such as neomycin to control or prevent any associated infection, as hydrocortisone has no antibacterial properties.

When injected locally, hydrocortisone has a more powerful anti-inflammatory action than cortisone, and as its activity is largely limited to the injected area, the general metabolic effects of the drug are rarely observed. Conversely the intense local action is of value in rheumatoid conditions, bursitis, and other conditions requiring local therapy.

In the treatment of acute adrenal insufficiency, during adrenalectomy, and in the crises of Addison's disease a very rapid action is required, and a water-soluble form of hydrocortisone (hydrocortisone sodium succinate or phosphate) is available for intravenous use. Hydrocortisone given intravenously is also of immense value in the treatment of severe shock. Pressor drugs are often used to restore low blood pressure due to shock, but in cases of severe blood loss the restoration of blood volume by plasma or other fluids is necessary if pressor drugs are to achieve their effect. Occasionally these measures fail to restore the blood pressure and in such circumstances the intravenous injection of 100 mg. of hydrocortisone or a related steroid may be life-saving. Hydrocortisone is also of value in the circulatory failure due to septicaemia. Here the hypotension is not due to an adrenal insufficiency, as the glands may in fact be secreting large amounts. Yet by some mechanism not yet clear, large doses of hydrocortisone may restore the cardiac output and increase the blood pressure. *Brand names :* Efcortesol, Efcortelan, Hydro-Adreson, Hydrocortisyl, Hydrocortone.

Prednisone † **and Prednisolone** † (dose, 10 to 100 mg. daily)

One of the chief disadvantages of cortisone therapy is the disturbance it causes in the salt and water balance of the body. This disturbance of the blood electrolytes can be serious in conditions such as acute rheumatic fever, where the pyrexia and pain respond rapidly, but the retention of salts and water may increase the load on the weakened heart. The more potent synthetic corticosteroids now available, such as prednisone and prednisolone, have a more selective action, and the increased glucocorticoid action is accompanied by a decrease in the mineralocorticoid activity.

Prednisone and prednisolone can be regarded as derivatives of cortisone and hydrocortisone respectively, but are about five times more active. They have the same general action, are used for the same conditions, are effective orally and are given in similar doses.

The reduced tendency of these drugs to cause salt and water retention is a considerable advantage in many conditions, but conversely, they are not suitable for use in Addison's disease. In that condition salt loss is already severe, and the use of a salt-retaining steroid such as cortisone or fludrocortisone is essential.

Prednisolone brand names : Decortisyl,† Deltacortone,† Di-Adreson,† Delta-Cortelan,† Deltacortril.†

Prednisolone brand names: Codelcortone,† Delta-Cortef,† Deltastab,† Di-Adreson-F,† Precortisyl,† Prednelan,†

Methyl prednisolone (Medrone,†) dexamethasone (Decadron,† Oradexon †), betamethasone (Betnelan,† Betnesol), triamcinolone (Adcortyl,† Ledercort †) and paramethasone (Haldrate,† Metilar †) are examples of other corticosteroids, effective in lower doses, and with reduced side-effects. An approximate indication of comparable doses is given in the following table.

Cortisone	25·0 mg.
Hydrocortisone . . .	20·0 mg.
Prednisone ⎫ Prednisolone ⎭ . . .	5·0 mg.
Methyl prednisolone . .	4·0 mg.
Triamcinolone . . .	4·0 mg.
Paramethasone . . .	2·0 mg.
Dexamethasone . . .	0·75 mg.
Betamethasone . . .	0·5 mg.

7

Mineralocorticosteroids

Cortisone and analogous compounds are known as glucocorticosteroids because their main effect is on carbohydrate metabolism. Other hormones of the adrenal cortex, represented by deoxycortone and aldosterone, have no such action, but are concerned with the maintenance of the electrolyte balance of the body. One synthetic compound, however, fludrocortisone, has glucocorticosteroid and a marked mineralocorticoid activity.

Fludrocortisone Acetate (dose, 0·1 to 1 mg.)

This compound is a fluorine-containing derivative of hydrocortisone, and is characterised by a marked increase in potency and salt-retaining properties. It has a powerful anti-inflammatory action when applied locally, and is also of considerable value in Addison's disease. In that disease the adrenal glands have been damaged or destroyed by tubercular infection, or have atrophied from other causes, and in consequence there is a deficiency of adrenal steroids. As a result of the absence of the sodium and water retaining factors, large amounts of salt and fluid are excreted, and if untreated will lead to hypotension and collapse. Fludrocortone, deoxycortone and cortisone reduce this electrolyte disturbance, and restore the blood pressure to normal, In severe cases fludrocortisone may be given in doses of 1 mg., but for maintenance therapy doses of 0·1 mg. daily may be adequate. The drug is often given in association with cortisone. *Brand name :* Florinef.†

Deoxycortone Acetate † (dose, 5 mg.)

Deoxycortone was once widely used in the treatment of Addison's disease, but with the introduction of cortisone and related drugs, which permit a wider degree of control, the use of deoxycortone has declined. The standard dose is 5 mg., given by intramuscular injection as an oily solution. It is occasionally of value when a patient cannot tolerate or accept oral treatment with fludrocortisone. *Brand name :* DOCA.†

Aldosterone † (dose, 0·1 to 0·2 mg.)

Aldosterone is the principal mineralcorticoid of the body and has no anti-inflammatory properties. It is sometimes used in

Addison's disease, when a rapid restoration of electrolyte balance is required and in crisis, doses of 0·5 may be given intravenously. *Brand name :* Aldocorten.†

GONADOTROPHIC HORMONES

These hormones of the anterior pituitary gland stimulate the gonads in both sexes. Two separate hormones are known, the follicle-stimulating hormone (FSH) and the luteinising hormone (LH).

In the female, the follicle-stimulating hormone initiates and controls the development of the ovarian follicles and the production of oestrogens; in the male it controls the development of spermatozoa. The luteinising hormone is concerned with the development in the ovary of the corpus luteum, and the formation of progesterone; in the male it controls the production of androgens. It has not proved possible to extract these hormones from anterior pituitary glands except in very small amounts, but larger quantities of hormones with very similar actions are obtainable from other sources. The blood of pregnant mares contains a hormone, termed serum gonadotrophin, which has a follicle-stimulating action, and the urine of pregnant women contains a hormone derived from the placenta, and referred to as chorionic gonadotrophin, which resembles the luteinising hormone. As some patients may be allergic to these gonadotrophins, a preliminary test dose should be given before commencing treatment.

Serum Gonadotrophin † (dose, 200 to 1000 units)

This product has been given by intramuscular injection twice weekly in amenorrhoea and functional uterine bleeding to stimulate the production and augment the action of oestrogen, but in general the results are variable and disappointing. It has also been used to induce ovulation, but the large doses required may cause overstimulation and multiple pregnancy. *Brand names :* Gestyl,† Gonadotrophin F.S.H.†

Chorionic Gonadotrophin † (dose, 500 to 5000 units)

The main use of chorionic gonadotrophin is the treatment of undescended testicle. In the absence of any anatomical abnormalities that might be responsible for the cryptorchidism, chorionic gonadotrophin may be given by intramuscular injection in doses of 500 units twice weekly. It has also been used for functional uterine bleeding and threatened abortion. *Brand names:* Pregnyl,† Gonadotrophin L.H.†

OESTROGENS

Following the development of the ovarian follicles under the influence of the gonadotrophic hormone (FSH), oestrogens are formed and released according to physiological needs. These hormones are concerned with the general development and maintenance of the female genital system, and with the marked changes in the uterine mucosa that occur during the first half of the menstrual cycle. Therapeutically they are of most value in the treatment of menopausal symptoms associated with the decline in the natural secretion of oestrogen   The aim of treatment is to relieve the flushes, palpitations and psychological disturbances of the menopause with the lowest effective dose of oestrogen, thus allowing the body to adjust itself to a lower hormone level more slowly. Oestrogens are also useful in relieving post-menopausal conditions such as senile vaginitis and pruritus vulvae.

Oestrogens are also useful in genital hypoplasia, primary amenorrhoea and delayed puberty, and in certain menstrual disturbances associated with ovarian deficiency. They are also used in the palliative treatment of post-menopausal mammary carcinoma and to relieve the pain associated with bony metastases.

Oestrogens are also valuable in the treatment of carcinoma of the prostate gland in the male. Androgens stimulate prostatic growth, but their action can be antagonised by large doses of oestrogens, with considerable symptomatic relief.

Oestradiol is the most important natural oestrogen, but several synthetic oestrogens such as stilboestrol are also available.

Oestradiol Monobenzoate † (dose, 1 to 5 mg. daily)

Oestradiol is not very effective orally, and for injection it has been given as an oily solution of oestradiol monobenzoate. It has been used in the treatment of menopausal symptoms, but it is not of great clinical value.

In the treatment of post-menopausal carcinoma of the breast

large doses have been given, and a marked, but usually temporary, remission of symptoms may follow. Several preparations containing oestadiol or the related oestrone are available for local use in the treatment of vaginitis and menopausal pruritus vulvae. *Brand names :* Kolpon,† Menformon.†

Ethinyloestradiol † (dose, 0·01 to 0·05 mg. daily)

A more powerful synthetic oestrogen, and better tolerated than stilboestrol. It is effective in controlling menopausal symptoms in doses as low as 0·01 mg. daily. It is also used in primary amenorrhoea, functional uterine bleeding and for the suppression of lactation. Large doses, up to 3 mg. daily, are given in mammary and prostatic carcinoma. *Brand names :* Lynoral,† Primogyn C.†

Stilboestrol † (dose, 0·1 to 5 mg. daily)

Also known as diethylstilboestrol, this drug is a synthetic oestrogen and although chemically unrelated to the natural hormone it has powerful oestrogenic properties. It is effective orally, and may be given in all conditions requiring oestrogen therapy. Nausea and vomiting are more common with stilboestrol than with associated drugs but these side-effects are sometimes due to the use of unnecessarily high doses.

Stilboestrol is also very effective in the palliative treatment of prostatic carcinoma, and very high doses, up to 100 mg. daily or more, may be given. Such high doses may cause hypertrophy of the breast and other side-effects, and attempts have been made to avoid these undesirable manifestations by the use of stilboestrol diphosphate (Honvan †). That compound does not have the general effects of stilboestrol, but in the prostate gland it is broken down by the enzyme acid-phosphatase to give a high local concentration of stilboestrol in the carcinomatous tissues. The drug relieves pain, and brings about a regression in the size of the tumour, accompanied by a considerable relief of symptoms. Relapse may occur after an initial response. Stilboestrol is also used to suppress lactation, and various dosage schemes are employed, some based on a high initial dose of 15 mg. daily, falling to 1 mg. daily over fourteen days, others on a steady dose of 2 mg. three times a day.

Hexoestrol,† dienoestrol,† chlorotrianisene (Tace †) and methallenoestril (Vallestril †) represent other synthetic oestrogens.

PROGESTOGENS AND RELATED SUBSTANCES

The hormones secreted by the corpus luteum are concerned with the maintenance of pregnancy, and during that period with the inhibition of ovulation and the development of lactation. Towards the end of pregnancy the secretion of the progestogens wanes. This influence on the maintenance of pregnancy led to the use of progestogens in the treatment of threatened abortion, but they are now chiefly employed in functional uterine bleeding for their action on the development of the endometrium. They are also useful when the delay or prevention of menstruation is required.

Progesterone † (dose, 20 to 60 mg. daily)

Progesterone is the natural hormone, and is given by intra-muscular injection as an oily solution. In functional uterine bleeding 5 to 10 mg. may be given daily for one week; in threatened abortion early and continuous treatment with daily doses of 10 mg. or more is required. The use of progesterone has declined as orally effective compounds have been introduced.

Primolut-Depot † is a long-acting derivative of progesterone, and is given in doses of 65 to 250 mg. at monthly intervals, usually in association with an oestrogen.

Ethisterone † (dose, 25 to 100 mg. daily)

Ethisterone is a synthetic progestogen, which also has some oestrogenic potency, but it has the advantage of being active when given orally. In general, daily doses five to ten times greater than those of progesterone are necessary, and the drug is best given as sublingual tablets. *Brand names :* Gestone,† Progestoral.†

Norethisterone † (dose, 10 to 30 mg. daily)

Although this compound is very closely related to ethisterone, it is very much more active, and oral response compares with that of injections of progesterone. It is well tolerated, and is used in the treatment of all conditions requiring progesterone therapy. *Brand names:* Primolut N, † Norlutin-A †.

Clomiphene Citrate † (dose, 50 to 100 mg. daily)

Clomiphene is not a progestogen, but is considered here because of its effects on ovulation. It is a synthetic compound chemically related to the oestrogen chlorotrianisene. It has no intrinsic oestrogenic properties, but appears to have a selective action on the pituitary gland, as its use brings about an increased output of gonadotrophin, which in turn stimulates the maturation of the ovarian follicle and the development of the corpus luteum. Clomiphene has been used for various menstrual irregularities, but its stimulating action on the ovary is of main value in the treatment of infertility due to ovulatory failure. In patients with some ovulatory function and adequate oestrogen production, clomiphene in doses of 50 mg. daily for five days may bring about ovulation, and produce an endometrium favourable to the establishment of pregnancy. If ovulation does not occur, the dose may be increased to 100 mg. daily for five days, but if conception does not occur after three courses of clomiphene, further treatment with the drug is unlikely to be successful. *Brand name :* Clomid.†

Norethynodrel † (dose, 5 to 30 mg. daily)

Norethynodrel is a progesterone-like steroid with a more specific action on the endometrium. Following oral administration it rapidly induces early changes in the endometrium, but development is then held at that level, and with adequate doses, subsequent bleeding does not occur during treatment. Withdrawal of the drug is followed after two to five days by a bleeding, resembling normal menstruation. The compound thus has value in menorrhagia, metrorrhagia, and other forms of functional uterine bleeding.

Norethynodrel also has applications in the treatment of dysmenorrhoea. That condition is associated with the ovulatory stage of the menstrual cycle. Norethynodrel suppresses ovulation, and the pain of dysmenorrhoea can be controlled by the administration of 5 mg. of the drug from the fifth to the twenty-fourth day of the menstrual cycle. Treatment should be repeated for three cycles. The general action of norethynodrel appears to be increased by the presence of small amounts of oestrogen, and proprietary products such as Enavid † contain a small dose of oestrogen for that reason.

VIRILISING EFFECTS OF PROGESTOGENS

The use of oral synthetic progestogens for the maintenance of pregnancy in early threatened abortion has raised problems owing to the androgenic properties of some of these drugs. Masculinisation of the female foetus in this way is a definite possibility if the foetus is subjected to androgenic influence before the twelfth week of pregnancy, but after that time the female characteristics are well differentiated, and unlikely to be affected.

Such masculinisation is usually limited to clitoral enlargement and some labial fusion. The internal genitalia are not affected, and develop normally. This side-effect may occur after treatment with progestogens derived from testosterone, such as ethisterone (ethinyltestosterone) and norethisterone. Other derivatives, including dydrogesterone (Duphaston) and allyoestrenol (Gestanin) are less likely to have masculinising effects, but the safest drugs are the esters of hydroxyprogesterone (Primulot) which are given by injection.

Fertility Control

The explosive rise in world population in recent years, particularly in underdeveloped countries, has led to large-scale investigations of the problems of controlling fertility and birth-rates. Any acceptable method must be simple, effective and free from long-term disadvantages.

It has long been recognised that the temporary suppression of ovulation would be effective, but the practical application proved difficult. Oestrogens can suppress ovulation, and lower doses can be used if a progestogen is also given. With the production of synthetic and highly active progestogens, acceptable products became available, and oestrogen-progestogen preparations can inhibit ovulation for long periods, apparently without influencing subsequent fertility. The use of hormones in this way has been described as physiological contraception, and oestrogen-progesterone products are given in daily oral doses, starting on the fifth day of the menstrual cycle, and continuing for 20 days. During the interval between courses, a bleeding occurs, and treatment is restarted on the fifth day of the next cycle. Alternatively, a sequential system may be used during which an oestrogen is taken for 10-14 days, followed by an oestrogen-progestogen mixture for 5-7 days, followed in turn by an interval of 7 days. The action of these hormones is complex, as they not only suppress ovulation, but appear to influence the endometrium, and make it unsuitable for the implantation of a fertilised ovum, and also affect the viscosity of cervical mucus. Many products are now available as oral contraceptives, formulated on the pharmacological basis outlined, and representative products include Anovlar,† Conovid,† Feminor,† Gynovlar,† Lyndiol,† Norlestrin,† Previson,† Sequens† and Volidan†. These products are in general well tolerated, but some nausea, acne, gain in weight, liver damage, and thrombosis may occur.

The possible relationship between thrombo-embolism and the use of oral contraceptives has caused some concern, and a Medical Research Council Report has confirmed that a causal relationship may exist. The magnitude of the risk is difficult to assess, as thrombosis and pulmonary embolism may occur in a woman of child-bearing age who is not taking oral contraceptives. Perhaps many of the problems will be solved when more is known about prostaglandins. The prostaglandins are a remarkable group of natural substances found in mammalian tissues, one of which has been used successfully by intravenous injection for the termination of pregnancy. The use of a locally acting prostaglandin to induce menstruation is under investigation.

ANDROGENS

The androgens are the male sex hormones secreted by the testes, and are responsible for the development and maintenance of the male sexual system. They also have powerful anabolic or tissue-building properties, and the rapid physical development of the male at puberty is associated with increased androgen activity. Therapeutically, the androgens are used mainly in testicular deficiency in the male, and in carcinoma of the breast in females. Their anabolic effects are useful in osteoporosis and wasting diseases, but their virilising action is a limiting factor when attempting to use the anabolic properties of androgens in the treatment of female patients. These two properties of the androgens can be separated to some extent by chemical modification of the hormones, and a number of modified androgens with a reduced virilising action are described later under ' Non-virilising Androgens.'

Testosterone † (dose, 5 to 25 mg.)

Testosterone is the most important natural androgen, originally obtained from the interstitial cells of the testes, but now prepared synthetically. In testicular deficiency it may be given by intramuscular injection, or by the subcutaneous implantation of sterile pellets. A subcutaneous dose of 500 mg. in this way will provide a slow but effective release of testosterone over a period of six months. For intramuscular injections, solutions of testosterone propionate in oil are preferred. Testosterone can depress the output of gonadotrophins, and in the female can suppress ovulation and the development of the endometrium. It is thus useful in some cases of functional uterine bleeding and may be given in doses of 10 mg. or more two or three times a week. Large doses of 100 mg. or more are given in the palliative treatment of carcinoma of the breast. *Brand names:* Neo-Hombreol,† Primoteston,† Sustanon,† Testoral.†

Methyltestosterone † (dose, 5 to 50 mg. daily)

Testosterone is inactivated by the liver when given orally, unless given as sublingual tablets and oral treatment has limited therapeutic value. Methyltestosterone largely escapes hepatic inactivation, and is more effective, and may be given orally to maintain or supplement the effects of testosterone injections. The drug is best given as sublingual tablets, and oral doses should be three to five times greater than those of testosterone by injection. *Brand name:* Perandren Linguets.†

Fluoxymesterone † (dose, 1 to 20 mg. daily).

Fluoxymesterone has the general effects of testosterone, but has the advantages of being active orally, and much more effective than methyltestosterone. Small doses of 1 to 2 mg. are given for its anabolic action in osteoporosis, but for carcinoma of the breast daily doses of 20 mg. may be required. *Brand name :* Ultandren.†

Non-virilising Androgens †

The tissue-building and protein-forming (anabolic) properties of the androgens are valuable in wasting diseases, in convalescence, the treatment of severe burns, and osteoporosis, but their clinical use is limited by their masculinising effects on female patients. In recent years a number of related compounds have been synthesised, which have an increased anabolic action, accompanied by markedly reduced virilising properties. The therapeutic use of these new compounds can be extended to the treatment of female patients and children, as in suitable doses the virilising effects, such as the growth of facial hair and deepening of the voice, are virtually absent. Most of these drugs are active orally, but others may be given by intramuscular injection, and have a longer action. Some compounds may cause hepatic disturbance or damage if given for long periods and intermittent treatment with a rest period may reduce this risk. As these drugs are androgen derivatives, they should not be given in prostatic carcinoma. Conversely, some compounds such as methandrenome (Dianabol) and drostanolone (Masteril) are useful alternatives to testosterone in the treatment of advanced carcinoma of the breast. The following are representative of a number of available products. *Brand names :* Adroyd,† Anabolex,† Anapolon,† Dianabol,† Durabolin,† Lysinex,† Nilevar,† Primobolan,† Stromba.†

THYROTROPHIC HORMONE

The activity of the thyroid gland is normally controlled by the thyrotrophic or thyroid stimulating hormone (TSH) of the anterior pituitary gland. This hormone is rarely used clinically, except in diagnosis, as in the treatment of deficiency states thyroxine is preferred.

Hyperthyroidism, which is due to an increased output of thyroxine, has long been regarded as basically a result of an excessive production of TSH. In some patients with Grave's disease only a low level of TSH is found, and it has been suggested that in such cases a long-acting thyroid stimulator (LATS) may exist. The source of this stimulator is not clear, but it is not derived from the pituitary gland, and so by-passes the normal control system governing thyroid activity. It appears to be an immunoglobulin, and to function as a thyroid auto-antibody.

THYROID GLAND

The thyroid gland is situated in the neck, on either side and in front of the trachea, and is one of the largest endocrine glands of the body. The main physiological function of the gland is to control the basal metabolic rate, which is mediated by the production of thyroxine. A high output results in hyperthyroidism; a low output and consequent slowing down of the metabolic processes causes a condition which in adults is termed myxoedema, and in children is known as cretinism.

The thyroid gland forms two iodine-containing hormones,

thyroxine and liothyronine. The iodine absorbed from the diet, and circulating in the blood, is selectively absorbed by the gland to form thyroxine, which appears to act as a reservoir from which the more rapidly acting liothyronine is formed and eventually liberated.

Thyroid Extract

In deficiency states, thyroid can be given orally as the dry gland, obtained from the ox, sheep or pig, but absorption may be variable, and thyroxine (*q.v.*) which is now prepared synthetically, is preferred by most clinicians. It should be noted that although thyroid is a metabolic stimulant it has no place in the treatment of obesity.

Thyroxine.† Thyroxine Sodium † (dose, 0·5 to 0·3 mg. daily)

Following oral administration the synthetic hormone evokes a more consistent response than the more variable dried thyroid gland, probably because of more efficient absorption. The effects are slow in onset, and may not reach a maximum until after ten days or so.

In myxoedema, treatment is commenced with small doses, slowly increased until a metabolic balance has again been achieved. Maintenance doses are about 0·2 mg. daily. The reason for these small initial doses is that the myocardium is often affected in myxoedema. Large initial doses of thyroxine may increase the heart rate, and add to the cardiac burden before the myocardium has had time to recover. In cretinism treatment should be commenced as soon as possible, as if delayed, mental damage may occur which cannot be reversed by subsequent thyroid treatment. The initial dose for a cretinous infant is about 0·02 mg., rising to maintenance doses in adults to 0·1 mg., and treatment must be continued for life. *Brand name :* Eltroxin.†

Liothyronine † (dose, 5 to 100 micrograms daily)

The latent period of ten days or so that elapses before thyroxine exerts a full effect is considered to be due to a slow conversion of the drug into liothyronine. This compound appears to be the form of the hormone which finally affects the metabolism of the tissues. Liothyronine is therefore used when a rapid action is required, as it is effective within a few hours. The action is correspondingly short, and the drug is not suitable for maintenance treatment.

In severe myxoedema, when coma may be imminent or present, liothyronine may be given by intravenous or intramuscular injection in doses of 100 micrograms. *Brand name :* Tertroxin.†

THYROID INHIBITORS *

Excessive activity of the thyroid gland, referred to as hyperthyroidism or thyrotoxicosis, is characterised by rapid pulse, loss of weight, raised metabolic rate, and enlargement of the thyroid. At one time surgical removal of much of the gland was the only effective treatment, but since the introduction of certain antithyroid substances, oral therapy has become an established method of control.

Carbimazole (dose, 5 to 60 mg. daily)

Carbimazole is the most effective and least toxic of the antithyroid drugs. These compounds suppress the formation of thyroxine and liothyronine by the thyroid gland by combining with the iodine absorbed from the blood. By this means the iodine necessary to form thyroxine is made unavailable, and carbimazole brings about an indirect lowering of the basal metabolic rate. As the uptake of iodine by the gland is not affected, these antithyroid drugs are better regarded as thyroid inhibitors rather than as thyroid antagonists.

Carbimazole is active orally, and the dose depends on the degree of thyrotoxicosis. An average initial dose is 30 mg. daily; maintenance doses are around 5 mg. daily. The effects are slow in onset as the thyroxine already formed and stored in the gland must be metabolised, and the raised basal metabolic rate may not return to normal until after three to five weeks. Toxic effects are uncommon, but are similar to those referred to under methylthiouracil. It should be noted that carbimazole and related drugs may appear in breast milk, and may depress the thyroid activity of a breast-fed infant. *Brand name :* Neo-Mercazole.

Methylthiouracil, Propylthiouracil (dose, 50 to 200 mg. daily)

These compounds also have an antithyroid action, but are more liable to cause toxic effects than carbimazole and are used less

* These are not hormones, but are considered here because of their therapeutic connection with thyroid.

frequently. The most serious side-effect is agranulocytosis, which may occur in the early stages of treatment; skin reactions, drug fever, hepatitis and some enlargement of the thyroid may also occur. Careful control of dosage of any antithyroid drug is essential, as treatment may have to be continued for long periods.

Potassium Perchlorate (dose, 200 mg. to 800 mg. daily)

Potassium perchlorate is an effective drug in the treatment of thyrotoxicosis, but its action differs sharply from that of carbimazole both in nature and rapidity of onset. Normally, iodine in the circulation becomes concentrated in the thyroid, and is used to form thyroxine. Carbimazole and related drugs inhibit the utilisation of iodine by the gland, but potassium perchlorate prevents the take-up of iodine by the thyroid, and thus inhibits the formation of thyroxine at an early stage. An average dose is 200 mg. four times daily for one month, subsequently reduced to 200 mg. twice daily. It is chiefly used in the treatment of children and young adults. The drug is usually well tolerated, especially when lower doses are used, although nausea may occur, but agranulocytosis, aplastic anaemia and purpura have been reported. Sore throat, rash or bruising are indications for the immediate withdrawal of the drug. *Brand name :* Peroidin.

Iodine

Although iodine in very small amounts is necessary for thyroid activity, larger doses can depress thyroid function for short periods, and temporarily relieve the symptoms of thyrotoxicosis. This action appears to be a blocking effect on the release of thyroxine from the gland. The effect of large doses is at a maximum after about two weeks, and iodine is often given to reduce the basal metabolic rate during the preparation of patients for thyroidectomy. It also reduces the hyperplasia and vascularity of the gland, making it smaller and firmer, and so making subsequent surgery more easy. It is usually given as Lugol's Solution (aqueous solution of iodine) in doses of 0·3 to 1 ml. three times a day for two weeks before operation, but larger doses are sometimes preferred. Potassium iodide in doses of 60 mg. three times a day is equally effective. Lugol's Solution has been given in doses of 2 ml. (after dilution with saline) by slow intravenous injection in thyrotoxic crisis. Radioactive iodine is occasionally used in the diagnosis of thyroid dysfunction, in the treatment of thyrotoxicosis resistant to other drugs, and in cancer of the thyroid.

OTHER ANTERIOR PITUITARY HORMONES

Lactogenic Hormone

This hormone, also known as prolactin, is concerned with milk formation. During pregnancy, premature lactation is suppressed by the relatively large amounts of oestrogen in the blood, but following delivery there is a sharp fall in the oestrogen level, and a release of prolactin. In the breast prepared during pregnancy, prolactin stimulates milk production at term, and sustains subsequent lactation. Oestrogens can suppress the action of the hormone, and this effect on the lactation process is exemplified by the use of stilboestrol (*q.v.*) to inhibit lactation.

Growth Hormone

Human growth hormone, which controls the formation of bone and other tissues, has been used to stimulate growth in dwarfed children, but the results are often disappointing because of the formation of antibodies.

Parathyroid Gland

These small glands have no relationship with the thyroid glands other than that of position. They are situated in the neck, near the thyroid, and their function is the control of calcium and phosphate metabolism. A deficiency of parathyroid activity, or an accidental removal of the glands during thyroidectomy, results in a lowering of blood calcium and an increase in the phosphate level. The former, if unchecked, leads to severe tetany. The intramuscular injection of parathyroid extract (Parathormone) can relieve the symptoms of parathyroid deficiency by mobilising calcium from the bones, and increasing the excretion of phosphates, but as tolerance and consequent lack of response soon develop because of the formation of antibodies, such extracts are of limited therapeutic value.

Tetany due to low blood calcium can also be relieved by the administration of calcium salts. For the acute attack, calcium gluconate solution (10 per cent.) can be injected intravenously or intramuscularly in doses of 10 to 20 ml., and treatment may be maintained by the oral administration of calcium gluconate or calcium lactate (dose, 1 to 5 G.). Vitamin D (calciferol) may also be given to promote the absorption of calcium. Recent work has indicated that the thyroid gland secretes a third hormone, referred to as calcitonin, which is also concerned with calcium balance, and may be useful in hypercalcaemia and osteoporosis.

Dihydrotachysterol (dose, 0·25 to 2·5 mg. daily)

This compound is not a hormone, as it is related to calciferol (*q.v.*), but has an action resembling that of the parathyroid hormone. It increases the absorption of calcium from the small intestine, promotes deposition in bone and restores the blood-phosphate level to normal. Dihydrotachysterol is therefore often given with calcium salts in the maintenance treatment of parathyroid deficiency, but the dose must be related to calcium level. It is available as an oily solution (0·25 mg. per ml.) and when the blood calcium level has been stabilised, doses of 1 to 7 ml. weekly may be sufficient for maintenance. Excessive doses lead to decalcification of bone, deposition of calcium in other tissues, and an increased excretion of calcium in the urine. *Brand name :* A.T.10.

INSULIN

The pancreas is the large gland that secretes trypsin and other digestive enzymes that enter the duodenum as pancreatic juice. It also secretes the hormone insulin which controls the metabolism of carbohydrates, and a deficiency of insulin causes the once fatal disease diabetes mellitus. Insulin is produced by small pockets of specialised tissue in the pancreas, termed the islets of Langerhans, and the extraction of the hormone from the pancreas is an illustration of the time-lag that may elapse between a discovery and its therapeutic application. Although it was demonstrated in 1890 that the pancreas was concerned with carbohydrate metabolism, it was not until 1922 that the active substance, insulin, was finally extracted from animal glands in a form suitable for clinical use. Insulin controls the uptake and use of glucose by the tissues, as well as its storage in the liver as glycogen, but in diabetes mellitus the body no longer produces an adequate amount of insulin and in consequence glucose soon accumulates in the blood. Part of this excess is excreted in the urine, and this forms the basis of the well-known tests for diabetes.

The large amounts of glucose in the urine act as a diuretic and increased amounts of electrolytes are also excreted. The polyuria is accompanied by severe thirst, and if untreated, dehydration and coma result. Owing to the deficiency of insulin, the energy-supplying glucose in the blood is virtually denied to the body, and so increased amounts of proteins and fats are used as sources of energy, leading to tissue breakdown and wasting. In health, fats are metabolised in the liver to simple acids, which are finally oxidised, but in diabetes other breakdown products are formed, referred to as acetone bodies or ketone bodies. These substances are acidic in nature, and although excreted in part in the urine they may gradually accumulate in the blood, eventually leading to diabetic acidosis and coma. The symptoms of diabetes mellitus can be controlled by the administration of insulin, and the diabetic patient is able to live a virtually normal life.

SOLUBLE INSULIN

Soluble insulin is the standard form of the drug, and it is usually given by subcutaneous injection. It is useless orally, as being a protein it is rapidly broken down by the gastric enzymes, but following subcutaneous injection it is rapidly absorbed, and a peak effect is reached in about three hours. With a suitable dose, the high blood-sugar level falls rapidly, the depleted glycogen reserves are restored, ketone bodies are oxidised, and as glucose is no longer excreted in the urine, the characteristic thirst and polyuria of diabetes are relieved. Soluble insulin is normally injected twice a day, but the dose depends upon the degree of insulin deficiency. The diet must be adjusted so that the intake of carbohydrate coincides with that of insulin, and frequent urine tests are necessary to control any variation in the severity of the disease. The use of soluble insulin has declined in recent years since the introduction of longer-acting forms, but it is still the drug of choice in the initial treatment of severe diabetes, and in diabetic emergencies. Its effects are prompt and predictable, and permit flexibility of dose as the condition is brought under control. Conversely, in stabilised patients the twice-daily injection of insulin can be a burden.

Protamine Zinc Insulin (P.Z. Insulin)

Many attempts have been made to extend the action of insulin, and P.Z. insulin is a combination of soluble insulin with protamine, a simple protein obtained from fish sperm, and a trace of zinc chloride. This modification is not soluble in water, but is supplied as a suspension, and the change in the physical state is reflected in the slow onset of action and prolonged effect. Following injection, the action of P.Z. insulin begins in about six hours, reaches a maximum in about eighteen hours, and may persist well over twenty-four hours. The effects thus resemble those of natural insulin, and a single daily dose is often sufficient to control the symptoms of diabetes when suitable dietary adjustments are made.

Some patients with severe diabetes require a product with a more rapid initial action, and this can be achieved by giving a mixed injection of soluble and P.Z. insulin, prepared at the time of use. Although P.Z. insulin is usually well tolerated, it sometimes causes local reactions, or a rash. These reactions are allergic in character and may be associated with the protamine, or possibly traces of animal protein. With the highly purified insulins now in use, these reactions are less common. Local reactions may also occur if the subcutaneous injection is made too superficially.

Globin Insulin, Isophane Insulin (NPH Insulin)

These are modifications of insulin that have an action midway between those of soluble insulin and P.Z. insulin. Globin insulin is occasionally useful in the treatment of patients who react very badly to P.Z. insulin; isophane insulin resembles globin insulin in the onset of action, but has a more prolonged effect.

INSULIN ZINC SUSPENSIONS

These preparations are better known as the lente insulins and their introduction marked a considerable advance in the treatment of diabetes. By a slight change in manufacture, using an acetate buffer, suspensions of zinc insulin can be prepared without the addition of any protamine, and with this modification of insulin, allergic reactions due to protamine have been eliminated. The rate of absorption of this modified insulin is markedly influenced by the particle size of the suspension. When the particles are extremely small (amorphous zinc insulin) absorption is rapid; if a crystalline form is used the absorption is slower, but the action more prolonged. The use of mixtures of each variety gives a product with a steady action of considerable therapeutic value. Three forms of these lente insulins are now in wide use :—

Insulin Zinc Suspension (Amorphous).

SEMI-LENTE INSULIN. Resembles soluble insulin in rapidity of effect, but has longer action (twelve hours).

Insulin Zinc Suspension (Crystalline).

ULTRA-LENTE INSULIN. Resembles P.Z. insulin, but the action may extend over thirty hours.

Insulin Zinc Suspension.

LENTE INSULIN. A mixture of three parts of semi-lente insulin and seven parts of ultra-lente insulin, with a twenty-four-hour duration of action.

These forms of insulin can be mixed with each other in proportions designed for a particular patient, and control of diabetes is usually possible with a single daily dose. Such insulins are intended for maintenance treatment only. They are not suitable for emergency use, neither should they be mixed with any other form of insulin.

The great majority of moderately severe diabetics can be controlled by a single morning injection of insulin zinc suspension. The effects of an injection begin in about half to one hour, reach a maximum in four to six hours, and slowly subside over a period of twenty-four hours. The dose must be adjusted to the individual, as patients with much the same apparent degree of diabetes may react differently to a similar dose of insulin. For the few for whom the insulin zinc suspension is unsuitable, special mixtures of the lente insulins can be prepared. The aim of treatment is to adjust the diet and dose of insulin so that the patient has enough calories whilst keeping the urine almost sugar-free. Insulin requirements are increased during illness, but in any case regular urine tests with Clinitest tablets are essential. Patients should be warned that insulin is available in more than one form and in more than one strength, and accuracy of dose is important. Thus soluble insulin is available in strengths of 20, 40 and 80 units per ml. respectively; the other types of insulin are issued in strengths of 40 and 80 units per ml. Each strength is distinguished by special coloured labels, and the dose should always be expressed in units and not by volume.

Overdosage with insulin results in an excessive lowering of the blood-sugar level (hypoglycaemia). Faintness and dizziness are initial symptoms, accompanied by sweating and confusion. In severe conditions coma results. Mild hypoglycaemia in diabetics is usually due to a temporary reduction in the carbohydrate intake, and can be relieved by the immediate taking of dextrose or sugar solution. In severe hypoglycaemia, the low blood-sugar may be raised very quickly by an injection of glucagon. Glucagon is a hyperglycaemic agent secreted by the alpha islet cells of the pancreas, and in doses of 0·5 to 1 mg. by injection (s.c., i.m. or i.v.) it brings about a dramatic mobilisation and output of glucose from the liver.

In diabetic coma, which must be distinguished from the insulin coma referred to above, large doses of soluble insulin are given, and the dehydration and loss of electrolytes relieved by the intravenous administration of sodium bicarbonate or lactate or Nabarro's solution (q.v.). With the large doses of insulin required, it is possible to pass from a diabetic or hyperglycaemic coma into an insulin or hypoglycaemic coma. It is therefore not unusual to give a ' protecting ' dose of dextrose solution during the early stages of treatment.

ORALLY ACTIVE ANTIDIABETIC DRUGS *

Tolbutamide †

Many attempts have been made to find orally active antidiabetic drugs, and thus avoid the need to inject insulin, but no real success was obtained until tolbutamide was discovered in 1955. Tolbutamide is chemically related to the sulphonamides, although it has no antibacterial properties, but following oral administration it produces a significant lowering of the blood-sugar level. Tolbutamide is not effective if the pancreas has been removed or destroyed, so that the effects of the drug are bound up in some way with the increased production or release of insulin by a functioning pancreas. It is therefore not an insulin substitute, but a pancreatic-islet stimulant, with the advantage of being

---

* These drugs are not hormones, but are considered here because of their therapeutic connection with insulin.

effective orally. It is most effective in middle-aged and elderly patients, who are well stabilised on low doses of insulin. Juvenile diabetics do not respond well to oral therapy with tolbutamide or related drugs.

Transfer from insulin to tolbutamide should be made slowly over a few days, and the initial doses of the oral drug depend to some extent on the dose of insulin being given. With small insulin requirements the changeover may commence with an initial tolbutamide dose of 1 G. three times a day, reducing steadily to a maintenance dose of 1 G. daily or less. Larger doses, or a reversion to insulin, may be necessary during illness and other periods of stress. Tolerance to tolbutamide may occur in a few patients after treatment for some months, necessitating a change of therapy.

Tolbutamide is well tolerated, but occasional side-effects may be noted, such as gastro-intestinal disturbances and skin rashes. It should be used with care in liver disease. Depression of bone marrow activity is uncommon, but an occasional and unexpected side-effect is an intolerance of alcohol, characterised by marked flushing of the face if alcohol is taken. *Brand names:* Artosin,† Rastinon.†

Chlorpropamide † (dose, 250 to 500 mg. daily)

Chlorpropamide is an oral hypoglycaemic drug similar in action to tolbutamide, but with a more prolonged effect owing to a slower rate of excretion. The maximum response may not occur for four to seven days, and adjustment of dose is then necessary. Many patients with low insulin requirements can be transferred to chlorpropamide and stabilised on a single daily dose of 200 to 500 mg. Some patients who fail or cease to respond to tolbutamide may also be controlled by chlorpropamide. The occasional toxic side-effects are those common to related drugs such as tolbutamide and acetohexamide. *Brand name:* Diabinese.†

Acetohexamide † (dose, 0·25 to 1·5 G. daily)

This compound, like chlorpropamide and tolbutamide, belongs to the chemical group of drugs referred to as sulphonylureas, and has a similar type of action.

It is given as an initial dose of 1·5 G., followed by average daily doses of 0·25 to 1 G. before breakfast. *Brand name:* Dimelor.†

Tolazamide (Tolanase) and glymidine (Gondafon) are examples of other orally-active hypoglycaemic drugs. Experimental work suggests that glymidine may stimulate the formation of more islet tissue and thus increase the production of insulin. Glibenclamide (Daonil, Euglucon) is a new compound, characterised by high potency and low toxicity. It is effective in lowering the blood sugar of many diabetic patients in doses of 2·5 to 20 mg.

Metformin † (dose, 1 to 3 G. daily)

Metformin is an orally-active hypoglycaemic drug that differs both chemically and pharmacologically from the sulphonylureas. It does not influence the islets of Langerhans to produce more insulin, but appears to act by increasing the utilisation of glucose by the tissues. Maturity-onset diabetes may be a disturbance of the sugar-regulating mechanism, and not a lack of insulin, and metformin may correct this disturbance. It is given in initial doses of 500 mg. two or three times a day, gradually increasing over a period of 10 days according to response to a maximum dose of 3 G. daily. Patients already receiving insulin should maintain that treatment for two days, and then reduce the insulin dose gradually. Metformin is well tolerated, and has no toxic effects on the liver, and is of value in the treatment of patients who fail to respond to the sulphonylureas, as well as mature and obese diabetics. *Brand name:* Glucophage.†

Phenformin † (dose, 25 to 150 mg. daily)

Phenformin is an antidiabetic compound not related to tolbutamide or chlorpropamide, and appears to have an action similar to that of metformin in stimulating the uptake of glucose. It may be used in association with other oral hypoglycaemic compounds and with insulin to secure more effective control, and it also has applications in the supplementary treatment of juvenile diabetics. Phenformin is given two or three times a day, with meals, in doses ranging from 25 to 150 mg. daily, or occasionally more. A sustained-release form (dose, 50 mg.) is also available.

Side-effects include nausea and diarrhoea, but the drug is generally well tolerated, and liver damage and jaundice is uncommon. *Brand name:* Dibotin.†

CHAPTER XIII

ANTIHISTAMINES

HISTAMINE is an unusual substance, as when injected it has a wide range of pharmacological activity, yet its physiological role is far from clear. It is a normal constituent of animal tissues, where it is held in a combined and inactive form, but in allergic conditions some of this combined histamine is released, and gives rise to a variety of symptoms including hay fever, urticaria, asthma, serum sickness and anaphylaxis.

It is considered that in allergic individuals certain tissues of the body acquire a sensitivity to various compounds, termed allergens, which are usually protein in nature, although almost any substance may on occasion act as an allergen. These allergens function as antigens, and provoke the formation of neutralising substances termed antibodies. Subsequent re-exposure to the allergen results in an antigen-antibody reaction, accompanied by the release of histamine and associated substances, with consequent clinical manifestations characteristic of an allergic attack.

In order to treat these allergic states, the chain-reaction of allergen→antibody→histamine-susceptible tissue must be broken at some point. If the allergen is a food, for example, it can be removed from the diet, and the causative substance eliminated at the source. Alternatively, the patient may be desensitised by a course of injections of weak solutions of the offending allergen. In some cases, as in hay fever, which is due to a clear sensitivity to grass pollens, desensitisation is often very successful. When a number of allergens are involved desensitisation is more difficult, and the results are often less satisfactory.

The allergic symptoms may also be relieved by the use of ephedrine, adrenaline and related drugs, but the most dramatic results have been obtained with the antihistamines, and the introduction of this group of drugs marked a new approach to the problem. These drugs do not attack and destroy histamine, or even prevent its release during an allergic attack, but appear to become attached selectively to the sensitised tissues. They thus block the access of released histamine to these tissues, and so inhibit the allergic response.

Antihistamines are therefore palliative drugs, which relieve the symptoms by protecting the susceptible tissues, and treatment must be continued during the period of exposure to the allergen. With the wide range of antihistamines now available a considerable degree of symptomatic control is possible. Urticaria and other allergic skin reactions usually respond well to the antihistamines, but the drugs appear to have little ability to bring about a relaxation of smooth muscle, and in allergic bronchospasm and asthma the results are often disappointing. Individual response to any one drug is also variable. Paradoxically, the antihistamines may themselves cause skin reactions if used locally, and the systemic treatment is much more satisfactory.

Besides their specific antihistamine action, many drugs of this group have mild sedative effects; some have useful anti-emetic properties, and are given in travel sickness, nausea and vomiting and also to reduce the symptoms of parkinsonism. It should be noted that the antihistamines do not antagonise the effects of injected histamine on gastric secretion. In the histamine secretion test (*q.v.*) to assess the acid-secreting powers of the stomach, an antihistamine is also given to control the other effects of histamine.

TOXIC EFFECTS.—Excessive doses of antihistamines have marked sedative effects, and may cause gastro-intestinal disturbances, but in small children the drugs have a stimulant action, and may cause convulsions. There is no pharmacological antidote to this group of drugs, and the treatment should be directed towards removing any unabsorbed drug from the stomach, with injections of a short-acting barbiturate to control any convulsions. Histamine is not an antidote, and may produce severe bronchospasm and circulatory collapse if so used. The following compounds are representative of the large number of available drugs :

Diphenhydramine (dose, 25 to 75 mg.)

Diphenhydramine was one of the first antihistamines and has a more sedative action than some of the later compounds. That sedative action can have advantages, especially in the treatment of itching skin conditions, but has corresponding disadvantages for car drivers and others who must remain alert. Diphenhydramine also has anti-emetic properties, and is given in the treatment of travel sickness. It is also used as a constituent of some cough preparations, and is occasionally of value in relieving some of the symptoms of parkinsonism. *Brand name :* Benadryl.

Promethazine (dose, 25 to 50 mg.)

Promethazine is one of the most effective and long-acting of the antihistamines. It is widely used in the oral treatment of hay fever and urticaria, although it is less effective in perennial rhinitis. Promethazine also potentiates the action of some analgesic drugs and it is sometimes given by injection with chlorpromazine and pethidine for pre-anaesthetic medication. The central effects of promethazine are also useful in the treatment of parkinsonism. *Brand name :* Phenergan.

Phenindamine (dose, 25 to 50 mg.)

Phenindamine has the general properties of the antihistamine group of drugs, but is exceptional in being virtually free from sedative effects. It is therefore of value for day-time use, particularly for car-drivers and people in charge of machinery. *Brand name:* Thephorin.

Chlorpheniramine (dose, 2 to 4 mg.)

Chlorpheniramine is one of the most potent of the antihistamines, and effective in doses of 4 mg. twice daily. A prolonged action tablet is also available. In severe conditions it may be given by intramuscular or slow intravenous injection. Small doses are sometimes added to blood or intravenous drip infusions to prevent reactions. *Brand name :* Piriton.

Antazoline (Antistin), mepyramine (Anthisan) and halopyramine (Synopen) are examples of the wide range of available antihistamines. Anti-emetic properties are exhibited by a number of antihistamines, and those drugs used mainly in travel sickness and the nausea following radiotherapy include promethazine theoclate (Avomine), chlorcyclizine (Histantin), dimenhydrinate (Dramamine) and meclozine (Ancolan). See also page 165.

Cyproheptadine (dose, 2 to 4 mg.)

Some allergic and pruritic conditions are not always controlled by antihistamines, and allergic reactions may be associated with the release of serotonin as well as histamine. Serotonin resembles histamine in its wide distribution in the tissues, and in the absence of any clear physiological function, although it appears to be

associated with the vascular aspects of migraine. It is also linked
in some way with certain allergic conditions, as serotonin antagonists can sometimes increase the response to antihistamines. Cyproheptadine has both antihistamine and antiserotonin properties,
and may be effective in allergic conditions not responding to conventional antihistamine treatment. It is given in doses of 4 mg.
three or four times a day, but may cause drowsiness. Quite apart
from its value in allergy, cyproheptadine has been found useful
as an appetite stimulant. *Brand name :* Periactin.

Sodium Cromoglycate

Antihistamines are not of great value in allergic asthma and
bronchitis, as spasmogens other than histamine may be involved.
In the prophylactic treatment of such conditions, sodium cromoglycate is frequently effective. The drug has an unusual action,
as it is not a bronchodilator, neither has it any anti-inflammatory
properties, but it interferes in some way with the release of pulmonary spasmogens following an antigen-antibody reaction. It
does not antagonise the spasmogen directly, so is used primarily
in prophylaxis. Sodium cromoglycate is not absorbed when given
orally, and is administered by inhalation of the dry powder from a
' spin-inhaler.' Each dose of 20 mg. is contained in a gelatin capsule. As some patients may experience transient bronchospasm
after the inhalation of a powder, the standard capsule also contains isoprenaline 0·1 mg. to offset any temporary local irritation.
Plain capsules without isoprenaline are also available. *Brand names :*
Intal, Intal Compound.

CHAPTER XIV

THE VITAMINS

EXPERIMENTS during the early part of the present century showed that artificial diets containing adequate amounts of protein, fats, carbohydrates, minerals and water could not maintain growth and health in laboratory animals. Some other factors present in normal diets were necessary, and these factors are now well known as vitamins. They differ very widely in chemical constitution, and although in some cases their exact function is still obscure, they appear to be closely concerned with the action of enzymes in the body cells. When first discovered their chemical nature was unknown, and they were identified by letters. Many have now been synthesised, and are referred to by their chemical names as well as by the older letters. Over twenty vitamins are known, but some are of little therapeutic importance, and reference will be made mainly to vitamins A, B, C, D, E and K.

A good mixed diet provides adequate amounts of vitamins and some are also formed by bacteria in the colon, so vitamin supplements are normally unnecessary. Restricted diets, or defective absorption or utilisation of food result in vitamin deficiencies which lead to a number of recognisable conditions, and require the administration of the appropriate vitamins. Other factors connected with vitamin deficiencies include anorexia and vomiting, gastrointestinal disease, liver damage and cancerous conditions. Deficiencies may also arise when natural demands for vitamins are increased, as in fevers, pregnancy and metabolic disorders such as diabetes. Drugs which have a bactericidal action on the organisms normally present in the intestines, such as some oral antibiotics, may also indirectly cause a vitamin deficiency.

In such circumstances relatively small doses of vitamins are adequate to rectify the deficiency, but in certain unrelated conditions some vitamins are given in large doses, and should then be regarded as therapeutic agents, and not as dietary supplements.

Vitamins present in food can be divided into two classes, the fat-soluble and the water-soluble vitamins. The fat-soluble vitamins include vitamins A, D, E and K; the water-soluble vitamins are represented by vitamins B and C. As many vitamins are now made synthetically, and water-soluble derivatives are often available, this distinction between fat-soluble and water-soluble vitamins has become blurred, and they will be considered here alphabetically.

Vitamin A

Vitamin A may be present in various foods as such, or as the closely related compound carotene, from which the vitamin can be formed in the body. Dietary sources of the vitamin include milk, butter, carrots and green vegetables. Fish liver oils contain large amounts together with vitamin D. Vitamin A is concerned with the growth and maintenance of the epithelial tissues, and is also concerned with vision, as it plays an essential part in the formation of visual purple. A deficiency may lead to night blindness and xerophthalmia.

Vitamin A has been used in the hope of preventing recurrent infections of the upper respiratory tract, and in various dermatological conditions. Its chief value is in deficiency states such as coeliac disease and sprue, or where absorption has been reduced by the excessive use of liquid paraffin as a laxative. It may be given as capsules of halibut liver oil, containing 4500 units as cod liver oil or as the pure synthetic vitamin. *Brand name :* Ro-a-Vit. Adexolin contains vitamins A and D.

Vitamin B Group

This group or complex includes several water-soluble vitamins that usually occur together in various foods, and are concerned with the metabolism of proteins, fats and carbohydrates. The term ' vitamin B ' was originally applied to what was thought to be a single substance; as later work showed that a number of substances were present, these were distinguished as vitamins B_1, B_2, B_6, B_{12}, etc. Since then more specific names have been introduced. Deficiency rarely occurs singly, and administration of all the main vitamins of the group is usually advisable.

Thiamine (dose, prophylactic, 2 to 5 mg. daily; therapeutic,
     25 to 100 mg. daily, orally or by intramuscular injection)

Thiamine, also known as vitamin B_1 and aneurine, is essential for the utilisation of carbohydrates and the nutrition of nerve cells. It is present in egg, liver, yeast and wheat germ, but is now made synthetically. Severe deficiency results in beri-beri, a condition characterised by peripheral neuritis, cardiac enlargement, oedema and mental disturbances. Nausea and vomiting occur during the early stages of thiamine deficiency, and thus lead to further losses of the vitamin. Administration of thiamine in doses of 50 mg. or more results in a rapid improvement. Maintenance doses are about 3 mg.

Thiamine is also given in the treatment of the various manifestations of polyneuritis, in gastro-intestinal disorders, and during the administration of wide-range antibiotics. Large doses are given by injection, in association with other vitamins of the B group, in alcoholism and severe deficiency states.

Brand names: Benerva, Dibexin.

Brand names of B-complex products: Becosym, Becovite, Benerva Compound, Beplex, Parentrovite.

Riboflavine (dose : therapeutic, 5 to 10 mg. daily; prophylactic, 1 to 4 mg. daily)

Riboflavine, also known as vitamin B_1, resembles thiamine in being necessary for carbohydrate metabolism. Natural sources include yeast, liver and vegetables, but for therapeutic purposes it is now made synthetically.

Riboflavine deficiency results in a well-defined syndrome, characterised by cracking of the lips and of the skin at the corners of the mouth (angular stomatitis), photophobia and other visual disturbances. Response to oral treatment is usually adequate.

Brand name : Beflavit.

Nicotinic Acid (dose, therapeutic, 50 to 250 mg. daily; prophylactic, 15 to 30 mg. daily)

Nicotinic acid is present in liver, yeast, and unpolished rice but the synthetic compound is used medicinally. Lack of nicotinic acid results in the deficiency disease known as pellagra, characterised by diarrhoea, dermatitis and dementia. The diarrhoea is associated with stomatitis and a red and swollen tongue, and the dermatitis occurs on those parts of the body exposed to light. These symptoms, as well as the mental confusion, respond rapidly to nicotinic acid and associated vitamins. The drug is effective orally, but in severe conditions it may be given by injection.

Nicotinic acid also has vasodilatory properties, and has been used in Ménière's disease, peripheral vascular disorders and chilblains. In large doses it reduces blood cholesterol levels, and has been used in the treatment of hypercholesterolaemia, but the marked vasodilator effects are often beyond the patient's tolerance. Nicotinamide is closely related to nicotinic acid, and is used in pellagra and other deficiency states when the vasodilator action of the acid is not desired or proves an embarrassment. It has no value in lowering blood cholesterol. Ronicol is related to nicotinic acid and has a similar vasodilator action, but has no vitamin properties.

Pyridoxine (vitamin B_6) (dose, 50 to 150 mg. daily)

Pyridoxine is concerned with the metabolism of proteins, amino acids and fats. It is present in a wide variety of foods, and deficiency is uncommon. When it occurs, the symptoms resemble riboflavine deficiency. Deficiency in infants may cause convulsions, which can be treated by pyridoxine in doses of 4 mg. per kg. daily. Pyridoxine has been used empirically in the nausea of pregnancy, in irradiation sickness and alcoholism but not with marked success. *Brand name :* Benadon.

Pantothenic Acid

This substance occurs in all living cells, and is regarded as a part of the vitamin B complex. It has been used by injection in doses of 50 mg. or more in the treatment of paralytic ileus and by local application to stimulate the healing of bed-sores and ulcers. *Brand name :* Bepanthen.

Cyanocobalamin (vitamin B_{12})

Cyanocobalamin is the anti-anaemia factor, and its use in pernicious anaemia is discussed on page 158. It has also been used in doses of 1000 micrograms in the treatment of polyneuritis, trigeminal neuralgia and herpes zoster. *Brand names :* Bitevan, Cytamen.

Ascorbic Acid (vitamin C) (dose : therapeutic, 200 to 500 mg. daily; prophylactic, 25 to 75 mg. daily)

Vitamin C is the well-known water-soluble vitamin present in oranges and other citrus fruits, blackcurrants and green vegetables. It is essential for the development of collagen, cartilage and bone, and is concerned in haemoglobin formation and tissue repair. Deficiency of ascorbic acid, if severe, results in the once dreaded disease of scurvy, characterised by subcutaneous haemorrhages, bleeding of the gums and into the joints. The bleeding is due to capillary fragility, and results in anaemia and a reduced resistance to infection. Scurvy was once common on sailing ships with restricted supplies of fresh fruit and vegetables, but it is now rarely seen. Mild deficiency states may occur during pregnancy and in patients on restricted diets, and infantile scurvy may sometimes occur in bottle-fed infants. Vitamin C requirements are increased during infections and following trauma, and the drug has been given to promote wound healing.

Ascorbic acid is rapidly absorbed when given orally, and injections are rarely necessary unless the vitamin deficiency is marked or the patient is unable to tolerate oral treatment. *Brand name :* Redoxon.

Calciferol (vitamin D_2) (dose : therapeutic, 5000 to 50,000 units daily; prophylactic, not more than 800 units daily)

The term vitamin D includes several related substances, of which calciferol (vitamin D_2) is the most important. Vitamin D is found mainly in dairy products, although fish liver oils are a rich source, but calciferol is now prepared synthetically. It is an essential factor in the absorption of calcium and phosphorus from the gastro-intestinal tract, and thus in the formation of bone. Breast-fed infants, as well as those receiving proprietary milk products, (which usually contain added calciferol) normally receive an adequate supply of vitamin D. In children, a deficiency of calciferol results in rickets, a disease characterised by weak bones, bowed legs and deformities of the chest, and was once so common that it was known abroad as 'the English disease.' Calciferol is used in dietary deficiency states, and also used in certain other conditions associated with calcium absorption, as in coeliac disease, and in the low blood calcium due to parathyroid deficiency. It has also been used in the treatment of tuberculous infections of the skin such as lupus vulgaris, but for that purpose has been largely replaced by specific antitubercular drugs.

In general, the vitamins are well tolerated even in very large doses, but calciferol is the main exception, as toxic effects may follow the prolonged administration of high doses. Thirst, drowsiness and gastro-intestinal disturbances, which may be severe, are among the symptoms of overdosage, and continued administration may result in calcium deposition in the tissues, kidneys and arterial vessels, causing renal damage and hypertension. When high doses of calciferol are used the calcium blood level should be checked at regular intervals, and the drug withdrawn if the level rises much above 12 mg. per 100 ml. (standard level, 9 to 11). It should be noted that Calciferol Tablets B.N.F. are *strong* tablets, and contain 50,000 units. They are intended for the treatment of hypoparathyroidism and other unusual metabolic states, and not for dietary deficiency. *Brand name :* Sterogyl.

Dihydrotachysterol (dose, 0·125 to 1·25 mg. daily)

Although this compound is related to calciferol it has no significant antirachitic properties, but has a powerful influence on blood calcium levels. It is used mainly in parathyroid deficiency, as it increases the absorption of calcium and decreases the excretion of phosphates. The dose is related to the degree of calcium deficiency, and must be carefully adjusted to individual need. The drug is referred to in the section on parathyroid (*q.v.*). *Brand name :* A.T.10.

Tocopherol (dose, 3 to 200 mg.)

Tocopherol, also known as vitamin E, is present in wheat germ, soya-bean, lettuce and other green leaves, but the synthetic drug is referred to as tocopherol acetate.

The vitamin has some general action on the metabolism of fats, carbohydrates and proteins and deficiency results in a number of widely different manifestations. Tocopherol has been used empirically in large doses in a wide range of conditions, including muscular dystrophy, angina, Dupuytren's contracture, vascular disease and other unrelated conditions, but the results are very variable, and often disappointing. *Brand name :* Ephynal.

Mixed Vitamin Products

A very large number of mixed vitamin products are now available, often containing mineral supplements. These mixtures are mainly of value in the treatment of deficiencies due to restricted diets but have no ' tonic ' properties. A few are useful during the prenatal period, but their value in other conditions where full diets are available is problematical.

Polyvitamin Preparations—

Abecedin	Multivite
Abidec	Paladac
Aquavit	Parentrovite
Dayamin	

Vitamin Products containing Mineral Supplements—

Complevite	Minacedin
Geriplex	Minadex
Gevral	Pregnavite

Vitamin K

Vitamin K is an essential factor in the formation of pro-thrombin, and it is thus closely connected with the blood-clotting system. Lack of vitamin K leads to hypoprothrombinaemia, or deficiency of prothrombin, resulting in delayed clotting of the blood and, if severe, to spontaneous haemorrhage. The natural vitamin is fat-soluble, and bile is essential for its absorption. A deficiency may therefore arise, even during an adequate dietary intake, in such conditions as obstructive jaundice or coeliac disease. Deficiency may also occur during treatment with anticoagulants, which reduce vitamin K metabolism, and with antibacterial drugs which interfere with the formation of vitamin K by intestinal bacteria. Salicylates, clofibrate and phenylbutazone may also decrease the availability of vitamin K. Synthetic water-soluble compounds with a similar but more controllable action are now frequently used instead of the natural vitamin.

Menaphthone (dose, 5 to 10 mg. daily)

An oil-soluble compound with vitamin K activity, given by intramuscular injection as an oily solution in obstructive jaundice, biliary fistula and neonatal haemorrhage. A water-soluble form is also available as menaphthone sodium bisulphite.

Acetomenaphthone (dose, 5 to 20 mg.)

An orally effective derivative of menaphthone, and used for similar purposes. In neonatal haemorrhage, doses of 1 to 2 mg.

8

are used. In association with nicotinic acid or nicotinamide, it has been used for the relief of chilblains.

Water-soluble Analogues of Vitamin K

These compounds have the advantages of oral activity without the addition of bile salts, and by virtue of their solubility they can be given by intramuscular or intravenous injection. They are suitable for use in all conditions requiring vitamin K therapy. Vitamin K analogues are also given in small doses to new-born infants to prevent neonatal haemorrhage. For the treatment of hypoprothrombinaemia following the use of phenindione and other synthetic anticoagulants, phytomenadione (q.v.) is preferred, as it has a more rapid action. It is of interest that one compound (Synkavit) has been used as a ' radiosensitiser.' It appears to be absorbed selectively by certain cancerous tissues, and to render them more susceptible to X-ray therapy. *Brand name:* Synkavit.

Phytomenadione (dose, 5 to 20 mg. orally, or by slow intravenous injection)

Phytomenadione is a natural form of vitamin K, and is also referred to as vitamin K_1. Its physiological action function is to maintain a normal level of prothrombin in the blood, but therapeutically it is used almost exclusively to counteract the haemorrhage that may occur during oral anticoagulant therapy. (It is not an antidote to heparin.) In such cases, phytomenadione acts more rapidly than the water-soluble synthetic drugs, and the action is more prolonged.

In severe haemorrhage, doses of 20 mg. may be given by slow intravenous injection. The action is prompt, as a rise in prothrombin levels and a reduction in clotting time may occur within fifteen minutes. The prothrombin level should be determined three hours later, and subsequent doses adjusted according to need. For less severe conditions, phytomenadione may be given orally in doses of 10 mg., or by intramuscular injection. In the prophylactic treatment of neonatal haemorrhagic disorders, the drug may be given to the mother by intramuscular injection in doses of 0·5 to 2 mg. before delivery. *Brand names:* Aquamephyton, Konakion.

CHAPTER XV

ANTHELMINTICS AND ANTIMALARIALS

AND DRUGS USED IN TROPICAL DISEASES

Worms and Anthelmintics

The worms which have selected man as their unwilling host rarely cause severe disease, but they can cause a great amount of chronic ill health, and are therefore of considerable economic importance. Infestation with parasitic worms is the most common disease in the world, and even when adequate medication is available, social conditions in some areas are such that reinfestation is almost impossible to prevent.

Human parasitic helminths or worms can be classified thus :—

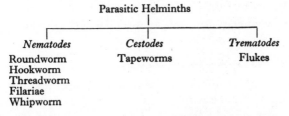

```
                        Parasitic Helminths
                               |
        ┌──────────────────────┼──────────────────────┐
    Nematodes                Cestodes              Trematodes
    Roundworm               Tapeworms                Flukes
    Hookworm
    Threadworm
    Filariae
    Whipworm
```

The life cycle of many of these parasites is very complex, and an intermediate host may be involved before development from egg to mature worm can occur.

Roundworms (*Ascaris lumbricoides*)

The adult worms are some 6 to 14 in. long, and are usually found in the small intestine. The females discharge enormous numbers of eggs, estimated at 200,000 daily, which are excreted in the faeces. Development occurs if the eggs are ingested by eating contaminated food, and larvae, about 0·25 mm. long, are released in the small intestine. They penetrate the intestinal wall, pass into the liver, and make their way to the lungs. A further stage in development then takes place and later the still immature worms reach the oesophagus, are swallowed, and develop into adult worms in the small intestine. *Strongyloides* is a small worm found in the mucosa of the upper small intestine. It causes abdominal disturbance, but may also give rise to pulmonary symptoms.

Hookworms (*Ancylostoma duodenale, Necator americanus*)

These small round worms are about $\frac{1}{2}$ in. long, and gain access to the body by penetrating the skin as larvae. They enter the veins, reach the lungs, pass into the bronchi, and eventually migrate to the alimentary tract. There they attach themselves, and feed on the blood of the host, eventually causing a severe secondary anaemia and general debility. The larvae also cause a local reaction during their penetration of the skin.

Threadworms (*Oxyuris vermicularis*)

The commonest intestinal worm, usually found in the caecum. The adult females are 8 to 13 mm. in length, and emerge from the anus to lay eggs on the adjacent skin. This causes an intense itching, with consequent scratching, and the infestation is maintained by transference of the eggs to the mouth by the fingers. A high degree of social cleanliness is an essential part of treatment.

Whipworm (*Trichocephalus trichiuris*)

This worm is common in warm humid countries, and is often associated with hookworm. It is usually found in the caecum ; eggs are passed in the faeces, and develop in the soil, and infestation occurs from contaminated food and water. The symptoms are often mild, but occasionally the worms penetrate the bowel wall, and cause peritonitis.

Filariae

These parasites are the cause of elephantiasis. That tropical disease is characterised by hypertrophy of the cellular tissues, and the legs in particular may attain a diameter of 12 in. or more. The hypertrophy is due to blocking of the lymphatic vessels by the adult worms, which are 3 to 4 in. in length. The females produce embryonic worms, which migrate to the peripheral vessels, where they are picked up by mosquitoes. When the insect bites another host at a later stage these immature parasites are released into the blood of the new victim where full development takes place.

Tapeworms

The most common are the beef tapeworm (*Taenia saginata*) and the pig tapeworm (*Taenia solium*), and infestation usually arises from eating undercooked meat containing the larva of the worm. The adult tapeworm, which develops in the intestines, is a segmented ribbon-like organism that may be several feet in length in the case of *T. saginata*, but the pork tapeworm is much smaller, being only some 2 ft. in length. The small head is firmly attached to the intestinal mucosa, and separation of the body from the head by an anthelmintic merely leads to regeneration of the worm.

Hydatid disease is due to the presence in the body of larval cysts of a tapeworm found in dogs. The larvae do not develop into worms, but the cysts may increase considerably in size, and cause symptoms suggestive of liver abscess and tuberculosis.

Flukes

Flukes are non-segmented flatworms, and the most important are the blood flukes, common in Egypt and some parts of Asia, and the cause of bilharzia or schistosomiasis. The adult flukes are found in the portal vein, and spined eggs are laid in the mesenteric and pelvic veins. The spines of the eggs damage the walls of the vein, which eventually ulcerates, and the eggs reach the bladder or intestines, and are excreted. The larval forms can only undergo further development in the body of a suitable snail, so the disease is restricted to those areas in which such snails are found. A free-swimming form of the parasite is liberated from the snail, and this organism can penetrate the skin of the human host, enter the blood stream, and eventually mature. Schistosomiasis may therefore be acquired by bathing in infected water.

ANTHELMINTICS

The types of substances used as anthelmintics show as great a diversity of structure as the parasites, as they include plant extracts and organic chemicals. In recent years new and more specific compounds have been introduced, and the treatment of worm infestation is now much more effective and reliable, although the problem of mass treatment to eradicate the parasites remains to be solved.

Antimony Lithium Thiomalate †

Antimony lithium thiomalate has the general action of antimony sodium tartrate (*q.v.*), but is less irritant to the tissues, and so can be given by intramuscular injection, and is less liable to cause coughing and vomiting. The standard dose is 1 ml. of a 6 per cent solution, given by intramuscular injection, gradually increased to 4 ml., and continued at that level with injections on alternate days until a total dose of 40 to 60 ml. has been given. *Brand name :* Anthiomaline.†

Antimony Sodium Tartrate † (dose, 30 to 120 mg.)

This soluble antimony compound when injected intravenously has a direct toxic action on the blood flukes causing schistosomiasis (and also on the protozoa causing leishmaniasis or kala-azar). A standard dosage scheme is the initial injection of 60 mg. as a 1 to 2 per cent. solution, followed at three-day intervals by doses of 90 mg. and 120 mg., and continued at that level until a minimum total dose of 1·2 G. has been given. Alternatively, an intensive course of four doses of 120 mg. at intervals of four hours may be given, but the method is not without risk. Toxic effects include nausea, collapse and convulsions. Antimony potassium tartrate is given by intravenous injection only, as intramuscular injections are painful and may cause necrosis, and oral therapy is impracticable as the drug is a gastric irritant and causes emesis.

Bephenium Hydroxynaphthoate (dose, 5 G.)

Bephenium is mainly effective against hookworms in the intestinal tract, although it is also active against roundworms. It is considered to be more effective than tetrachloroethylene, and is better tolerated. The drug is available as dispersable granules, and is given as a single dose of 5 G. on an empty stomach. *Brand name :* Alcopar.

Dichlorophen (dose, 6 G.)

Dichlorophen is used in the treatment of infestation by the beef tapeworm, *Taenia saginata*, and unlike the older remedies, it has a direct toxic action on the worm so that no previous purging or other preparation of the patient is necessary. The average adult dose is 6 G. daily for two days. Children should be given doses of 2 to 4 G., which may be given either as a single dose or in three divided doses at eight-hourly intervals, Divided doses ensure a longer contact of the drug with the parasite. Nausea and colic may occasionally occur with dichlorophen.

Following the administration of dichlorophen, the worms are killed and then disorganised by digestive action so that they are not eliminated in a recognisable form as with other anthelmintics. No search for the head or scolex is necessary, and the criterion of cure is the absence of segments of the worm in the stools after an interval of sixteen weeks. Should the scolex survive, the beef tapeworm grows to the point at which segments are again passed in the stools within about twelve weeks, and their continued absence is regarded as an adequate indication of successful treatment. *Brand name :* Anthiphen.

Diethylcarbamazine Citrate (dose, 150 to 500 mg. daily)

Diethylcarbamazine is one of the few compounds effective in the treatment of the various manifestations of filariasis. The drug is effective orally, and a standard dose is 4 to 6 mg. per kg. body-weight daily in divided doses for three to four weeks. Following the death of the organisms and their breakdown in the body some of their proteins are released and may cause allergic reactions. Such side-effects may be controlled by the administration of antihistamines and their incidence reduced by the use of small doses of the drug during the early stages of treatment. *Brand names :* Banocide, Hetrazan.

Hexylresorcinol (dose, 1 G.)

Hexylresorcinol, originally introduced as an antiseptic, is a wide-range anthelmintic, effective against hookworm, dwarf tapeworm, intestinal flukes, roundworm and threadworm. The average adult dose is 1 G. as a single dose ; children under 10 years, 100 mg. per year of age. This dose is followed by a saline purge. In hookworm and dwarf tapeworm infestation treatment should be repeated at intervals of three days. Other anthelmintics are now preferred for the removal of round worms and threadworms. Hexylresorcinol is well tolerated, but has an irritant effect on the oral mucosa, and should be given as enteric-coated tablets or capsules.

Lucanthone (dose, 0·5 to 1 G.)

Unlike other drugs used in schistosomiasis, lucanthone is a purely organic compound, and does not contain antimony. Although not equally effective against all varieties of blood flukes (it is of little value against *S. japonicum*), it has the great advantage of being active when given orally. It is therefore very suitable for the mass treatment of infected communities. The standard intensive dosage scheme is 1 G. twice daily for three days, but lower doses of 500 mg. may be given daily for twenty days. *Brand name :* Nilodin.

Male Fern

An extract of the underground parts of the male fern (*Filix mas*) has long been the standard remedy for tapeworm. The extract is a thick dark-green liquid with an unpleasant taste, and may be given as an emulsion with water as Male Fern Extract Draught (B.N.F.). The extract does not kill the worm but loosens its hold on the intestinal mucosa, so that it may be removed by subsequent purging.

Removal of the head of the worm is essential, as otherwise it will grow again, no matter how many segments of the worm may have been eliminated during treatment. Following preliminary fasting and purging, a single dose of 3 to 6 ml. of the extract is given, followed in two to four hours by another saline purge. A search should be made for the head of the worm and, if not found, treatment should be repeated after an interval of some weeks. Saline purges are an essential part of the treatment. Castor oil should not be used as it promotes absorption of the male fern extract, and toxic effects such as visual disturbances and jaundice may result. The use of male fern has declined as more reliable synthetic anthelmintics have become available.

Mepacrine (dose, 1 G.)

This antimalarial drug is effective in removing tapeworms and is a useful alternative to other forms of treatment. After preliminary purging, doses of 100 to 200 mg. as an aqueous suspension are given at five-minute intervals up to a total dose of 1 G. Two hours later a saline purge is given. The drug has a very bitter taste, and when given as a suspension may cause nausea. This effect may be minimised by premedication with chlorpromazine, or alternatively, the suspension may be given by duodenal tube.

Niclosamide (dose, 2 G.)

This compound is effective against the beef, pork, fish and dwarf tapeworms and, like dichlorophen, has a rapid killing action on the parasites. The average adult dose is 1 G., taken on an empty stomach, followed by a similar dose after one hour. Proportionate doses may be given to children. A purge may be given later if required. As with dichlorophen, the killed worms disintegrate, and there is no immediate proof of cure. The drug is well tolerated, and side-effects are not common. *Brand name :* Yomesan.

Niridazole (dose, 25 mg. per kg. daily)

Niridazole is a synthetic drug, unrelated to other anthelmintics, and is now considered the treatment of choice in schistosomiasis. It is given orally in a dose of 25 mg. per kg. daily (in two doses) for seven days. Side-effects include gastro-intestinal disturbance and skin reactions. *Brand name :* Ambilhar.

Piperazine (dose, 1 to 4·5 G.)

Piperazine is effective in the expulsion of both roundworm and threadworm, and is now the standard treatment. For the treatment of roundworm infestation in adults a single dose of 4·5 G. is given ; children's doses are relatively large, and a dose of 120 mg. per kilogram body-weight may be given up to a maximum of 4 G. The drug paralyses the worms, and they are removed by the peristaltic movements of the intestines and excreted in the faeces. As the worms are not killed, a purge may be necessary to ensure expulsion before the effects of the drug wear off.

In threadworm infestation a course of treatment for one week is given. Adults may be given doses of 1 to 2 G. daily in divided doses ; children 4 to 6 years half doses, and infants 9 to 24 months quarter doses. A second course may be given if required after the interval of a week. Threadworm infestation is easily spread, and it may be necessary to treat all members of a family at the same time to ensure eradication. Piperazine is well tolerated, but some giddiness may be experienced by a few patients on full doses. Proprietary preparations may contain piperazine adipate, citrate, phosphate or other derivative, and one product (Pripsen) is issued as granules containing senna extract, thus providing the anthelmintic and purge in a single preparation. *Brand names :* Antepar, Entacyl, Pripsen.

Stibophen Injection † (dose, 1·5 to 5 ml.)

Stibophen is a less toxic alternative to antimony sodium tartrate and is given by injection as a 6·4 per cent. solution. It is effective in schistosomiasis mainly against *S. haematobium*, and is given in doses of 5 ml. by intravenous or intramuscular injection to a total dose of 40 to 75 ml.

Tetrachloroethylene (dose, 1 to 3 ml.)

A clear colourless liquid with a characteristic odour, and is an effective anthelmintic for hookworm infestation. It is given as a single dose of 3 ml. on an empty stomach, either as capsules, mixture, or occasionally by duodenal tube. A saline purge should be given after two to three hours. Tetrachloroethylene has some toxic action on the liver, and a high-protein, high-carbohydrate diet should precede treatment. Children's doses can be calculated on the basis of 0·2 ml. per year of age up to a dose of 3 ml. When mass treatment is attempted, both drug and purge should be given together.

Thiabendazole (dose, 50 mg. per kg.)

Thiabendazole is a newer compound, mainly effective against *Strongloides*, but also active against roundworms, threadworms and hookworms. It is given in doses of 25 mg. per kg. in the evening, followed by a similar dose next morning after breakfast. If the infestation is severe, treatment should be continued for two or three days, or longer as required. Large single doses are often effective, but side-effects such as dizziness and diarrhoea are correspondingly severe. *Brand name :* Mintezol.

Viprynium (dose, 5 mg. per kg. body-weight)

Viprynium is a single-dose anthelmintic, highly effective in threadworm infestation. The drug is not absorbed to any extent when given orally, and in general is well tolerated, although occasionally it causes gastro-intestinal disturbance. Chemically it is a cyanine dye, and stains the faeces red. It is suitable for administration to infants as well as adults, and the single-dose treatment has considerable advantages when treating all the members of a family. If necessary, a second dose may be given after an interval of two to three weeks. *Brand name :* Vanquin.

ANTIMALARIALS AND OTHER DRUGS USED IN TROPICAL DISEASES

Those who live in temperate climates often find it difficult to realise that malaria is one of the greatest killing diseases in the world, and is responsible for more than a million deaths annually. Malaria was once rarely seen outside tropical and subtropical countries, but it is now met with more frequently as a direct consequence of high-speed travel from infected areas.

Malaria is a febrile disease, due to the presence in the blood of one or more species of the protozoal organism *Plasmodium.* These organisms are transferred to the unfortunate human victim by the bites of infected female mosquitoes of the genus Anopheles. The forms of the parasite present in the salivary glands of the mosquito, and injected into the host, are termed sporozoites. These organisms migrate to the liver and other tissues where they undergo further development, and during this initial period of the disease the parasites are rarely found in the blood. The liver or tissue stage of development is known as the exo-erythrocyte stage.

After a few days the organisms leave the tissues and enter into the red cells of the blood. Here they increase in number by division to form merozoites, and when division is complete and the cell nutrient is exhausted the cells burst, and the merozoites are set free to infect other red cells and so repeat the process. When the number of infected red cells approaches about 250 million or more, this bursting of the red cells and release of the merozoites results in the rise in temperature, rigor and sweating which characterise a malarial attack.

While this development in the erythrocytes is taking place some of the merozoites develop into the sexual forms (gametocytes). These gametocytes circulate in the blood, and if drawn up by an anopheline mosquito in the act of biting, develop in the stomach of the insect, and finally form more sporozoites. These in turn migrate to the salivary glands of the mosquito, ready to be passed on to another victim.

Three main varieties of the parasite are commonly associated with malaria, and they are differentiated mainly by the time taken for development and release of the merozoites in sufficient numbers to cause a malarial attack. The varieties are :—

Plasmodium vivax, which takes about forty-eight hours to develop, and causes benign tertian malaria.

Plasmodium falciparum, which also develops in about forty-eight hours and causes malignant tertian malaria.

Plasmodium malariae, which takes about seventy-two hours to develop, and causes quartan malaria.

The first two are the most common.

The diagram below indicates the general outline of the life cycle of the malarial parasites, and the points of attack of various drugs.

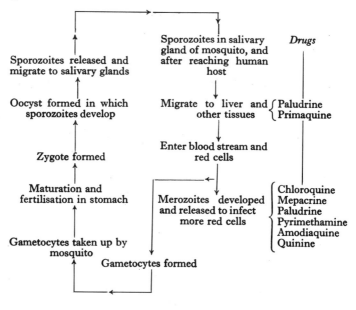

No drug has yet been found that will kill the sporozoites as injected by the mosquito, and treatment and prophylaxis must be directed against the organisms at a later stage of development. Drugs which act upon the parasites in the red blood cells are known as schizontocides, and those that attack the organisms in the tissues are referred to as tissue schizontocides. The following drugs are of therapeutic importance, and are divided into two groups—those used mainly in the treatment of an acute attack of malaria, and those used both to suppress attacks and for prophylaxis. Some drugs have properties common to both groups.

Amodiaquine (dose, 400 to 600 mg.)

Amodiaquine is an antimalarial compound resembling chloroquine in action and general properties. For treatment of acute attacks of both forms of tertian malaria an initial dose of 600 mg. may be given, followed by 400 mg. daily for two days. It also has a powerful suppressant action, and for prophylaxis a weekly dose of 400 mg. is adequate. Toxic side-effects are not common, although transient nausea may occur. Very prolonged treatment may cause corneal deposits. *Brand name :* Camoquin.

Chloroquine (dose, 300 to 600 mg.)

Chloroquine, available as phosphate or sulphate, is one of the most effective drugs used in the suppression and treatment of malaria. It is rapidly absorbed when given orally, and in general is well tolerated. In the treatment of an attack, an initial dose of 600 mg. is given, followed by doses of 300 mg. daily up to a total of about 1·5 G. Chloroquine is effective against all the erythrocytic forms of the parasite at every stage of development, with the exception of the gametocytes. These organisms, however, play no part in the malarial attack, and from the treatment point of view are of no significance. Adequate doses of chloroquine will cure malignant tertian malaria, as in that form of the disease all the organisms leave the tissues to enter the blood and so become vulnerable to attack. In the other forms of malaria there is a further release of sporozoites from the liver and tissues at intervals, so that relapses will occur unless suppressive treatment is given. For such suppression chloroquine may be given in doses of 300 mg. weekly, but pyrimethamine (*q.v.*) is often preferred. Resistance to chloroquine is not unknown and may become an increasing problem. Chloroquine is usually well tolerated, apart from occasional gastrointestinal disturbance and pruritus, but full and extended treatment may cause corneal opacity and changes in pigmentation. The drug is also useful in amoebic abscess and amoebic hepatitis.

It should be noted that malignant tertian malaria is so called because the attacks may take a fulminating and rapidly fatal course.

This complication is due to the obstruction of the small blood vessels, notably those of the brain, by merozoite-containing blood cells. In such circumstances chloroquine may be given by slow intravenous drip infusion in doses of 200 to 300 mg., repeated after eight hours. Intramuscular injections are also effective. Quinine dihydrochloride (*q.v.*) may also be given intravenously in the treatment of cerebral malaria. *Brand names :* Avloclor, Nivaquine, Resochin.

Mepacrine (dose, 100 to 500 mg. daily)

Mepacrine was once the most widely used of the synthetic antimalarials, but less toxic alternatives are now preferred. It is effective against the merozoites, and also against the gametocytes of *Plasmodium vivax* and *P. malariae*. In suppressive treatment of relapses in *P. vivax* infection, doses of 100 mg. daily for prolonged periods may be given. Occasionally such long treatment may cause anaemia, a yellow coloration of the skin and psychosis. For the curative treatment of an attack of malaria, mepacrine is given in doses of 300 mg. three times a day for one day, 300 mg. twice a day on the second day, with maintenance doses of 100 mg. daily for five days. *Brand name :* Quinacrine.

Primaquine (dose, 15 to 60 mg.)

Primaquine differs from most other antimalarials in acting upon the sporozoites in the liver and tissues, and on the gametocytes. It has little action on the erythrocytic forms of the parasites, and so is of no value alone in the treatment of acute malaria, but given after a course of chloroquine, which kills off the erythrocytic stages, primaquine will eradicate the remaining malarial parasites, particularly *P. vivax*. It is thus of value in the definitive treatment (radical cure) of malaria in those people returning from infected areas, who are unlikely to be exposed to the risk of further infection. The dose for such patients is 15 mg. of primaquine daily for two weeks, after a standard course of chloroquine.

Quinine (dose, 60 to 600 mg.)

Quinine is an alkaloid obtained from cinchona bark, and is of historical interest as the first effective drug for the treatment of malaria. It suppresses the development of the malarial parasites in the blood, but has no action against those in the tissues. It has now been replaced almost entirely by the synthetic antimalarials, but the emergence of malarial parasites resistant to the synthetic drugs may cause a return to quinine in some areas. It is occasionally used by intravenous injection in fulminating and cerebral malaria in doses of 600 mg. as quinine dihydrochloride.

SUPPRESSIVE TREATMENT

In areas where malaria is common, reinfection may occur so easily after treatment that the prolonged use of a drug that will prevent the development of the disease is essential. Chloroquine and amodiaquine, already described, and used mainly in the treatment of malarial attacks, are also used as suppressive agents in single weekly doses of 300 to 400 mg., but the most useful prophylactic drugs are proguanil and pyrimethamine.

Chlorproguanil (dose, 20 mg. weekly)

Chlorproguanil is an antimalarial compound with the general properties of proguanil, but it is more powerful, and has a much longer duration of action. This increased potency is reflected in the low dose of 20 mg. weekly, which should be continued for three weeks after exposure to the risk of malaria has ceased. *Brand name :* Lapudrine.

Proguanil (dose, 100 to 300 mg. daily)

Proguanil inhibits the development of the malarial parasites at several points, but in practice this action is too slow to be of value in the treatment of malarial attacks. Conversely, this slow action is of great advantage in suppressive treatment, and a daily dose of 100 mg. will confer immunity on susceptible patients. Regular dosing is essential, as both *P. falciparum* and *P. vivax* may acquire a resistance to the drug if inadequate doses are given. *Brand name :* Paludrine.

Pyrimethamine (dose, 25 to 50 mg. weekly)

Pyrimethamine resembles proguanil in general properties, but is more effective. A weekly dose of 25 mg. gives protection against all three varieties of *Plasmodium*, and it is one of the best drugs available for the mass control of malaria. Regular administration is essential, but side-effects are few and slight. Pyrimethamine is also suitable for children. Those under 5 years can be given a weekly dose of 6·25 mg., those from 5 to 15 years can be protected by 12·5 mg. weekly. Pyrimethamine does not kill the gametocytes, but it inhibits their growth, and they do not develop normally in the mosquito. Combined treatment with chloroquine is sometimes used to prevent the emergence of resistant strains of the parasites, and a mixture of pyrimethamine and chloroquine is available as Daraclor. *Brand name :* Daraprim.

TRYPANOSOMIASIS

This disease, also known as African sleeping sickness, is due to the presence in the blood of a flagellate parasite, either *Trypanosoma gambiense*, or *T. rhodesiense*. These parasites are transmitted from infected animals by the bite of the tsetse fly. In the early stages of the disease the organisms are mainly present in the blood, but later they penetrate into the lymphatic and cerebrospinal fluids and into the brain and other organs. The disease is characterised by a prolonged intermittent febrile condition, followed by a slow progressive mental and physical deterioration, ending in coma and death. The range of effective drugs is very limited, and early treatment is necessary.

Pentamidine Isethionate (dose, 150 to 300 mg. daily)

This organic chemical is effective in the early stages of trypanosomiasis, but as it cannot cross the blood-brain barrier it is of much less value once the central nervous system has been invaded by the parasites. It is given by intramuscular or intravenous injection in doses of 300 mg. daily or on alternate days, up to a total of ten injections. The course is repeated after a rest period of some weeks. For prophylaxis, a dose of 300 mg. may be given every three months. The intramuscular injection is painful, but is the preferred method, as intravenous injection may cause temporary hypotension, nausea and dizziness.

Suramin (dose, 1 to 2 G. weekly)

Suramin resembles pentamidine in general purposes, and is most effective in the earlier stages of trypanosomiasis. The average dose is 1 G. by intravenous injection at weekly intervals for five weeks. In the later stages of the disease it may be used in association with tryparsamide (*q.v.*). Suramin may cause vomiting and paraesthesia, and tolerance should be checked by a preliminary dose of 500 mg. *Brand name :* Antrypol.

Tryparsamide † (dose, 1 to 3 G. weekly)

Tryparsamide differs chemically from both pentamidine and suramin, as it is an organic arsenical compound, and contains 25 per cent. of arsenic. It is effective in the treatment of the late stages of the disease, as it penetrates easily into the nervous tissues, and is therefore of great value when the central nervous system is involved. Tryparsamide is given by intravenous injection at weekly intervals for some weeks, and is usually well tolerated. Some disturbances of vision may occur even with low therapeutic doses, and the drug should then be withdrawn.

Tryparsamide is sometimes used in association with pentamidine or suramin in the early stages of trypanosomiasis, in order to prevent any subsequent involvement of the central nervous system.

Melarsoprol † (dose, 3·6 mg. per kg. body weight daily)

Melarsoprol is an arsenic-derived trypanocide used mainly in patients who have become resistant to tryparsamide and where the parasites have invaded the C.S.F. The drug is given by intravenous injection daily for three days, repeated after a rest period of ten days. The injection solution is very irritant to the perivenous tissues. Side-effects are common, and may exhibit as pyrexia due to death of the parasites, or as reactive encephalopathy.

AMOEBIC DYSENTERY

This disease, also known as amoebiasis, is due to the presence in the intestines of the protozoal organism *Entamoeba histolytica.* The disease is usually acquired by the ingestion of food or fluids contaminated with amoebic cysts, and can be spread by symptomless human carriers. The cysts escape digestion in the stomach, but develop in the intestines and release active amoebae. These penetrate the mucosa of the lower intestines and set up an ulceration and chronic diarrhoea. In severe conditions large areas of the bowel become ulcerated, with consequent bleeding and sloughing of tissues. Amoebic dysentery is often complicated by a secondary bacterial infection. In some patients the disease runs a mild course, with apparent recovery. Some of these patients still harbour the cysts, and may transmit the disease to others, and are referred to as ' carriers.' Occasionally some organisms reach the liver, and may cause amoebic hepatitis. In such cases chloroquine (*q.v.*) may be given in doses of 300 mg. twice a day for two days, followed by doses of 300 mg. daily for one to two weeks.

Emetine † (dose, 30 to 60 mg.)

Emetine is the principal alkaloid of ipecacuanha, and is the standard drug in the treatment of acute amoebiasis. Emetine has an emetic action when taken orally, and for systemic use it must be given by injection as emetine hydrochloride. Following the subcutaneous or intramuscular injection of doses of 60 mg. daily for not more than ten days, relief of symptoms is rapid, and motile amoebae and cysts disappear from the faeces. Bed rest is necessary during treatment, as the drug has toxic effects on the heart. Complete cure, however, is not common with emetine alone, as many patients continue to pass cysts after symptoms have been relieved, and they are then a potential danger as carriers of the disease. Subsequent treatment with an organic arsenic compound such as carbarsone † (250 mg. twice daily for ten days) is usually necessary to eradicate the disease. Secondary bacterial infection of amoebic ulcers should be treated with one of the poorly absorbed sulphonamides.

Emetine hydrochloride has also been used in the treatment of amoebic hepatitis and amoebic abscess. In the latter, weak solutions (0·04 to 0·1 per cent.) are used for irrigation after the aspiration of pus, in addition to the systemic injections of the drug. (Emetine should never be injected intravenously, as it may cause dangerous cardiac arrhythmia.)

Emetine Bismuth Iodide † (dose, 60 to 200 mg, daily)

This red compound is an insoluble form of emetine, but is broken down in the intestines to release free emetine. It is used to supplement the action of injected emetine hydrochloride, but the side-effects, including nausea and vomiting, limit its usefulness, and other orally effective amoebicides are often preferred.

Diloxanide Furoate (dose, 1·5 G. daily)

Diloxanide furoate has a specific action against *E. histolytica*, and is effective in the treatment of acute intestinal amoebiasis and in the control of cyst-passing carriers of the disease. The drug is well tolerated and no special precautions during treatment, such as bed rest, are necessary. The standard adult dose is 0·5 G. three times a day for ten days, and the reduced toxicity makes the drug suitable for the treatment of ambulant patients. In conjunction with chloroquine, it is also of value in hepatic amoebiasis. It has no antibacterial properties, and supplementary treatment is necessary in mixed infections. *Brand name :* Furamide.

Metronidazole (dose, 1 to 2 G. daily)

Metronidazole, originally introduced for trichomonas infections of the genito-urinary tract, is also of value in amoebic dysentery. In severe conditions it is given in doses of 800 mg. three times a day for five days; in milder conditions, and for symptom-less carriers of the disease, doses of 400 mg. three times a day may be adequate. *Brand name :* Flagyl.

Paromomycin † (dose, 250 mg.)

Paromomycin is an antibiotic effective against *E. histolytica* and a number of organisms associated with enteric infection. It is not absorbed to any extent when given orally, and high concentrations in the intestinal tract are easily achieved and maintained. The dose of paromomycin depends to some extent on the severity of the infection to be treated. In amoebiasis a dose of 25 to 100 mg. per kg. body weight is given daily in divided doses, an average adult dose being 250 mg. four times a day for five to six days. Larger doses are given in acute intestinal bacterial infections. As paromomycin is not absorbed, it is of no value in hepatic or tissue amoebiasis. *Brand name:* Humatin.†

Other drugs used in the treatment of amoebiasis are represented by carbarsone (Leucarsone), di-iodohydroxy-quinoline (Diodoquin, Embequin) and phanquone (Entobex).

LEISHMANIASIS

This disease, also known as kala-azar, occurs in Africa, China, India and some Mediterranean countries. It is due to protozoal organisms such as *Leishmania donovani*, which enter the blood stream and later become localised in the spleen, bone marrow, liver and other organs. The condition is characterised by an irregular but recurrent fever, enlarged liver and spleen, anaemia and other constitutional disturbances. Therapy includes the administration of organic antimony compounds and pentamidine.

Sodium Stibogluconate † (dose, 0·6 to 2 G.)

This compound contains about 33 per cent. of antimony and is given by intravenous or intramuscular injection as a 30 per cent. solution in doses of 6 ml. daily for six days. A further course may be given after a rest period. Some forms of kala-azar are resistant to antimony compounds, but may respond to pentamidine isethionate (*q.v.*) which is used in the treatment of trypanosomiasis.

CHAPTER XVI

TISSUE FLUIDS AND ELECTROLYTE BALANCE

THE metabolic processes of the body can only function normally when adequate supplies of tissue fluids of suitable constitution are available. In health, the composition of the plasma and cell fluids is controlled by the kidneys within very narrow limits, and this control is capable of dealing with very variable physiological demands.

Some 70 per cent. of the body weight consists of water and dissolved electrolytes. Electrolytes are metallic salts which dissociate in solution to form ions, which may be positively or negatively charged. The principal electrolytes of the body are sodium, potassium, calcium and magnesium, present as chlorides, bicarbonates, sulphates and phosphates. In solution the metals or bases form positively charged ions or cations, and the non-metallic radicals form negatively charged anions.

Of the body water, some 40 to 50 per cent. exists within the cells, and is termed intracellular fluid ; the balance, which is present in the blood, lymph and tissue spaces, is termed extracellular fluid. The electrolyte composition of these fluids varies, as the intracellular fluid contains most of the potassium and phosphate, whereas the extracellular fluid contains the bulk of the sodium and bicarbonate. Normally, there is a dynamic balance between the concentration of the ions in these fluids, but this balance can be seriously disturbed by any severe loss of water and electrolytes. Loss of mineral salts is more serious than loss of water, which can be replaced easily. Thus prolonged vomiting causes a loss of chloride, potassium and sodium as well as water. Diarrhoea results in a loss of water and bicarbonates.

In an attempt to maintain the electrolyte balance of the body in such conditions, marked changes in the relative proportions of the intracellular and extracellular water may occur. Water may leave the subcutaneous tissues and large amounts of dilute urine may be excreted in order to maintain the concentration of remaining electrolytes. In severe conditions such as diabetic coma this excretion of electrolytes, especially potassium, may lead to respiratory and circulatory collapse, and rapid restoration of the fluid and electrolyte balance are essential therapeutic measures.

Ideally, the composition of the replacement fluid should be based on the actual degree and nature of the electrolyte disturbance. This is not always easy to achieve, and for a long time reliance was placed on a determination of the amount of urinary chlorides as an indication of the degree of imbalance. The introduction of the flame photometer, which permits a rapid and accurate estimation of the blood electrolytes to be made, has placed electrolyte therapy on a more rational basis, and replacement treatment can now be related to the actual degree of electrolyte deficiency.

At the same time a number of standard electrolyte replacement solutions are in use, designed to correct a number of common deficiency conditions. Such products include Darrow's, Hartmann's, Le Quesne's and Nabarro's solutions (named after their originators), and solutions of sodium lactate and bicarbonate. The latter are of particular value in acidosis, where chlorides are already in excess and alkali is particularly required.

The composition of these replacement solutions, once expressed in percentages, is now expressed to an increasing extent in terms of milliequivalents per litre (mEq./litre).

This term, although confusing at first, is basically much more illuminating than strengths expressed in the more familiar percentage notation.

As already indicated, there must be a balance between the cations and anions of the body fluids, and in cases of imbalance the replacement fluid should help to restore the balance. In a simple deficiency normal saline may be given, which is itself a balanced solution. It contains 0·9 per cent. of sodium chloride (NaCl) or 9000 mg. per litre. The molecular weight of sodium chloride is 58·5 (Na=23, Cl=35·5) and normal saline contains $\frac{9000 \times 23}{58 \cdot 5}$ =3540 mg. Na per litre, balanced by 5460 mg. Cl. The ionic balance between the amounts of these two constituents is, however, very far from clear, but becomes obvious when milliequivalent terms are used. In this system, amounts are expressed as milligramme equivalents of the molecular weight per litre. Thus the molecular weight of sodium is 23 ; that of chlorine is 35·5 ; therefore a milliequivalent solution of sodium contains 23 mg. per litre. As normal saline contains 3540 mg. of sodium per litre, it also contains $\frac{3540}{23} = 155$ milliequivalents (mEq.) of sodium per litre. Similarly, normal saline contains $\frac{5460}{35 \cdot 5} = 155$ mEq. of chloride per litre, and the ionic balance becomes clear. A further example is the approximate composition of the plasma expressed both in terms of weight and as milliequivalents :—

	Mg./100 ml.	mEq./litre
Sodium . . .	330	142 ⎫
Potassium . . .	15	5 ⎪ 155
Calcium . . .	10	5 ⎬
Magnesium . .	2·5	3 ⎭
Chloride . . .	360	103 ⎫
Bicarbonate . .	150	28 ⎪ 155
Phosphate . . .	3·5	6 ⎬
Protein, etc. . .	...	18 ⎭

The following are the milliequivalent strengths of some solutions used in the treatment of electrolyte disturbances :—

Constituents	Darrow's Solution	Hartmann's Solution	Nabarro's Solution	1/6 Molar Sodium Lactate
Sodium . .	123	124	20	166
Potassium . .	35	5·2	30	...
Calcium . .	...	3·6	...	...
Magnesium . .	...	...	5	...
Chloride . .	105	110	45	...
Phosphate . .	...	...	10	...
Lactate . .	53	22	...	166

Considerable care must be taken in the preparation of all intravenous drip injections, as well as in the speed and rate of administration, if reactions are to be avoided. The water used must be freshly distilled, and the solution must be prepared and sterilised within a few hours. Bacteria soon develop in unsterilised aqueous solutions, and some of their metabolic products, termed pyrogens, if present in an injection solution, may cause a rise in temperature, rigor and other side-effects. These pyrogens are not destroyed during sterilisation, but their development may be prevented by careful preparation of the injection solution. All these preparations can be nullified by the increasing tendency to add various drugs to infusion solutions, and some thought should be given to the risks of bacterial contamination and drug interactions. Not more than one bottle with additions should be made at a time, and with as few additives as possible. Penicillin and heparin may be inactivated by dextrose solutions, and vitamin concentrates may react with tetracyclines. Many of these difficulties could be avoided by injecting additives through the drip tubing, and not by addition to the infusion bottle.

Hyaluronidase

Normal saline and other electrolyte solutions are normally given by intravenous drip infusion. In young children and in older patients where intravenous injection presents difficulties, subcutaneous injection is a practical alternative when hyaluronidase is used to facilitate absorption.

Hyaluronidase is a mucolytic enzyme obtained from animal testes, and it has the power of causing a temporary decrease in the viscosity of the ' ground substance ' or ' cement ' of the tissue spaces. This reduction in viscosity permits a considerable degree of diffusion into the tissues of any subcutaneous injection, and facilitates its absorption. The standard dose of hyaluronidase is 1500 units, and as the enzyme soon loses activity in solution it must be dissolved immediately before use. The enzyme solution may be given subcutaneously directly into the injection site, or added to 500 to 1000 ml. of the injection solution. Absorption of the injection solution takes place at the rate of about 100 ml. per hour. Hyaluronidase is also used occasionally to facilitate the local absorption of other injection solutions. *Brand name :* Hyalase.

Plasma

In cases of severe burns, the exudate from the damaged tissues brings about a marked fall in the plasma protein level and a reduction in the osmotic pressure of the blood. If intravenous fluids are given they tend to pass out of the venous system very quickly, and their effect is largely lost, unless the osmotic pressure is restored by the injection of blood plasma. Plasma is normally prepared from the pooled blood of several donors, but occasionally a delayed hepatitis follows its use, due to the presence of a virus. For that reason, and other difficulties associated with the administration of plasma, some alternative products have been introduced, exemplified by dextran.

Dextran

Dextran is a polysaccharide, formed in sugar solutions by a non-pathogenic coccus, *Leuconostoc mesenteroides*. Polysaccharides may be regarded as aggregations of sugar molecules linked together to form large units, and the physical properties of products such as dextran depend on the size and molecular weight of these large aggregate units. Solutions of certain fractions of dextran have some of the physical properties of plasma, and have been employed as temporary substitutes for blood in conditions of severe blood loss. The suitability of dextran fractions for use as blood plasma substitutes depends on the molecular weight of the aggregate unit. Solutions containing low molecular weight units soon pass out of the circulation after injection, and so are of little value in maintaining blood volume. Solutions containing polysaccharide units of excessive molecular weight are effective, but the dextran remains in the circulation too long, and may cause antigenic reactions.

For therapeutic use, special fractions of dextran are available, which have an immediate action as blood volume expanders when given by slow intravenous injection. These fractions are referred to as dextran 150 and dextran 110, and the standard solutions contain 6 per cent. of dextran in normal saline or 5 per cent. dextrose solution. They are used in haemorrhage, traumatic shock, and burns in doses of 500 to 1000 ml., with a total dose in shock of 2000 ml., and up to 3000 ml. in severe burns. Care should be taken to avoid overloading the circulation in renal damage or heart failure. *Brand names :* Dextraven, Macrodex.

Low Molecular Weight Dextrans

Although the low molecular weight dextrans are eliminated from the circulation more rapidly than the standard dextran solutions, they are of value in improving blood flow in cases of intravascular aggregation or ' sludging ' of blood cells. The use of these solutions increases peripheral circulation, improves blood supply to crushed or damaged tissues, and may be of value in embolism and other conditions where a decrease in blood viscosity and an improved blood flow is required. The dose range is from

500 ml. initially to 1000 to 2000 ml. daily by slow intravenous injection. *Brand names :* Lomodex, Rheomacrodex.

Amino Acids

In conditions of severe protein deficiency due to defective absorption, or after abdominal operation, it is sometimes necessary to by-pass the digestive system, and to supply nitrogen and calories by the intravenous route. This can be achieved by the administration of protein hydrolysates, or of solutions of the amino acids essential for protein synthesis. Protein hydrolysates contain amino acids and peptides, and are obtained by the action of acids or enzymes on casein and other protein substances. Dextrose is usually added to such products as an additional source of calories, and to permit the amino acids to be used for protein synthesis. In the absence of dextrose, the protein hydrolysates or mixed amino acids would be utilised as a source of energy and not for protein building. Alternatively, fructose or alcohol may be added to increase the caloric value. *Brand names :* Aminosol-Vitrum, Trophysan, Vamin.

Intravenous Fat

Carbohydrate in the form of dextrose is often given intravenously to provide calories, but in severe burns and other conditions a very high caloric intake is required. Fats provide a rich source of calories, but an emulsion suitable for intravenous use is not easy to make, and early products caused severe side-effects. These difficulties have now been overcome, and emulsions of cotton seed oil suitable for intravenous drip infusion are now available. Antibiotics or other drugs must *not* be added to these intravenous fat emulsions. *Brand names :* Intralipid-Vitrum, Lipiphysan.

Peritoneal Dialysis

Peritoneal dialysis is often used in the treatment of poisoning to aid the removal from the body of toxic substances, but it can also be used to correct electrolyte and fluid imbalance. The peritoneum is a semipermeable membrane of great size, as in area it exceeds the glomerular filtration surface of the kidney. It is semipermeable in that it permits the movement of salts and other freely soluble substances (sometimes referred to as crystalloids) and water through the membrane in either direction, but proteins and other large molecules are retained. Any fluid in the peritoneal cavity can thus be linked with the extracellular fluid of the tissues, and differences between the two fluids tend to reach a balance by the transfer of salts, metabolites and water across the peritoneal membrane. This exchange has great therapeutic value, particularly where kidney function is impaired or where there is marked electrolyte imbalance.

At the same time, care must be taken to avoid the absorption of water from the solution used for peritoneal dialysis, and thus over-hydrating the patient. It will be remembered that much of the body potassium is contained in the intracellular fluid, so the solutions used for peritoneal dialysis are usually potassium-free, but contain varying amounts of dextrose to meet the particular need.

A standard peritoneal dialysing solution has the following composition :—

Sodium	141 mEq/Litre
Calcium	3·5 mEq/Litre
Magnesium	1·5 mEq/Litre
Chloride	101 mEq/Litre
Lactate	45 mEq/Litre
Dextrose	1·5 to 7 per cent.

Potassium is not included as peritoneal dialysis is often used in cases of hyperkalaemia. On the other hand, when there is no gross disturbance of the potassium level, as in barbiturate poisoning, a potassium-containing solution may be used for dialysis.

The technique of dialysis is relatively simple. After the usual preoperative skin preparation for laparotomy, and local infiltration of the area with lignocaine solution, an incision is made and a trocar is inserted into the peritoneal cavity. The stylet is removed, and a plastic catheter is then inserted through the trocar. The catheter should penetrate well into the peritoneal cavity, and the end should be unobstructed to permit the free flow of the dialysing solution. The catheter is then connected to the bottle of dialysing solution, which should have been previously warmed to body temperature. One or two litres of solution should be allowed to run into the peritoneal cavity fairly rapidly (5 to 10 minutes) and allowed to remain for 20 to 30 minutes. The almost empty bottle should then be taken down, with the tubing still attached, and the fluid allowed to drain out of the cavity and back into the bottle by a simple siphon effect. The flow at first should be rapid, but as it slows down after some minutes, gentle pressure on the abdomen may assist in the draining of the remaining fluid.

This process of infusion and drainage may be repeated continuously as required, and as much as thirty to fifty litres of solution, or even more may be used. The method is of value in the treatment of acute and chronic renal failure with a rising blood urea, intractable oedema, barbiturate poisoning, and hepatic coma. The method is not entirely free from risk, but the greatest danger, peritonitis, can be minimised by a closed circuit technique, and the addition of 250 mg. of tetracycline or other broad-spectrum antibiotic to each litre of dialysing solution, and the limitation of the procedure to a maximum of 36 hours. Heparin is sometimes added to the dialysing solution to reduce the risk of blood clots.

When a solution containing the higher proportion of dextrose is used, the volume of water extracted from the tissues may lead to a lowering of blood pressure. This can be corrected by using a solution with less dextrose, and awaiting the restoration of plasma volume by a physiological adjustment, but if the lowering of the blood pressure results in a shock-like state, the infusion of human albumin, plasma or blood may be necessary.

CHAPTER XVII

BIOLOGICAL PRODUCTS

VACCINES, SERA AND RELATED PREPARATIONS

WHEN pathogenic organisms gain access to the body, some of the products of their metabolism, referred to as toxins, pass into the blood. Such foreign substances are known as antigens, and the body defends itself against such antigens by the formation of specific antidotes, termed antibodies. Tetanus antitoxin is a well-known example of an antibody preparation. The formation of antibodies in response to infection is termed ' active immunisation ' and may be naturally acquired or artificially induced.

Natural Immunity

Naturally acquired immunity follows recovery from infection, and the degree and duration of the immunity varies with the nature of the invading organism. Thus recovery from diphtheria is accompanied by a high and prolonged degree of immunity, whereas the immunity that follows recovery from tetanus is brief and of low intensity. A natural immunity may also be acquired from an infection so mild as to escape notice. Such immunity may not be very high in itself, but it sensitises the reticulo-endothelial system, and increases its powers to produce antibodies, and in the event of a subsequent infection the rapid production of antibodies in quantity can cut the infection short. Occasionally, although the patient recovers, the infecting organisms are not killed off, and the individual then becomes a carrier of the disease.

Induced Active Immunity

Immunity can be acquired artificially by several means, and is a very valuable prophylactic measure. It is this form of immunisation that is meant when the term ' active immunisation ' is usually employed. The products used to induce active immunity can be divided into two main groups—the vaccines, and products containing modified bacterial toxins. Vaccines can be further divided into bacterial vaccines, which are suspensions of dead bacteria, such as typhoid (T.A.B.) vaccine, pertussis vaccine ; viral vaccines, in which the virus has been inactivated by formaldehyde (some forms of poliomyelitis vaccine) ; and products containing living organisms which have been rendered harmless (B.C.G. vaccine, smallpox and yellow fever vaccine). In products containing bacterial toxins the activity of the toxin has been reduced by treatment with formaldehyde, and these modified products are termed toxoids. Diphtheria toxoid and tetanus toxoid (tetanus vaccine) are familiar examples.

All these products, when injected, function as antigens, and induce the formation of antibodies. The response to an initial injection is usually weak, but it acts as a trigger to the antibody production mechanism, and a second injection, given some days or even weeks later, evokes a powerful response and large amounts of antibodies or antitoxins are produced. Should a subsequent infection occur the circulating antibodies can prevent or minimise the development of the disease. The active immunity thus acquired may persist, in some cases for many years, and even if the degree of immunity falls to low levels in time, a further injection rapidly restores the original level of antitoxin.

As with these products there is a definite time-lag between the original injection and the maximum level of antibody, they are of chief value in prophylaxis. In the treatment of established infections products conferring immediate protection are required. Such temporary protection is referred to as passive immunity.

Passive Immunity

A transient immunity or protection to certain infections can be obtained by the use of serum which already contains antibodies. The injection of such a product results in the immediate presence of antibodies in the blood, and before antibiotics were available, such temporary immunity was of considerable value in the treatment of established disease, and for the protection of contacts. Passive immunity can be very effective, and occasionally lifesaving, but is a short-term measure, as the immunity thus conferred does not last more than two or three weeks. Immunological products of this type include diphtheria and tetanus antitoxins, and are prepared from the blood of horses. The animals are injected with small doses of toxin or toxoid, and develop the corresponding antitoxins. When an adequate amount of antitoxin has been produced some of the blood is withdrawn, the plasma is separated, concentrated and refined for therapeutic use.

Gamma Globulin

Human gamma globulin is a fraction of plasma containing protein and the various antibodies present in the blood of normal adults. It is used occasionally in doses of 250 to 500 mg., or more, by intramuscular injection to confer temporary protection on children and others who have come into contact with measles and rubella, and who are unlikely to have developed adequate antibodies of their own. It is also useful for the protection of contacts of poliomyelitis and infective hepatitis. Gamma globulin is also of value in the treatment of generalised vaccinia that may follow smallpox vaccination. Early injection after contact is important, but the protection is usually short-lived, and rarely lasts more than four to six weeks.

SERUM REACTIONS

Products for passive immunisation are derived from animals and although highly refined, contain some protein, and may cause severe reactions in susceptible patients. The most severe reaction is serum anaphylaxis, which comes on within a few minutes of injection, and is characterised by collapse and low blood pressure. The treatment is the immediate intramuscular injection of 1 ml. of adrenaline solution (1-1000), followed by doses of 0·5 ml. every thirty minutes if the blood pressure remains below 100 mm. Hg. Hydrocortisone (100 mg.) by intravenous injection may be given to supplement the action of the adrenaline, and an antihistamine by intramuscular injection if urticaria or oedema occurs.

A delayed reaction, referred to as serum sickness, may occur four to twelve days after the injection. An urticarial rash, joint pains and fever may also occur.

These reactions are most likely to occur in asthmatic subjects, and in those who have previously received injection of serum. With such patients, a test dose of 0·1 ml. of the antitoxin or vaccine may be given by subcutaneous injection, followed by the full dose intramuscularly if no reaction occurs within half an hour. Allergic patients should receive 0·1 ml. of a 1-10 dilution, and if that dose is tolerated, 0·1 ml. of undiluted serum may be given and if again there is no reaction after half an hour, the standard dose may be given by intramuscular injection.

Diagnostic Products

In a few cases, serological products are available which can be used to detect those individuals who lack a natural immunity.

Schick Test

This test is occasionally used to detect susceptibility to diphtheria, and is carried out by the intradermal injection of 0·2 ml. of a weak solution of diphtheria toxin. A positive reaction is shown by the development of a red area 10 to 50 mm. in diameter. A negative response is not an absolute test of immunity as young children are rarely immune, and the test is used mainly for older children and young adults.

Mantoux (Tuberculin) Test

The Mantoux test fluid is a solution of tuberculin, and is used to detect infection with the tubercle bacillus. It is available in three standard strengths—1-10,000, 1-1000 and 1-100—and the test is carried out by the intradermal injection of 0·1 ml. of the required strength. Many workers prefer to begin with the 1-1000 solution. The test is read after forty-eight to seventy-two hours, and a positive reaction is shown by a raised indurated area at least 6 mm. in diameter. A red area without induration is of no significance. An alternative method, which avoids the need for an injection, and so is very suitable when many tests have to be carried out, is the Heaf multiple-puncture gun.

A positive reaction indicates that the individual has been infected at some time with the tubercle bacillus, but it does not distinguish between past infection and present disease, except in young children. A positive reaction in a young child is an indication of an active infection that requires immediate treatment. In adults the diagnostic value of a positive test is of much less significance, but a reaction in a person known to have been a non-reactor is an indication of a new infection. Tuberculin testing is essential before B.C.G. vaccine (q.v.) is used prophylactically, as only tuberculin-negative patients should be so treated.

The following list of immunological products includes those in common use :—

Vaccines (including Toxoids) for Active Immunisation or Prophylaxis

Bacillus Calmette-Guérin vaccine (B.C.G.). Dose, 0·1 ml. as a single intracutaneous injection.

Cholera vaccine. Dose, 0·5 ml. initially by subcutaneous or intramuscular injection, followed by 1 ml. one to four weeks later.

Diphtheria vaccines :—
Alum-precipitated toxoid (A.P.T.). Dose, 0·2 to 0·5 ml. by intramuscular or deep subcutaneous injection, followed by 0·5 ml. after an interval of not less than four weeks.

Toxoid-antitoxin floccules (T.A.F.). Dose, 0·5 ml. by intramuscular or deep subcutaneous injection, followed by 0·5 ml. after an interval of not less than four weeks.

Purified toxoid aluminium phosphate (P.T.A.P.).

Influenza vaccine. Dose, 1 ml. by deep subcutaneous injection.

Measles vaccine. Two types of measles vaccine are available, the ' live ' vaccine, and the ' killed or inactivated ' vaccine. The killed vaccine is given in three doses of 0·5 ml. at monthly intervals by intramuscular injection. It is well tolerated, and reactions are uncommon. The live vaccine is given as a single dose by subcutaneous injection, but may cause a febrile reaction. This reaction may be reduced by giving an initial injection of killed vaccine, followed by a dose of live vaccine four to six weeks later.

Pertussis vaccine. Dose, 0·5 ml. by subcutaneous or intramuscular injection, repeated twice at intervals of four weeks.

Poliomyelitis vaccine (inactivated). Dose, 1 ml. by subcutaneous or intramuscular injection, followed by a second dose after four to six weeks, and a third dose after eight to twelve months.

Poliomyelitis vaccine (oral).

Rubella vaccine. Dose, 0·5 ml. by subcutaneous injection only.

Smallpox vaccine. Dose, 0·02 ml. by scarification of the skin.

Tetanus vaccine (tetanus toxoid). Dose, 0·5 to 1 ml. by subcutaneous or intramuscular injection.

9

Typhoid-paratyphoid vaccine (T.A.B.). Dose, 0·5 ml. initially by subcutaneous or intramuscular injection, followed by 1 ml. one to four weeks later. Combined with Cholera vaccine as T.A.B.C.

Yellow fever vaccine.

Vaccination Scheme

Certain of the above vaccines are available as mixed products, and give protection in childhood against several common infectious diseases with a minimum number of injections. Other vaccines can be given at later intervals, and the following scheme represents an average course of such immunising injections.

Age	Prophylactic	Interval
Not before 3 months, preferably about 6 months	Diphtheria, tetanus, pertussis and oral polio vaccine (First dose) Diphtheria, tetanus, pertussis and oral polio vaccine (Second dose) Diphtheria, tetanus, pertussis and polio vaccine (Third dose)	Preferably after an interval of 6-8 weeks Preferably after an interval of 6 months
1-2 years	Measles vaccination Smallpox vaccination *	After an interval of not less than 3-4 weeks After an interval of not less than 3-4 weeks
School entry	Diphtheria, tetanus and oral polio vaccine or Diphtheria, tetanus, polio vaccine Smallpox revaccination	
10 and 13 years	B.C.G. vaccine	For tuberculin-negative children
15-19 years	Polio vaccine (Oral or inactivated) Tetanus toxoid Smallpox revaccination	

* Vaccination against smallpox should not be undertaken within two weeks of the prior injection of poliomyelitis vaccine or diphtheria, tetanus and pertussis vaccine; at least three weeks should elapse before either of the other vaccines is injected after smallpox vaccination.

Antitoxins and Antisera for Passive Immunisation or Treatment :

Diphtheria antitoxin. Dose, 500 to 2000 units by subcutaneous or intramuscular injection for prophylaxis; 10,000 to 100,000 units by intramuscular or intravenous injection for treatment.

Gas-gangrene antitoxin. Dose, 25,000 units by intramuscular or intravenous injection for prophylaxis ; not less than 75,000 units by intravenous injection for treatment.

Tetanus antitoxin. Dose, not less than 1,500 units by subcutaneous or intramuscular injection for prophylaxis : not less than 50,000 units by intravenous or intramuscular injection for treatment.

NOTE.—Vaccines are usually prepared from laboratory cultures of the various organisms. Occasionally, special vaccines are prepared from organisms obtained from the patient requiring treatment. Such vaccines are known as autogenous vaccines. The so-called desensitising vaccines, used in the treatment of certain allergic conditions, are not true vaccines. They are weak solutions of various protein products known to be associated with allergic reactions, and are referred to on page 205.

CHAPTER XVIII

THE DRUG TREATMENT OF MALIGNANT DISEASE

NORMAL growth is a process of ordered multiplication, differentiation and integration of cells. The built-in control system of the body is so finely adjusted that growth, development and replacement of cells continues for years, and ageing is but the slow breakdown of the regenerative powers of the body.

Sometimes, for reasons still not understood, certain cells of the body escape from the normal rigid control. When such escape occurs the rate of growth and degree of development of the cells may change profoundly. The integration of growth with that of other cells is soon lost, specific differences of structure and function become blurred, and the rate of undifferentiated and haphazard growth may become rapid. As a consequence of this rapid growth, invasion or penetration of abnormal cells into adjacent normal tissues occurs, and sometimes these renegade cells travel via the blood or lymphatic system to other parts of the body, and set up new centres of abnormal growth. Such secondary growths are termed metastases.

These uncontrolled cells, referred to generically as tumours, cancers or neoplasms, do not all conform entirely to the same pattern. Some neoplasms do not form metastases, some grow very slowly, some develop very fast, and may cause considerable pain. But whatever their individual variations may be, they are all characterised by a continued undifferentiated growth that is inimical to the health of the body.

Treatment

For many years surgery, radiotherapy, or a combination of both, were the only means available to alleviate, and occasionally cure, malignant disease. With the advances in pharmacology, hopes have long been held that a new approach to the problem would be found. In order to have a therapeutic effect a drug is required that has a selective action on all abnormal, rapidly dividing cells found in cancerous conditions, but no toxic effects on normal cells. What is wanted is some kind of guided missile with a homing device that can seek out the cancer cell and destroy it, yet have a minimum spread of effect on other tissues. Such a substance is unknown and may long remain a pharmacologist's dream. Yet the possibility of killing infective bacteria in the body was once thought equally remote until the discovery of the sulphonamides, and there is little doubt that the problem will eventually be solved.

That the successful attempts to kill bacteria in the body by chemotherapeutic agents have not been extended to neoplastic cells is not surprising. Bacteria and somatic cells differ widely in their nature and energy requirements, whereas the metabolic processes of both normal and neoplastic cells are so closely related that it is unlikely that a specific anti-neoplastic drug will be found until more is known about the fundamentals of cell growth and differentiation. The drugs now available for the treatment of malignant disease tend to attack normal growing cells as well as cancerous cells, and are therefore limited in scope, and their toxic effects, especially those on the blood-forming elements of the bone marrow, limit their therapeutic use. Careful assessment of dose in relation to the condition of the disease, and the duration of treatment, are essential factors when considering the chemotherapy of malignant disease.

Chemotherapy

The drugs used in the treatment of cancer fall into three groups, the alkylating agents, the anti-metabolites, and chromosome inhibitors, and are sometimes referred to generally as cytotoxic drugs. The mode of action of each group differs, as the alkylating agents attack and damage the nucleo-proteins of the cells, antimetabolites prevent the take-up and utilisation of certain essential substances such as folic acid, and some plant extracts, exemplified by colchicine and vinblastine, inhibit the movement of the chromosomes during cell division. The final result is the inhibition of growth of the malignant cell. Such cytotoxic drugs will also attack normal dividing cells, and in practice a balance must be struck between the therapeutic and toxic effects of these drugs. They are most effective when the malignant cells are slow in recovering from the effects of the drug, and the cells of the bone marrow remain relatively undamaged. In many cases, the neoplastic cells recover more quickly than the cells of the haemopoietic system, and in some conditions, notably bronchial carcinoma, the malignant cells appear almost unaffected by doses that bring about a profound and sometimes irreversible depression of the bone marrow.

It must be remembered that all drugs which affect dividing cells are toxic, and many side-effects must be expected when cytotoxic drugs are used therapeutically. Nausea, vomiting, gastro-intestinal ulceration, stomatitis, and anorexia are common side-effects, as is alopecia. More serious are the effects on bone marrow, with a rapid fall in the leucocytic count, and a general depression of bone marrow activity. Cytotoxic drugs, by their nature, are extremely toxic to embryonic tissues, and should therefore not be given during pregnancy.

In order to avoid some of these dangerous side-effects, new techniques are being developed, such as isolation perfusion. By this method certain tumours can be temporarily isolated from the general circulation, and a relatively large dose of drug may be given in high concentration to the tumour, thus localising and increasing the cytotoxic effect. This technique shields the normal cells of the body to a great extent against cytotoxic damage, and sometimes brings about a remission that could not be achieved by more conventional methods.

In general, cytotoxic drugs are most effective in the leukaemias, in Hodgkin's disease, malignant lymphomata, and are useful in the control of myelomatosis, and mammary and ovarian carcinoma. The hormone treatment of mammary and prostatic carcinoma is referred to on pages 186 and 187. The following drugs represent the types now in use.

Mustine Hydrochloride † (dose, o·1 mg. per kg. body-weight)

Mustine, also known as nitrogen mustard, is used mainly in the treatment of Hodgkin's disease, especially when the condition has become resistant to irradiation therapy. It is also useful in lymphosarcoma and related conditions, but it is contra-indicated in acute leukaemia. The drug is very irritant, and is usually given by intravenous drip infusion as a solution in normal saline. The maximum daily dose is about 8 mg. which may be repeated daily or on alternate days to a total dose of o·4 mg. per kg. body-weight. Care must be taken not to allow any of the solution to escape into the perivenous tissues, or on to the skin. The drug may cause nausea and vomiting, and sedation and treatment with anti-emetics may be necessary. Mustine is also useful in bronchial carcinoma, when it is given by intrapleural injection to promote the absorption of pleural effusions. Uramustine, or uracil mustard, is an orally active derivative used mainly in the treatment of chronic lymphocytic leukaemia.

Azathioprine † (dose, 1·5 to 4 mg. per kg. daily)

Azathioprine is a derivative of mercaptopurine (*q.v.*) and has a similar pharmacological action, as it is metabolised in the body to form the parent drug. The action is therefore slow in onset, and prolonged in duration, and has a more steady and consistent effect than mercaptopurine. Quite apart from its antimetabolic properties, azathioprine has a powerful immunosuppressive action, and prevents homograft reactions. This effect has been made use of in suppressing tissue reactions during transplantation of kidneys, where it facilitates the function and survival of renal transplants by inhibiting rejection of the grafts. This surgical procedure is a complex but rapidly developing one, in which drugs such as azathioprine can play a very important part. The drug, by its nature, depresses the bone marrow, and decreases resistance to infection, and supportive treatment with high doses of corticosteroids is essential. The dose, which is larger than that used for leukaemia, must be adjusted according to the condition of the patient and may range from 2 to 5 mg. per kg. daily. An adequate immunosuppressive response may sometimes be obtained without marked change in the leucocyte count. *Brand name :* Imuran.†

Busulphan † (dose, 2 to 4 mg. daily)

This compound, although not chemically related to the nitrogen mustards, has a similar though more selective cytotoxic action. Busulphan acts chiefly on the myeloid cells, and is of considerable value in the treatment of chronic myeloid leukaemia. It is given in daily doses of 2 to 4 mg. orally, and prolonged treatment is necessary. The drug is also effective in those patients who have become resistant to other forms of treatment. Busulphan brings about a marked reduction in the excessive number of immature white cells, an increase in the haemoglobin level, and a considerable subjective improvement. Following remission, maintenance doses of 0·5 to 2 mg. may be given. It is of no value in the acute leukaemias, Hodgkin's disease or malignant lymphoma. *Brand name* : Myleran.†

Chlorambucil † (dose, 0·2 mg. per kg. daily)

Chlorambucil is an orally active derivative of mustine, and is of value in the long-term treatment of Hodgkin's disease and various lymphomas. The response to treatment is similar to that following X-ray therapy, but the drug appears to cause less damage to the bone-marrow. The average daily dose varies from 5 to 10 mg. daily and an initial course of treatment may last two to three weeks until remission occurs. Further suppressive courses with lower doses may also be given, but a rest period may be necessary if the blood picture shows signs of marked depression of bone-marrow activity.

Nausea may occur occasionally with chlorambucil, but is much less frequent than with mustine. It should be noted that although the drug has properties similar to those of mustine, it is of no value in bronchial carcinoma. *Brand name* : Leukeran.†

Cyclophosphamide

Cyclophosphamide can be regarded as a derivative of mustine, in which toxicity and activity have been reduced by combination with a phosphorus-containing organic compound. Potency is restored when the phosphorus link is broken by enzyme action to release the active fragment. Such breakdown occurs readily in malignant cells, which are rich in enzymes, and the drug thus has a more localised anti-tumour action than mustine, melphalan or related drugs. Cyclophosphamide is not irritant, and may be given orally or by intramuscular or intravenous injection, or injected directly into body cavities. It is used in the treatment of malignant diseases of the blood-forming system, in Hodgkin's disease, lymphosarcoma, carcinoma of the breast, lung and ovary, and inoperable broncho-carcinoma. Treatment may be commenced with a daily intravenous dose of 100 mg. increasing to 200 to 300 mg. daily, until a total dose of 6 to 8 G. has been given, limited by the depression of the bone marrow as shown by the white cell count. Following a satisfactory response, oral maintenance doses of 100 to 300 mg. daily may be given. For the treatment of malignant pleural effusions, a dose of 600 mg. may be injected intrapleurally. *Brand name* : Endoxana.†

Cytarabine

Cytarabine is a synthetic compound, chemically related to cytidine, which is one of the breakdown products of nucleic acid. Experimentally, cytarabine is markedly toxic to many mammalian cells, but it is used therapeutically to induce remission in acute myeloid leukaemia. It is also effective in the treatment of some solid tumours. Cytarabine may be given by rapid and continuous intravenous injection, or intermittently, with several days between the injections, and the dose varies accordingly from 2 mg. to 5 mg. per kg. Nausea and vomiting may be severe. For maintenance treatment, subcutaneous injections may be given. In common with other cytostatic agents cytarabine depresses bone marrow activity. *Brand name :* Cytosar.

Mannomustine † (dose, 100 mg.)

Many attempts have been made to reduce the toxicity of mustine by combination with other substances, and in mannomustine the drug is combined with the sugar-like substance mannitol. The compound is markedly less irritant than mustine, and is used in the treatment of chronic myeloid and lymphoid leukaemia, as well as in the palliative treatment of other cancerous conditions but it is not as effective as mustine in Hodgkin's disease. Doses vary from 50 to 100 mg. by slow intravenous injection on alternate days to a total dose of 0·8 to 1 G. It is also given orally in doses of 100 to 150 mg. weekly for maintenance. A rest period of three months should elapse before another course is commenced. *Brand name:* Degranol.

Melphalan †

Melphalan represents a combination of mustine with an amino acid. The latter acts as a carrier for the mustine, and the compound has the general cytotoxic properties of the nitrogen mustard group, with certain differences in action.

The drug is effective orally, and is given in doses of 10 mg. daily for seven days in the treatment of multiple myelomatosis. That disease is characterised by an excessive formation of plasma cells by the bone marrow, and this excess is not only damaging in itself, but may erode bone, and bring about skeletal changes. Melphalan can suppress this proliferation of cells by a general depression of bone marrow activity, and repeated courses of treatment may be necessary to obtain the maximum response. A rest period between each course is necessary to allow the blood count to recover. Melphalan may also be given by intravenous injection in a dose of 1 mg. per kg., repeated if necessary after a rest period of eight weeks.

Melphalan is also used by the isolated perfusion technique in the treatment of malignant melanoma. By this method a large dose of the drug, from 70 to 100 mg. may be circulated through the tumour, and the drug has the further advantage of having a much longer action in such circumstances than mustine. *Brand name :* Alkeran.†

Mercaptopurine † (dose, 2·5 mg. per kg. body-weight daily)

Mercaptopurine is related to adenine, a constituent of nucleic acid, and appears to act by entering malignant cells and interfering with the synthesis of nucleic acid, and in consequence with the development and proliferation of the cancer cells. It has a valuable suppressive action in acute leukaemia and chronic myelogenous leukaemia, particularly in children, but it is of no value in other malignant conditions. Mercaptopurine is given orally, and there may be a time-lag of three weeks before any effect can be detected. It produces a remission of the disease of varying duration, but the response to a second course of treatment may be less dramatic and repeated treatment leads eventually to a refractory state unresponsive to further therapy. Mercaptopurine should therefore not be used until after treatment with other drugs has been fully exploited. *Brand name :* Puri-Nethol.†

Methotrexate (dose, 2·5 to 10 mg.)

Methotrexate is an antagonist of folic acid. That acid plays an essential part in the metabolism of the cell nucleus, and folic acid antagonists can block the metabolic process and inhibit further development.

Methotrexate is used mainly in the treatment of acute leukaemia and Hodgkin's disease, and it is usually more effective in children than in adults. The initial dose is 2·5 to 5 mg. daily followed by maintenance doses of 5 to 10 mg. weekly. Methotrexate is absorbed orally, but may be given by intramuscular or intravenous injection if a very rapid action is required. The response to treatment is slow, and the drug should be given for several weeks before assessing the response. Methotrexate should not be used in pregnancy as it may cause malformation of the foetus.

Procarbazine † (dose, 50 to 300 mg. daily)

Procarbazine is a cytotoxic drug used mainly in the treatment of Hodgkin's disease. The drug is given orally with a commencing dose of 50 mg. increasing slowly to a maximum of 300 mg. daily until remission occurs, when the dose is reduced to a maintenance level. The total dose is about 6 G. The drug may be effective when resistance to other treatment occurs. *Brand name :* Natulan †

Thio-tepa

Thio-tepa is chemically and pharmacologically related to mustine, and has a marked toxic effect on rapidly dividing cells. It has been used in a wide variety of neoplastic diseases, but the most consistent and reliable results have been obtained in the treatment of mammary and ovarian carcinoma, and in sarcoma and various lymphomas. Good results have been obtained by intra-pleural injection to control effusions due to neoplasms, and the drug is sometimes useful in chronic myeloid leukaemia. Thio-tepa is less irritating than mustine, and may be given by intramuscular injection, but the dose must be carefully assessed on an individual basis. An average initial dose is 0·2 mg. per kg. for two or three doses daily, and subsequent doses, which are given at weekly intervals and based on blood counts, may vary from 5 to 30 mg. These doses should be reduced by half if the drug is given intra-venously. The response to treatment may be slow, but once the maximum response has occurred, reduced maintenance doses should be given at intervals of one to three weeks. Thio-tepa is sometimes given orally, and tablets containing 15 mg are available.

Tretamine (dose, 0·5 to 2·5 mg.)

Tretamine, also known as triethylenemelamine or TEM, has a cytotoxic action resembling mustine, but the drug is active orally as well as by injection. It is used mainly in the treatment of myeloid and lymphatic leukaemia, Hodgkin's disease, polycythemia vera, and other neoplastic conditions, but it is of no great value in acute leukaemia. Initial doses of 2·5 mg. daily for a few days may be followed by maintenance doses of 0·5 to 2·5 mg. every two to seven days. The drug is slow in action, and initially appears to be well tolerated, but it may have an increasingly toxic effect on the bone marrow, and for the early stages of treatment mustine is the preferred drug.

Triaziquone

Triaziquone is one of the most potent cytotoxic drugs available as it is active orally or by injection in doses of 0·2 to 0·5 mg. It is effective in many malignant blood disorders, in ovarian and mammary carcinoma, and in the treatment of effusions ; but is of little value in tumours of the gastro-intestinal tract. Triaziquone is given by intravenous injection in doses of 0·2 mg. daily up to a total dose of 7 mg., and depending on the response and blood picture generally, treatment may be continued with oral doses of 0·5 mg. daily or less frequently. The solution is irritant, and care must be taken to avoid perivenous leakage during intravenous administration. *Brand name :* Trenimon.†

CYTOTOXIC ANTIBIOTICS AND ALKALOIDS

Antibiotics in general have no cytotoxic properties, but there are a few exceptions, and the following are in current therapeutic use.

Actinomycin C †

Actinomycin C is one of a mixture of antibiotics obtained from cultures of *Streptomyces antibioticus*, and is used mainly in the treatment of Hodgkin's disease, and some forms of leukaemia. It is given by slow intravenous drip infusion in doses of 200 micrograms daily, up to a total dose of 10,000 to 15,000 micrograms. Supportive treatment with vitamins B and C is necessary. Solutions of actinomycin C are unstable, and should be freshly prepared, and protected from light. *Brand name :* Sanamycin.†

Actinomycin D †

Actinomycin D is used in the palliative treatment of some sarcomas of the soft tissues, such as rhabdomyosarcoma, which may not respond to irradiation therapy. It is also effective in Wilm's tumour (a malignant tumour of the kidney) and tumours of the testes and uterus. The standard adult dose is 0·5 mg. daily by intravenous injection for a maximum of five days. A second course may be given after an interval of four weeks.

Actinomycin D is very irritant to the tissues, and extravasation may cause severe local damage. The drug is also toxic, and gives rise to gastro-intestinal disturbances, skin eruptions and marked bone marrow depression. *Brand name :* Cosmegen.†

Daunorubicin †

Daunorubicin is an antibiotic with some antibacterial potency, but is of interest because of its marked activity against some experimental tumours. Clinically, the drug has been used with some success in acute myeloblastic and lymphoblastic leukaemia, but because of its toxicity, it is employed only in the treatment of conditions that have become resistant to other drugs. Daunorubicin is given by intravenous injection in doses varying from 0·5 to 3 mg. per kg. It is very irritant to the tissues if extravasation occurs. With the lower doses, injections may be made daily, but higher doses must be given at intervals of a week or more. The drug is cardiotoxic, and a total dose of 20 mg. per kg. should not be exceeded. *Brand name :* Cerubidin.†

Mithramycin

Mithramycin is an antibiotic with useful cytostatic properties, and is used mainly in the treatment of inoperable testicular tumours. It is given by slow intravenous infusion in doses of 25 micrograms per kg. daily for eight to ten days. The drug is toxic, and severe haemorrhagic side-effects may occur. Mithramycin is also effective in Paget's disease of bone, and in the hypercalcaemia associated with malignant disease. A short course of treatment over three or four days both lowers the blood calcium level and reduces the high rate of calcium excretion in the urine. *Brand name :* Mithracin.

Vinblastine Sulphate

Vinblastine is an alkaloid obtained from the flowering herb periwinkle, and represents a new type of anticancer drug. The mode of action is still obscure, but the drug appears to arrest division of the neoplastic cells. At present the main therapeutic use of vinblastine is in the treatment of generalised Hodgkin's disease, especially those patients who have not responded to other forms of treatment. The drug is given by intravenous injection in initial doses of 0·1 to 0·15 mg. per kg. followed at intervals of not less than seven days by doses of 0·2 mg. per kg. increasing to 0·4 mg. per kg. as two doses of 0·2 mg. per kg. on successive days, according to the white cell count. The side-effects of vinblastine are related to the size of dose, and include nausea, vomiting, depression and epilation. *Brand name :* Velbe.

Vincristine Sulphate

Vincristine is found together with vinblastine in the periwinkle, and has similar antineoplastic properties, but therapeutically it is used only for the treatment of acute leukaemia in children. The drug is given by intravenous injection at weekly intervals in doses of 0·05 to 1·5 mg. per kg. Side-effects are common with the higher dosage range, and include alopecia, constipation and neuromuscular disorders. *Brand name :* Oncovin.

RADIUM AND RADIOACTIVE ISOTOPES

The atoms of a chemical element consist essentially of a stable nucleus of protons and neutrons, surrounded by shells of electrons. A few elements, of which radium is the most familiar example, have unstable nuclei, and some of these nuclei undergo changes at intervals, and in doing so emit energy as alpha and beta rays or particles and gamma rays, the latter being very similar to X-rays.

This radioactive or disintegration process continues over a period of time until the element finally attains a different and stable form. Some normally stable elements, such as gold and iodine, can also be made radioactive by bombardment in a nuclear reactor, and such modified elements are known as radioactive isotopes.

These radioactive isotopes also emit energy in the form of rays, much in the same way as radium, but those isotopes used medicinally differ markedly from radium in having a relatively short period of activity, as the modified and radioactive atoms soon revert to a stable and inactive form. The period of activity is based on the ' half-life ' of the isotope, and is the time taken for the radioactivity or emitted energy to fall to half the original value.

The rays emitted by radium and radioactive isotopes have a

damaging effect upon the metabolism of the body tissues, and the most highly specialised and rapidly multiplying cells are most susceptible to such radiation. This selective action can be employed therapeutically in the diagnosis and treatment of tumours and other abnormal conditions. The following substances are of interest :—

Radium

Radium has been used extensively in the treatment of some forms of cancer, but its use is declining for some purposes as more easily handled radioactive isotopes have become available. In use radium is applied as radium needles or tubes, made of platinum or other metals. For surface treatment these containers are applied to the skin by means of plastic applicators ; for deeper or less superficial treatment the needles are inserted into the tissues to be treated. In all cases the number, position and distance of the needles or other containers must be carefully controlled, to ensure that a uniform amount of radioactivity is applied to the tissues under treatment.

Radio-gold

Radioactive gold is used mainly in the treatment of pleural and other effusions associated with malignant disease. It is supplied as a colloidal suspension of the metal in solutions of gelatin or dextran, and after tapping the effusion, the radioactive material is injected into the fluid remaining in the cavity. The rate of formation of the effusion can sometimes be reduced very considerably, and a second dose may not be necessary for some weeks.

Radio-iodide

Radioactive iodine has been used as sodium radio-iodide in the diagnosis of thyroid disease, and the treatment of certain forms of thyrotoxicosis. This isotope, being selectively taken up by the gland and metastatic tissue, has a local destructive effect, and is useful in the palliative treatment of carcinoma of the thyroid.

Radiophosphorus

Radioactive phosphorus, used as sodium radiophosphate, is taken up rapidly by actively growing tissues such as the bone marrow, liver and spleen. It is therefore of value in the treatment of disturbances of the blood-forming system such as polycythema vera and chronic myelogenous leukaemia. Sodium radiophosphate has also been used in the diagnosis and location of intra-ocular and brain tumours, and for uptake studies of metabolism.

All radioactive substances, including those used medicinally, are potentially dangerous to the tissues, as already indicated. Nurses and others who handle radioactive compounds, or who are concerned with the care of patients treated with such drugs, must take suitable protective measures to prevent exposure to excessive radiation. Considerable care must also be taken in disposing of the excreta of patients undergoing radioactive treatment.

The risk is greatest during the therapeutic use of radium, as a relatively large amount of radioactive material is used and patients may require nursing attention in circumstances that may make protection difficult. The risks can be reduced by limiting the time during which the patient may require close attention, and limiting the frequency of exposure. Thus the use of anaesthetics with a brief recovery rate, and the use of portable lead screens, can play an important part in reducing the period of exposure of nursing staff to the influence of radiation. In all cases when the possibility of such exposure to radiation exists, all the staff concerned should wear photographic monitoring devices, in order that the degree of radiation received can be measured at frequent intervals, and any unusual amounts detected at a very early stage.

CHAPTER XIX

DRUGS USED IN OPHTHALMOLOGY

THE drugs used in ophthalmic work fall into two main groups, (*a*) those applied locally, and (*b*) those used systemically. The former group can be further divided, and will be considered under the following headings:—

Mydriatics and Cycloplegics

Mydriatics are drugs that dilate the pupil ; and cycloplegics are those that paralyse the accommodation. Some drugs have both effects.

Dilatation of the pupil is necessary for retinoscopy and to immobilise the iris and ciliary muscle, and eye-drops of atropine sulphate are widely employed for this purpose. Atropine is the most powerful and persistent of the mydriatics used therapeutically as the effects may extend over several days. There is always the risk with older patients that atropine may precipitate an attack of glaucoma, and several alternative drugs are now available. Homatropine is related to atropine, but has a more rapid and less prolonged action, as the mydriatic effect fades after about twenty-four hours. Hyoscine also produces a more rapid mydriatic response than atropine with a correspondingly brief duration. Occasionally some patients have, or develop a sensitivity to atropine and associated alkaloids, and in such cases a synthetic drug, lachesine, may be used. Oxyphenonium (Antrenyl) is also useful in cases of atropine irritation.

Occasionally a drug is required, particularly in examination of the fundus, that has the mydriatic but not the cycloplegic effects of atropine, and so will dilate the pupil without paralysing the accommodation. Phenylephrine is often used in this way, in strengths ranging from 1 to 10 per cent.

When a drug with a rapid action is required, cyclopentolate may be used. This synthetic compound, also known as Mydrilate and Cyclogyl, is used as a 0·5 to 1 per cent. solution when a rapidly-acting drug for refraction is required.

Miotics

Miotics are drugs that cause the pupil to contract, and they are widely employed to reduce intra-ocular tension in the treatment of glaucoma. The contraction of the pupil facilitates drainage of the anterior chamber into Schlemm's canal, and so relieves the intra-ocular pressure, and physostigmine (Eserine) as a 0·5 per cent. solution is in frequent use, as the effects are rapid and sustained for about twelve hours. Pilocarpine nitrate (1 per cent.) is used in a similar way, but the action is less prolonged. When a long action is essential, compounds such as ecothiopate iodide (Phospholine iodide) and demecarium (Tosmelin) may be used. These substances have a more powerful and prolonged action, and one drop daily in the eye may be sufficient to produce an adequate lowering of intra-ocular pressure.

Adrenaline also reduces intra-ocular tension, but ordinary solutions are too irritating in use to be of real value. These difficulties have been overcome in the proprietary product Eppy, which is a stabilised, non-irritant and virtually neutral solution of adrenaline. It is widely used in simple or wide-angle glaucoma, and can be used in association with miotics or drugs such as acetazolamide.

Guanethidine (q.v.), the antihypertensive drug, has a useful though limited place in the treatment of chronic glaucoma. It not only reduces intra-ocular pressure but also the lid retraction associated with thyrotoxicosis.

A reduction in intra-ocular pressure may also be achieved by the oral use of certain drugs. Acetazolamide (Diamox) brings about a reduction in the volume of aqueous humour by a process of enzyme inhibition, and is given in doses of 250 mg. six-hourly. Dichlorphenamide (Daranide) has a similar action, and is effective in doses of 25 to 50 mg. once to four times a day.

Anaesthetics

Cocaine has long held a premier place as a local anaesthetic in ophthalmology, as it is very effective, and has the advantages of causing dilatation of the pupil and blanching of the conjunctiva. It is usually employed as a 2 per cent. solution, often in association with homatropine (q.v.). The intense anaesthetic effect of cocaine is not always necessary, and as an alternative amethocaine hydrochloride (1 per cent.) may be used.

Antibacterial Drugs

The sulphonamides have been used both locally and systemically in many ophthalmic conditions. Locally, sulphacetamide drops and eye-ointments have been used very extensively, as the solutions (10 to 30 per cent.) are neutral and non-irritant. Resistance to sulphacetamide may occur, and the action of the drug is reduced by the presence of pus. Other sulphonamides used locally in eye infections include sulphafurazole (Gantrisin) and Sulfomyl. The sulphonamides can also be used systemically, and adequate intra-ocular levels of the drug can be obtained by the oral administration of sulphadimidine and similar compounds. Certain antibiotics also have value in infections of the eye. Chloramphenicol is widely used as drops (0·5 per cent.) and ointments (1 per cent.), and neomycin drops (Nivemycin), framycetin (Soframycin, Framygen) gentamicin (Genticin) represent other antibiotics used in ophthalmology. Neomycin and framycetin are wide-range antibiotics that may be used locally or by subconjunctival injection, and rarely cause sensitivity reactions. Polymyxin and gentamicin represent those antibiotics with a narrower range of activity against gram-negative organisms, including *Pseudomonas pyocyanea.*

The tetracyclines are used chiefly as eye ointments.

Corticosteroids

Corticosteroids are used in ophthalmological practice in the treatment of a number of inflammatory conditions such as keratitis, uveitis and spring catarrh. For local use hydrocortisone as drops or ointment (1 per cent.) is satisfactory, but frequent use of the drops is necessary. Some patients find that the suspension of hydrocortisone causes a feeling of ' grittiness ' in the eye, and in such cases a solution of prednisolone phosphate (Predsol) or with the addition of neomycin (Predsol N, Codelsol) may be more acceptable. Subconjunctival injections may be required in severe infections.

Corticosteroids are also used in association with pyrimethamine (Daraprim) orally in doses of 25 mg. daily for the treatment of toxoplasmosis. That condition is due to a protozoal parasite, and is associated with uveitis. The pyrimethamine kills off the parasites, but the associated inflammation may be controlled by corticosteroid eye drops.

Antiviral Drugs

The virus of herpes may attack the eye, at first causing a superficial punctate keratitis, characterised by minute white plaques on the cornea. In severe cases the erosions coalesce to form a shallow ulcer, and an extensive keratitis may develop. In such severe cases it was formerly necessary to denude the affected epithelium by cauterising the eye, after anaesthetic, with iodine (7 per cent.) and potassium iodine (5 per cent.) in alcohol. More specific treatment is the use of the antiviral drug idoxuridine. Thymidine appears to be an essential metabolite for the virus, and idoxuridine, sometimes referred to as I.D.U., resembles thymidine in chemical structure, and by replacing thymidine in the metabolic process, can prevent development of the virus. The drug is effective only by local application, and frequent use as eye drops (0·1 per cent. solution) is necessary to achieve the necessary high local concentration. The response to treatment is often striking, and the use of idoxuridine has largely replaced such radical measures as cauterisation and debridement. *Brand names :* Dendrid, Kerecid.

Lime Burns

Lime (calcium oxide) has caustic properties, and as it is used in the building trade, lime burns of the eye are not uncommon. Immediate irrigation is essential, but when the burns are severe, and lime particles are still present, the lime may be dissolved by sodium versenate solution 0·4 per cent. Sodium versenate is a chelating agent, and dissolves metallic salts and removes them from the tissues as a soluble complex. In lime burns the eye is first anaesthetised, and the solution of sodium versenate is then dropped on the denuded surface. Opacities due to calcium deposits soon dissolve, and subsequent corneal healing is rapid.

Corneal Staining

It is occasionally necessary to determine the nature and extent of damage to the corneal epithelium, and this can be done by staining with fluorescein solution (2 per cent.). Fluorescein is a yellow dye, and any areas of the cornea that have become denuded of epithelium by abrasions or ulcers, even if quite invisible to the naked eye, take up the dye, and are stained green. The undamaged epithelium remains unstained. Bengal Rose solution (1 per cent.) may also be used. This dye stains damaged and devitalised cells a red colour. Fluorescein is also given by intravenous injection as a 5 per cent. solution to facilitate examination of the retinal vessels.

Eye drops and Sterility

Infections of the eye are always potentially serious, particularly when due to *Pseudomonas pyocyanea*. As a precautionary measure, eye drops are now supplied as sterile solutions, but the possibility of subsequent contamination during use remains an ever-present risk. It has been recommended that eye drop bottles should no longer be supplied complete with dropper, and that a separate sterile disposable dropper should be used for each application of the drops, particularly when the eye has been damaged. As an extension of this safety measure, pre-filled single-use eye-droppers are being developed, exemplified by the Opulet and Minims products. The range of drugs available in these special droppers is still limited, but the use of the conventional and unsatisfactory eye drop bottle may decline as the range of drugs is extended.

CHAPTER XX

ANTISEPTICS AND DISINFECTANTS

FEW subjects in the field of practical medicine have been associated with such a variety of practice and products as antiseptics, disinfectants and sterilisation. This confusion has been due to many factors. Without a clear understanding of the purpose of antisepsis and an appreciation of the limits imposed on its achievement in actual practice, the value of available methods cannot be assessed. The subject of antiseptics in particular has been bedevilled by a confusion of terms and a profusion of products of widely different composition.

The terms antiseptic, bacteriostat, disinfectant, germicide and bactericide are in common use, but are often more easily understood than defined. Strictly speaking the descriptions antiseptic or bacteriostat should be applied to substances which inhibit the growth of bacteria, whereas disinfectants, germicides and bactericides have a definite lethal action, but antiseptics are now usually expected to have germicidal properties, and it is in that sense that the word will be used in this book.

Many attempts have been made to evaluate antiseptic substances and to compare the efficiency of various compounds, but in practice it has proved extremely difficult. Some antiseptics are relatively specific in their action, and are very much more effective against some groups of organisms than others. Other antiseptics are affected by changes in pH, others by the presence of blood or pus.

The position is complicated still further by the fact that some bacteria pass through a stage in the life cycle when ' spores ' are formed. These spores are a dormant phase, and usually form when conditions for growth become unfavourable. Such spores are very resistant to the action of antiseptics, and can survive prolonged exposure, but may develop later when conditions again become favourable. The claims made for any antiseptic product therefore require careful investigation, but the following are among the essential properties that should be possessed by any substance used for its antiseptic properties :—

1. Wide range of activity in a wide range of strengths.
2. Not affected by other substances likely to be present in antiseptic creams, lotions and other products, or by wound exudates.
3. Non-irritant and of low toxicity.
4. High degree of penetration and rapidity of action.
5. Physically acceptable, and available at an economic price.

Nurses often ask how long an antiseptic or disinfectant solution takes to act, and it can be said at once that no hard-and-fast rules can be given. The killing of bacteria by antiseptics is not an instantaneous process, but takes time. The more bacteria there are to be killed the longer the process. Conversely, when fewer bacteria are present sterilisation will be achieved more rapidly. This point has particular application to the sterilisation of instruments, as a high standard of social cleanliness of such instruments increases the rapidity and effectiveness of sterilisation methods.

PHENOL ANTISEPTICS

Phenol

This substance is of historical interest, as it was introduced into medicine in 1867 as carbolic acid by Lister, and the remarkable results achieved by Lister and his followers in reducing postoperative infection paved the way to the present era of aseptic surgery. A 1-20 solution of phenol has certain antiseptic properties, but has now been replaced for most purposes by more active and less toxic compounds.

Cresol

Phenol is but one of several related compounds with antiseptic properties, and has the advantage of being freely soluble in water. Cresol is a more powerful germicide, but is less soluble in water. It dissolves in soap solution, and Solution of Cresol with Soap, better known as lysol, is a widely used cresol antiseptic. Lysol has a powerful action against a very wide range of organisms, including spores, but its caustic nature is a distinct disadvantage. It has been used for sterilising instruments, cleaning and disinfecting baths, and for general disinfectant purposes. For instruments heat sterilisation is now preferred where possible.

The caustic nature of cresol antiseptics can be reduced by

using special fractions of coal tar phenols. With this type of product, exemplified by Sudol and Printol, the range of activity is comparable with that of lysol, with a marked reduction in the corrosive effects on tissues.

Cresol and related phenols are also present in a range of general disinfectant products, usually classified as 'black fluids' and 'white fluids.' Black fluids contain various phenols dissolved in soap solutions ; when diluted with water they form white emulsions, and are used to disinfect floors and drains, and for other domestic purposes. White fluids are emulsions of similar composition but are less liable to stain linen, etc., when used for terminal disinfection.

Chlorocresol

This compound is a more powerful but less soluble derivative of phenol, and is used mainly as a bacteriostat to preserve the sterility of injection solutions. It will be appreciated that when injections are supplied in multiple-dose containers (*i.e.* rubber-capped bottles), from which successive doses can be withdrawn at intervals as required, there is a risk that the unused contents may become contaminated by faulty technique or the accidental use of an unsterile needle. A preservative is therefore added to such solutions to inhibit bacterial growth, and chlorocresol is widely used for that purpose in a strength of o·1 to o·2 per cent. Chlorocresol is also used in some instrument storage solutions, as in Sodium Benzoate and Chlorocresol Solution, B.P.C. The sodium benzoate is added to inhibit the corrosion of instruments during storage. It should be noted that this solution is intended for the storage of previously sterilised instruments ; it should not be regarded as a sterilising solution.

Chloroxylenol and Dichloroxylenol

Chloroxylenol is a powerful bactericide, widely employed in a variety of medical and domestic antiseptic products. In suitable concentrations it is non-irritant to the tissues, but the degree of activity varies considerably and it is less effective against staphylococci and some gram-negative organisms than against streptococci. Dichloroxylenol has similar general properties, but has a wider range of activity and is more effective against staphylococcal organisms. Products of the chloroxylenol type are widely used as general antiseptics in surgery and obstetrics ; the official preparation is Chloroxylenol Solution.

Some brand names : Dettol, Hycolin, Ibcol, Prinsyl, Streph, Supersan.

Thymol

Thymol is a phenolic compound that occurs naturally in oil of thyme and other aromatic oils. It is mainly used in antiseptic mouth-washes such as compound glycerin of thymol, and other preparations for local use.

Thymol iodide, once known as Aristol, is a reddish-brown powder with absorbent and protective properties. It is still in limited use as an antiseptic dusting powder.

Cetrimide

Cetrimide represents a class of substances sometimes referred to as surface-active agents. Such compounds not only have the ability to spread and penetrate easily into tissue crevices, but have useful emulsifying, detergent and antiseptic properties. Solutions containing 0·1 per cent. of cetrimide are used for general antiseptic purposes ; stronger solutions up to 1 per cent. are used for cleaning dirty wounds and for pre-operative skin preparation. Although cetrimide has a fairly wide range of activity against gram-positive organisms, it is much less effective against gram-negative organisms, particularly *Pseudomonas pyocyanea.* Cetrimide solutions are often found to be contaminated with *Ps. pyocyanea*, particularly if corked bottles are used, and ideally cetrimide and similar products should be supplied as sterilised solutions in screw-capped bottles. *Brand name :* Cetavlon.

Chlorhexidine

Chlorhexidine is a complex phenyl derivative with a powerful bactericidal action against a wide range of organisms, and that action is retained even in very dilute solutions, as well as in the presence of blood and other body fluids. For general antiseptic purposes it may be used as a 1-2000 solution ; for bladder irrigation a 1-5000 solution is effective. For rapid pre-operative sterilisation of the skin a 1-200 solution in 70 per cent. alcohol has been recommended. An aerosol spray product for skin disinfection is also available, which contains a dye to indicate the area treated.

Chlorhexidine cream (1 per cent.) is also used for obstetric and general antiseptic purposes. As with cetrimide, contamination with *P. pyocyanea* may occur, and bladder irrigation solutions in particular should be sterilised. *Brand name :* Hibitane.

Savlon (*Brand name*)

This product is a general-purpose antiseptic, and is supplied as a concentrate containing chlorhexidine (1·5 per cent.) and cetrimide (*q.v.*) (15 per cent.) Whilst cetrimide has certain antiseptic properties its range of activity is limited, and it is best regarded as an antiseptic detergent. In Savlon the advantages of both cetrimide and chlorhexidine are utilised, and the product is characterised by a very wide range of activity and a rapid effect, allied with penetrating, non-irritant detergent properties. For general antiseptic purposes, including equipment, masks and linen, a 1-200 dilution of Savlon is used ; for the treatment of wounds, hand-rinsing, etc., a 1-100 dilution, and for pre-operative skin sterilisation a 1-30 dilution in alcohol is effective. Savlon (1-20 in alcohol) can be used for the emergency sterilisation of instruments and rubber articles, but it is not suitable for the prolonged storage of previously sterilised articles. For that purpose a 1-5000 solution of chlorhexidine is preferred. As with cetrimide and chlorhexidine, cork closures must be avoided, as contamination and inactivation by *Pseudomonas pyocyanae* may occur.

NON-PHENOLIC ANTISEPTICS

Iodine

Iodine is one of the oldest, best known, and most effective of antiseptics, as unlike many newer antiseptics it is not selective in action. A 2 per cent. solution in alcohol is one of the best pre-operative skin preparations available, as it is highly effective, penetrates well and, by virtue of the deep brown colour of the solution, it has the advantage of acting as an indicator and marks the area that has been treated. Iodine is also used occasionally as the so-called tincture of iodine as an antiseptic application to wounds, but the action is brief, as iodine is rapidly inactivated by combination with tissue proteins and other substances. Sensitivity to iodine is not unknown, and a general skin reaction may follow the use of iodine in those who have an idiosyncrasy to the drug.

Iodine is also used as a solution in glycerin (Mandl's paint) for application to mucous surfaces in the treatment of tonsillitis.

Povidine-Iodine

Iodine can be taken up by various organic substances to form a complex known as an iodophore. In these complexes the iodine is held in a loose combination from which it is slowly liberated when in contact with the skin and mucous membranes. In povidone-iodine, the antiseptic is combined with polyvinylpyrrolidine, and the product is useful for skin preparation, and as a douche or lotion. *Brand names :* Betadine, Wescodyne.

Iodoform

Iodoform is a lemon-yellow powder with a marked odour and contains iodine in organic combination. It was once used extensively as an antiseptic wound dressing, as it decomposes slowly to liberate small amounts of free iodine, and now survives only as the antiseptic constituent of B.I.P.P. (bismuth, iodoform and paraffin paste) occasionally used with gauze as a packing for sinuses and abscesses.

Chlorinated Lime

Chlorinated lime, or bleaching powder, is a powerful germicide and deodorant, and has been widely used for general disinfectant purposes and to disinfect excreta. It contains calcium hypochlorite and is of chief interest as a means of preparing various hypochlorite solutions and for the chlorination of swimming baths.

Eusol

Eusol is a solution of calcium hypochlorite and boric acid, and contains the equivalent of about 0·25 per cent. of chlorine. It is widely used as a general antiseptic dressing, but the solution soon loses strength, and should not be used when more than two weeks old. Eusol also has a solvent action on protein, and is useful in the removal of pus and debris from wound surfaces.

Dakin's Solution

Dakin's solution is similar to eusol but contains sodium carbonate instead of boric acid. Both eusol and Dakin's solution have now been largely replaced by stabilised sodium hypochlorite solutions, prepared by electrolysis.

Electrolytic Sodium Hypochlorite Solution

When an electric current is passed through a solution of sodium chloride under suitable conditions, sodium hypochlorite is produced. Such solutions can be stabilised, and retain their activity over long periods, and have great advantages over the older and unstable hypochlorite solutions. Milton is a well-known electrolytic sodium hypochlorite solution, widely used as a well-tolerated general antiseptic product.

OXIDISING AGENTS

The chlorine antiseptics owe their action, in part at least, to the fact that the hypochlorites finally decompose to liberate oxygen. A number of other substances are also used as antiseptics by virtue of their oxygen-liberating properties, and the following are in use :—

Hydrogen Peroxide

Hydrogen peroxide (H_2O_2) is easily decomposed in the presence of oxidisable matter to yield oxygen and water. It is mainly used to treat infected cavities and dirty wounds, as the tissue enzymes cause a rapid release of oxygen, and the gas has the added mechanical action of loosening cell debris in the tissue crevices. It is also used, when diluted with water, as an antiseptic mouth wash, but continued use may make the gums soft and the tongue sore. Solutions of hydrogen peroxide are often described as ' 10 volume ' or ' 20 volume ' strength. The numbers refer to the volume of oxygen yielded by one volume of the solution.

Zinc Peroxide

A white powder, resembling zinc oxide in appearance. Zinc peroxide slowly decomposes to yield free oxygen and zinc oxide, and its action therefore resembles that of hydrogen peroxide, but is much more prolonged. It is used as a suspension in water, or as an aqueous cream in the treatment of infected wounds and necrotic ulcers. It is sometimes combined with urea in order to promote granulation.

Potassium Permanganate

Dark purple crystals which rapidly decompose in contact with organic matter, and have powerful antiseptic and deodorising properties. A 1-5000 solution is used for suppurating wounds and abscesses, and weaker solutions are employed for bladder and vaginal irrigation. Potassium permanganate is also used in dilute solution (1-5000) as a mouth-wash, and for mycotic infections of the skin. As the drug rapidly decomposes during use its action is brief, and the decomposition products may cause brown stains on the skin, fabrics and utensils. When potassium permanganate is mixed with formaldehyde solution, there is a very rapid release of formaldehyde gas. The release is made use of in the formaldehyde disinfection of rooms.

ANTISEPTIC DYES

A number of synthetic dyes have antiseptic properties, but the therapeutic use of such substances has declined as more active chemotherapeutic drugs have become available for the treatment of infections. The following substances are still in use, but often to a steadily diminishing extent.

Proflavine

Proflavine and acriflavine are orange-red dyes with a powerful action against gram-positive and gram-negative organisms. The germicidal activity is not affected to any extent by serum or pus, and the compounds are therefore valuable in the treatment of suppurating wounds. The standard strength of proflavine and acriflavine solutions is 1-1000, either in water, normal saline, or as an emulsion with a liquid paraffin base. Weaker solutions are used for infections of the eye and ear.

Crystal Violet (gentian violet)

This dye has powerful but selective antiseptic properties, and is effective chiefly against gram-positive organisms. It is used occasionally as a 0·5 to 2 per cent. solution for chronic ulcers and fungus infections of the skin, and as pessaries for vaginal moniliasis. A solution containing 0·5 per cent. of crystal violet and brilliant green in 45 per cent. alcohol (sometimes known as Bonney's blue) is used for pre-operative preparation of the skin.

Brilliant Green

A useful antiseptic dye, used as lotion (1-1000), as a paint or ointment (1-2 per cent.). It has the advantage of stimulating granulation and is used in the treatment of indolent ulcers. It is also used with crystal violet for skin preparation.

Scarlet Red

Scarlet red has mild antiseptic properties, but is chiefly used to stimulate clean but indolent ulcers, burns, and other damaged areas which are slow to heal. The standard ointment contains 5 per cent. of scarlet red, but weaker ointments are often preferred.

Mercurochrome †

Mercurochrome is a mercury-containing derivative of fluorescein. It forms dark-red solutions which have been used locally as antiseptics, but the action is weak and unreliable.

HEAVY METAL ANTISEPTICS

Certain compounds of mercury, silver and zinc have long been used as antiseptics but they have definite limitations, and their use has declined as more active and less toxic products have become available. Some, however, are still in use in some places, and the following compounds should be known :—

Mercuric Chloride †

Mercuric chloride has been used as a skin antiseptic, and for the disinfection of excreta. For application to the skin, a 1-1000 solution is suitable, and 1-10,000 solutions have been employed for bladder and vaginal irrigation. Mercuric chloride, like other soluble salts of mercury, is very poisonous, and by tradition solutions are coloured blue as a safety measure.

Mercuric Oxycyanide †

A mercury compound with antiseptic properties resembling those of mercuric chloride. It does not react with body fluids and proteins, and is better tolerated. It is used as 1-10,000 solution for bladder irrigation, and in conjunctivitis. It should be noted that soluble salts of mercury attack many metals, and their solutions are not suitable for the storage of instruments.

Other Mercury Compounds †

Mercuric iodide dissolved in potassium iodide solution forms the product known as 'biniodide.' Its efficiency as an antiseptic is open to doubt.

Mercuric oxide and ammoniated mercury are insoluble salts of mercury, used for external application as ointments. The former is mainly used for conjunctivitis, and the ointment is popularly known as ' golden eye ointment.'

Phenylmercuric Nitrate †

The toxic and irritant action of the mercury antiseptics can be reduced by combining the metal in the form of an organic complex, and some organic mercurial antiseptics retain their bacteriostatic properties even in high dilution. Phenylmercuric nitrate is a well-known example of this type of antiseptic, and is used as a 1-15,000 solution for irrigation of wounds. It is also used to preserve the sterility of injection solutions as an alternative to chlorocresol (q.v.). Phenylmercuric nitrate is also used in fungicidal creams and powders for mycotic infections of the skin. Merthiolate (thiomersal) and Penotrane are examples of related compounds. Mercurochrome is referred to on page 276.

Silver Compounds

Silver salts have powerful antiseptic properties, but in practice their therapeutic applications are few. Silver nitrate solution (1 per cent.) was once used extensively as eye-drops as a prophylactic against ophthalmia neonatorum, but has now been replaced by antibiotics. Solid silver nitrate is used as a caustic to destroy warts.

The reactive properties of silver can be controlled to some extent by combining silver oxide with gelatin, albumin or other protein substances. These products are less active than silver nitrate, but are non-irritant and have a prolonged action. They are useful in conjunctivitis and for infections of the nose and throat.

The strength of solutions used may vary from 2 to 10 per cent. *Brand names* : Argyrol, Argotone.

OTHER ANTISEPTICS

Alcohol

Alcohol in the form of methylated spirit has been used for many years as an antiseptic, particularly for skin preparation, but is not very effective or reliable. Isopropyl alcohol has similar general properties, but is more powerful, and may be used both for pre-operative cleansing of the skin, and for surgical instruments.

Formaldehyde

This powerful antiseptic is a gas, but is usually employed as a 40 per cent. aqueous solution referred to as ' formalin.' It is too irritant for general use, but is useful for the disinfection of apparatus and the preservation of specimens. In association with potassium permanganate (*q.v.*) it is used for the disinfection of rooms.

Glutaraldehyde

The problem of disinfection increases as more complex instruments and apparatus are used. Many such instruments cannot be sterilised by conventional methods, and may be damaged beyond repair if heat sterilisation is attempted. Further, as many disinfectants cannot be relied upon to kill spores, there is need for an antimicrobial substance that is sporicidal, prompt in action, non-corrosive, and suitable for the sterilisation of a wide range of materials.

Glutaraldehyde has the necessary range of activity, as it can kill bacteria, spores, viruses and fungi, and does not attack plastics, rubber or metals. The compound is normally slightly acid in solution, but the antimicrobial and sporicidal action is increased when the solution is slightly alkaline; but such solutions are less stable. In practice, a 2 per cent. solution of glutaraldehyde is activated before use by the addition of alkaline activating and buffering agents, and can be expected to retain its full potency for two weeks. It should then be discarded and replaced with freshly prepared solution. *Brand name* : Cidex.

CHAPTER XXI

DIAGNOSTIC AGENTS

AN increasing number of substances is now employed in medicine for diagnostic rather than therapeutic purposes. Many of these are used as X-ray contrast agents to outline body cavities and organs, others are used as tests for liver and kidney function and for various other investigations. The contrast agents form the largest single group. Serological products used as diagnostic agents are referred to on page 246.

X-ray Contrast Agents

These are substances of high atomic weight, and are therefore relatively opaque to X-rays. They appear as shadows on X-ray films, and are invaluable in outlining various tissues in order to detect abnormalities. With the exception of barium sulphate, the substances used as contrast agents are almost invariably complex iodine-containing organic compounds.

Barium Sulphate

Barium sulphate is a very heavy, dense white powder, used for the visualisation of the gastro-intestinal tract. It is given as a suspension in water, orally or as an enema, according to the area to be examined. When so used, barium sulphate forms a temporary coating of the alimentary tract, and abnormalities can be outlined and detected. Large doses, varying from 100 to 250 G. may be given, and it is important to obtain a complete and even coating of the mucosa. A number of proprietary preparations of barium sulphate, specially formulated for X-ray use, are available, and Micropaque, Raybar and Barosperse are representative products.

It should be noted that soluble salts of barium are very poisonous. Barium sulphate, however, is one of the most insoluble substances known, and is non-toxic by virtue of its insolubility.

Iodine Compounds

Iodine as such is far too reactive and toxic to be used as a contrast agent, but by suitable organic combination non-toxic contrast agents can be formed and are in wide use. Such compounds can be divided into four main groups : (1) Oily or other viscous products used to outline body cavities, (2) those used to indicate the gall-bladder and bile ducts, (3) compounds intended to outline the urinary tract, and (4) those used in the investigation of the arterial system. Some compounds are suitable for several types of investigation. A detailed consideration of this valuable and interesting group of drugs is beyond the scope of this book, but the following table indicates some of the main applications, and the various products in use.

Contrast Agents

Angiography	Arteriography	Bronchography	Choleocystography
Diodone Sodium acetrizoate Sodium iothalamate Sodium metrizoate	Diodone	Iodised oil	Calcium ipodate Iopanoic acid Phenbutiodil Iodipamide

Cystography	Myelography	Pyelography	Salpingography
Diodone Iodoxyl	Iophendylate	Diodone Iodoxyl Sodium acetrizoate Sodium diatrizoate Meglumine iothalamate Sodium metrizoate	Diodone Sodium acetrizoate

Brand names :

Calcium ipodate—Solu-Biloptin.
Diodone—Uriodone.
Iophendylate—Myodil.
Iodipamide—Biligrafin.
Iodised oils—Lipiodol, Neo-Hydriol.
Iodoxyl—Uropac.
Iopanoic acid—Telepaque.

Meglumine iothalamate—Conray.
Phenbutiodil—Biliodyl.
Sodium acetrizoate—Hypaque, Urografin, Gastrografin.
Sodium iothalamate—Conray.
Sodium metrizoate—Triosil.

RENAL FUNCTION TESTS

Indigo Carmine

Indigo carmine is a blue dye, and when given by intravenous or intramuscular injection, it is excreted so rapidly that the appearance of a blue colour in the urine is a useful test of renal efficiency. The dye is used as a 0·4 per cent. solution, and is given in doses of 5 to 10 ml. If a catheter is passed at the beginning of the injection the time taken for the dye to appear at the ureteral orifices can be determined. In normal subjects the dye appears in the urine in about ten minutes. Methylene blue is also used as a renal function test, and may be given by intramuscular injection of a 2·5 per cent. solution. With a normal kidney, excretion of the dye in the urine begins about thirty minutes after injection.

Phenolsulphonphthalein

Also known as Phenol Red, phenolsulphonphthalein is given in doses of 6 mg. by intramuscular or intravenous injection, and the urine is collected later at intervals. The colour is then compared with that of a standard solution. Some 25 per cent. of the dye is normally excreted in fifteen minutes, and over 50 per cent. at the end of one hour, and any marked delay is an indication of the degree of renal dysfunction.

Urea

In health the kidney can excrete large amounts of urea without difficulty, but that ability is markedly reduced when renal damage has occurred. Urea has been used as an index of renal function by giving a dose of 15 G., and collecting the urine after one hour. The concentration of urea in each specimen of urine is normally 2 to 5·3 per cent.; a concentration below 2 per cent. indicates renal inadequacy.

LIVER FUNCTION TESTS

One of the most important functions of the liver is the detoxification of foreign substances, and the degree of ability of the liver to metabolise or excrete such substances can be used as a test of its efficiency.

Sulphobromophthalein

This compound is a red dye, and following intravenous injection it is taken up by the liver and excreted in the bile. Normally most of the dye is removed from the blood within thirty minutes, and the drug is therefore of value in assessing hepatic activity. The dose is 5 mg. per kg. body-weight, and it is given as a 5 per cent. solution by intravenous injection. Samples of blood are taken 45 minutes later and the amount of sulphobromophthalein present in the plasma, normally about 7 per cent., is measured by comparison with standard solutions of the dye. Cardio-Green is also given intravenously to determine liver damage.

Sodium Benzoate

The use of sodium benzoate as a liver function test is based on the fact that benzoates are combined in the liver with an amino acid (glycine) to form hippuric acid. A healthy liver has an adequate amount of glycine available for such combination, but when the liver is damaged a deficiency of glycine occurs, and the reduction in the amount of hippuric acid formed is an indication of the degree of damage. In the oral test, 6 G. of sodium benzoate is given and the amount of hippuric acid excreted during the next four hours is determined by the laboratory. The normal amount so excreted is 2·5 to 3·5 G., and an excretion as low as 1·5 G. is indicative of severe hepatic dysfunction. Alternatively, an intravenous dose equivalent to 1·5 G. of benzoic acid may be given, and an estimation made of the amount of hippuric acid excreted over the next hour. In health, 1 to 1·4 G. of hippuric acid would be excreted under the test conditions. Other liver function tests depend on the rate of absorption and excretion of various sugars.

GASTRIC FUNCTION TESTS

Histamine has a powerful stimulant action on the acid-secreting cells of the stomach, and is used in the investigation

of achlorhydria.   Following the subcutaneous injection of 0·5 to
1 mg. of histamine acid phosphate, samples of gastric juice are
withdrawn at intervals of ten minutes, and the degree of acidity
checked.   Except in pernicious anaemia, the samples have a higher
acidity than normal.   In the ' augmented histamine test,' the dose
of histamine is 0·04 mg. per kg., but the systemic effects of such a
large dose must be controlled by the previous injection of an antihistamine.   A dose of 100 mg. of mepyramine by intramuscular
injection is often used.   Alcohol is also used occasionally for
fractional test meals, and is given as a single dose of 50 ml. of a
7 per cent. solution.

Diagnex is a proprietary product used in the diagnosis of
achlorhydria.   It contains a blue dye combined with a synthetic
resin, and in the presence of acid the dye is released and colours
the urine.

Pentagastrin

Gastrin is a hormone secreted by the stomach, and it is considered that the main physiological action is to stimulate the
gastric glands to secrete acid and pepsin.

Pentagastrin is a synthetic compound, related chemically to
part of the gastrin molecule, and it has a similar stimulating effect
on acid secretion.   It is given by subcutaneous or intravenous
injection in doses of 6 microgrammes per kg., and the response is
similar to that following an injection of histamine, but with fewer
side-effects.   Pentagastrin is thus useful in the clinical testing of
gastric secretory activity.   *Brand name :* Peptavlon.

CIRCULATION TIME

Many substances have been used by rapid intravenous injection to determine blood circulation time, and the test is carried
out by timing the interval between the injection and the response.
The information that such tests give is limited, and more sophisti-
cated and reliable electrical machine tests are now available.
Soluble saccharin is still occasionally used, and a dose of 2·5 G.
dissolved in 2 ml. of water may be injected into the antecubital
vein.   The time is recorded when the patient notes a sweet taste,
which normally occurs in nine to sixteen seconds.

PANCREATIC AND GALL-BLADDER FUNCTION TESTS
Secretin

Secretin is an enzyme obtained from duodenal mucosa that stimulates the pancreas to produce a large volume of alkaline pancreatic juice. Pancreozymin, a related enzyme obtained from the same source, increases the output of enzymes by the pancreas. The combined use of these enzymes is thus of considerable value in assessing pancreatic function. Several tests are in use, which differ in detail, but essentially the test is carried by first aspirating a sample of the duodenal juice, and then giving secretin in doses of 1 to 2 mg. by intravenous injection. Further specimens are aspirated at intervals, and after half to one hour, pancreozymin is also given intravenously. Comparative tests on the activity of the various specimens indicate the nature of any pancreatic dysfunction.

Pancreozymin

In addition to its stimulant effect on the pancreas, pancreozymin also influences gall-bladder contraction, and so augments the flow of bile. It is given in doses of 100 units by intravenous injection to cause rapid contraction of the gall-bladder during cholecystography. An intravenous injection of morphine (6 mg.) should be given immediately after the pancreozymin to reduce spasm. In the combined secretin-pancreozymin test, the presence or absence of bile in the aspirated duodenal juice is also of diagnostic value.

OTHER TEST COMPOUNDS
Azovan Blue

This dye, also known as Evans Blue, is used to estimate the volume of the blood plasma. It is given as a 0·5 per cent. solution in doses of 5 ml. by intravenous injection, and as it becomes bound to the plasma proteins, excretion of the dye is delayed. Samples of blood are withdrawn at intervals of twenty, forty and sixty minutes. The amount of dye in the samples can be measured by suitable apparatus, and the total volume of blood in the body can be calculated. Coomassie Blue is also used as a 2 per cent. solution for the determination of blood and plasma volumes.

Congo Red

In amyloid disease, a waxy substance termed amyloid is deposited in the vessels of the spleen, liver and kidneys. This substance has the ability to absorb congo red, and that property is made use of in the diagnosis of amyloid disease. Congo red is given by intravenous injection as a 1 per cent. solution, in doses of 0·25 ml. per kg. body-weight, and the amount of the dye remaining in the circulation after one hour is determined. Normally 70 to 90 per cent. of the dye is still present in the plasma, but in amyloid disease the greater part has been taken up by the waxy deposit, and less than 10 per cent. of the injected dose may remain in circulation.

ALLERGY TESTS

The full diagnosis of allergic disease depends on the identification of the causative allergen, and skin tests to confirm sensitivity to a suspected allergen are of considerable value, particularly where inhalant allergens such as pollens, animal hair and feathers are concerned. These tests are intended to confirm a diagnosis, as some subjects may exhibit a positive skin test, yet have no allergic symptoms. These skin tests are of very little value when the allergen is a foodstuff. Special extracts containing small amounts of the allergens are used as skin test solutions and may be applied as prick tests, scratch tests or intradermal tests.

In the prick test, a drop of the solution is applied to the arm or other area and a needle is passed through the drop into the skin. In the scratch test, a small area of skin is scarified, a drop of test solution applied and rubbed in gently.

The intradermal test is more sensitive, and a much weaker solution is injected into the skin in a dose of 0·01 to 0·02 ml. The result of any form of the test is read after fifteen minutes, and is assessed by the degree of erythema and size of wheal produced by the test solution. A control test with a control solution is usually carried out to eliminate false-positive reactions. Patch tests are used when testing for allergens which cause contact dermatitis, and are useful in confirming sensitivity to drugs.

CHAPTER XXII

THE TREATMENT OF POISONING

THE increasing use of potent drugs and the widening range of toxic chemicals used for industrial purposes has increased the risk and also the incidence of poisoning. The term ' poison ' is a relative one, as many substances not usually regarded as poisons may prove toxic if taken in sufficient dose, or if swallowed by children.

Many cases of accidental poisoning can be traced to careless handling or storage of the drugs and chemicals, and every effort should be made to impress on patients, relatives and all users of potentially toxic substances the importance of keeping all such products under proper control. The familiarity with drugs acquired by nurses, pharmacists and doctors is also apt to blunt the awareness of the dangers of mishandling potent substances and the ever-present possibilities of error. With drugs, as with other things of potential danger as well as value, constant vigilance is the only safeguard. No drug should ever be used from an un-labelled container, neither should a product be used unless the label is clear and unambiguous, and conveys the required information. Many drugs have both a brand name and an approved or non-proprietary name, and in all cases of doubt the identity of the product should be checked before it is used. Belief is not an adequate substitute for certainty where drugs are concerned.

In the treatment of poisoning the first steps to be taken are general ones, and should be instituted at once. When the poison has been inhaled the patient should be removed immediately to fresh air and oxygen or artificial respiration given as required. Other measures include warmth and circulatory stimulants. When the poison has been taken by mouth, any unabsorbed material should be removed from the stomach as completely as possible by gastric lavage. This should be done repeatedly, using a stomach tube about $\frac{1}{2}$ in. in diameter, and about 5 ft. long, with at least two side-orifices of adequate size. About 500 ml. (1 pint) of water, warmed to body temperature, should be used for each lavage. There is no point in using much more water at a time, as a larger volume may cause fluid and gastric contents to pass into the duodenum. After about six such washings, assuming that no more material is being recovered, a solution of magnesium sulphate (30 G. in 300 to 500 ml. of water) should be left in the stomach to act as a purge, and is of particular importance when the poison is a slowly absorbed compound. The few cases in which gastric lavage should not be carried out, or only attempted with great care and a knowledge of the risks involved, are cases of poisoning by strong acids and alkalis. Such substances are corrosive and may weaken the walls of the stomach, and attempts at gastric lavage may result in perforation.

Emetics are also useful first-aid measures in the treatment of poisoning, and may be tried whilst preparations for gastric lavage are being made. Mechanical stimulation of the back of the mouth by the fingers is an effective method of inducing vomiting, as is a solution of common salt or mustard (1 to 10 oz. water), but the most effective compound is apomorphine. That substance is, as the name implies, a derivative of morphine, and has a specific stimulant action on the vomiting centre of the brain medulla. It is given by subcutaneous injection as a single dose of 2 to 8 mg., and vomiting should occur in ten to fifteen minutes. Apomorphine is a powerful drug and, like other emetics, should not be given to unconscious patients or in poisoning by corrosive substances. It should be noted that apomorphine may decompose on storage and lose its emetic power. Injection solutions and hypodermic tablets should be protected from the light, and any products that have developed a green colour should be rejected.

All stomach washings, vomit and any medicines or other substances possibly associated with the particular poisoning should be set aside for subsequent inspection and investigation.

Acids

Corrosive Acids, *i.e.* hydrochloric acid, spirits of salt, nitric acid, sulphuric acid, oil of vitriol (and oxalic acid).

SYMPTOMS.—Burned lips and mouth, thirst, gastric pain, vomiting and collapse.

TREATMENT.—Cream of magnesia, milk, olive oil. Chalk or sodium bicarbonate may be used with care to neutralise the acid, but are best avoided as the gastric distension caused by the released carbon dioxide may cause perforation if the stomach has been severely damaged.

General measures include demulcents, morphine for pain, atropine for spasm and circulatory stimulants as required. When the poisoning is due to oxalic acid, sodium bicarbonate should not be used, but a solution of magnesium sulphate, calcium chloride or other soluble calcium salt should be given to precipitate the acid as the insoluble calcium or magnesium salt.

Alcohol

SYMPTOMS.—Confusion, dilated pupils, dizziness, tottering gait, lips livid, breath alcoholic, stupor and coma.

TREATMENT.—Immediate gastric lavage, fluids for dehydration, oxygen if respiration is depressed, and artificial respiration as required.

Alkalis (caustic), including caustic potash, caustic soda, soap lyes, strong ammonia, etc.

SYMPTOMS.—Pain in mouth, throat and abdomen; lips and tongue swollen, vomiting, diarrhoea, skin cold and clammy, pulse rapid and weak, shock.

TREATMENT.—Use stomach tube with caution if at all. Give diluted vinegar or lemon juice or solutions of citric or tartaric acids to neutralise the alkali. Follow with milk, oil and other demulcents, stimulants, morphine for pain.

Amphetamine, Dexamphetamine and related stimulants

SYMPTOMS.—Excitement, hallucinations, convulsions, cyanosis, coma.

TREATMENT.—Gastric lavage followed by intravenous thiopentone sodium, oral or rectal barbiturate, chloral hydrate or paraldehyde, oxygen, or oxygen-carbon dioxide mixture for cyanosis.

Antihistamines

SYMPTOMS.—Drowsiness, inability to concentrate, headache, tinnitus, vertigo, inco-ordination, blurred vision, dryness of mouth, convulsions and coma.

TREATMENT.—Histamine is *not* an antidote, and must not be used. Emetics and gastric lavage with sodium bicarbonate solution, leaving some in stomach. If drowsiness is excessive, injections of methylamphetamine or other stimulants; if convulsions occur give intramuscular paraldehyde or intravenous thiopentone, but care must be taken if the respiration is already depressed.

Antimony Compounds (including tartar emetic, butter of antimony, etc.)

SYMPTOMS.—Burning and choking in throat, severe pain in abdomen, thirst, nausea, violent vomiting, purging, cramp, urine scanty or suppressed, skin cold, clammy and cyanotic, profuse perspiration, delirium, paralysis and collapse.

TREATMENT.—Gastric lavage with weak tannic acid solution repeated until cessation of vomiting ; milk and egg albumen, morphine to relieve pain, noradrenaline or metaraminol for shock as required. Injections of dimercaprol four-hourly.

Arsenical Compounds (including arsenical weedkiller, sheep dip, horticultural sprays, etc.)

SYMPTOMS.—Burning pain in throat and stomach, intense thirst, vomiting (often blood-stained), profuse diarrhoea, urine scanty or suppressed, cramps, cyanosis, pulse small, frequent and feeble, collapse, convulsions.

TREATMENT.—Ferric hydroxide as soon as possible, prepared by adding $1\frac{1}{2}$ oz. ferric chloride solution to $\frac{1}{2}$ oz. sodium carbonate dissolved in half a tumberful of water. Follow by gastric lavage and a saline purge. Injections of dimercaprol four-hourly, morphine for pain, oil and demulcents orally, stimulants.

Aspirin and Other Oral Salicylates

SYMPTOMS.—Nausea with or without vomiting, dizziness, tinnitus, mental confusion, visual disturbances, profuse perspiration, pulse rapid and feeble, breathing laboured, sleepiness, coma. The urine gives a strong reaction with ferric chloride for salicylate and may contain acetone and acetoacetic acid.

TREATMENT.—Prompt and repeated gastric lavage with water or sodium bicarbonate solution. Copious fluids containing dextrose and sodium bicarbonate orally. If acidosis is severe give sodium lactate or bicarbonate by intravenous drip infusion. Oxygen if required. Large doses of vitamin K_1 by injection if prothrombin time is low.

Barbiturates (including barbitone, phenobarbitone, buto-barbitone, etc.)

SYMPTOMS.—Giddiness, mental confusion, delirium, marked fall in blood pressure, depression of respiration, pupils moderately dilated, absence of corneal reflex, cyanosis, suppression of urine, prolonged coma.

TREATMENT.—Gastric lavage with water or weak potassium permanganate solution. Alkaline solutions should not be used. Catheterisation if required, artificial respiration or airway if necessary ; penicillin, 250,000 to 500,000 units every six hours, to prevent bronchopneumonia; oxygen, dextrose-saline intravenously together with noradrenaline or metaraminol if blood pressure is very low. Forced diuresis with injections of mannitol.

Belladonna (atropine, hyoscine and related alkaloids)

SYMPTOMS.—Dryness of mouth, great thirst, pupils dilated (double vision), skin flushed and dry, temperature raised, rapid bounding pulse, breathing slow and stertorous, scanty urine, restlessness, delirium, coma.

TREATMENT.—Gastric lavage with weak tannic acid solution, paraldehyde intramuscularly or thiopentone sodium intravenously to control excitement, oxygen, artificial respiration.

Bleaching Solutions

SYMPTOMS.—Inhalation of fumes causes severe pulmonary irritation with coughing and choking; ingestion causes irritation and corrosion of mucous surfaces; oedema of pharynx and larynx.

TREATMENT.—Gastric lavage or emesis using sodium bicarbonate solution ($\frac{1}{2}$ oz. to 1 pint). Follow with sodium sulphate, 1 oz., and sodium bicarbonate, $\frac{1}{4}$ oz., in $\frac{1}{2}$ pint of water as cathartic.

Boric Acid, Borax

SYMPTOMS.—Nausea and vomiting, diarrhoea, rash, shock accompanied by subnormal temperature and cold sweat, eventual collapse.

Absorption of boric acid can occur through continual use as an ointment, lotion or powder. Infants are particularly susceptible. Boric acid powder should never be applied undiluted to infants, and dusting powders should not contain more than 5 per cent. of boric acid.

TREATMENT of acute boric acid poisoning by ingestion is by emesis or gastric lavage. The patient should be kept warm and treated for shock. Severe poisoning may require intravenous normal saline solution or dextrose-saline.

Camphor

SYMPTOMS.—Face flushed then pale, excitement and dizziness, vomiting, colic, tinnitus, pulse quickened, respiration difficult, characteristic odour of breath, anuria, skin clammy, delirium, convulsions.

TREATMENT.—Gastric lavage; control convulsions with thiopentone sodium intravenously or paraldehyde intramuscularly; magnesium sulphate solution as purgative.

Cantharides

Has been used in hair lotions, but owing to high toxicity the use of the drug is no longer recommended.

SYMPTOMS.—Burning pain in throat and stomach, swollen blistered tongue, salivation, intense thirst, colic, vomiting, bloody diarrhoea, raised temperature, respiration depressed, burning pain in bladder and urethra, incessant desire to micturate, delirium, collapse.

TREATMENT.—Gastric lavage; if throat is blistered use emetics; give white of egg, milk, charcoal, barley water; pethidine or morphine for pain, anaesthetics to control convulsions, oxygen, artificial respiration. Do not give oils.

Carbon Monoxide (including coal gas and exhaust fumes)

SYMPTOMS.—Headache, nausea, giddiness, tinnitus and throbbing of the heart, coma. There may be convulsions and incontinence of urine and faeces. Bright red coloration of the skin and mucosae.

TREATMENT.—Remove patient to fresh air, ensure airway. If respiration has failed institute artificial respiration immediately. Oxygen by oronasal mask for an hour or more. Keep patient warm and quiet.

Carbon Tetrachloride

SYMPTOMS.—In mild cases of poisoning following ingestion there is nausea, dizziness, headache, vomiting (often haematemesis) and feeble pulse ; in more severe cases there is diarrhoea and mental confusion. Respiration may be laboured. Toxic hepatitis, and fatty degeneration of the liver and toxic nephritis may follow.

TREATMENT.—Following inhalation of vapour, remove patient to fresh air. Artificial respiration, if necessary, and administration of oxygen.

Treatment of poisoning following ingestion is gastric lavage, fluids by mouth, hypertonic dextrose, mannitol or plasma solutions parenterally to increase diuresis, and oral or intravenous calcium gluconate. Blood transfusion may be necessary if there has been extensive haemorrhage. Oils and fats must be avoided.

Cocaine and Synthetic Local Anaesthetics

SYMPTOMS.—Excitement, confusion, nausea, vomiting, dilated pupils, rapid pulse, slow respiration, convulsions.

TREATMENT.—Gastric lavage with weak potassium permanganate solution, thiopentone sodium intravenously for convulsions, warmth and oxygen.

Copper Salts

SYMPTOMS.—Salivation, vomiting, diarrhoea, giddiness, headache, pulse rapid, shallow respiration, skin cold and clammy, suppression of urine, delirium, convulsions, coma.

TREATMENT.—Milk in quantity, followed by gastric lavage or an emetic; 10 G. of potassium ferrocyanide in water repeated at intervals as necessary; demulcents, stimulants, pethidine or morphine for pain.

The excretion of copper may be increased by the administration of disodium calcium edetate intravenously or injection of dimercaprol (B.A.L.) intramuscularly.

Cyanides (including prussic acid, cherry laurel water, bitter almond oil, etc.)

SYMPTOMS.—Characteristic smell of bitter almonds; respiration rapid and vigorous, becoming slow and gasping; slow imperceptible pulse, glassy protruding eyes, dilated pupils, convulsions, skin clammy and cold.

TREATMENT.—Immediate action is imperative : inhalations of amyl nitrite for fifteen to thirty seconds at a time at short intervals; artificial respiration if time permits; intravenous injections of sodium nitrite (0·3 G. in 10 ml. water) followed through same needle by sodium thiosulphate (25 G. in 50 ml.), then nikethamide (2 to 5 ml.) intravenously or intramuscularly. If available, inject intravenously, and as soon as possible, 40 ml. of Kelocyanor, followed immediately by 50 ml. of hypertonic glucose saline. (Kelocyanor contains 1·5 per cent. of dicobalt tetracemate.)

Digitalis (Foxglove)

SYMPTOMS.—Headache, giddiness, abdominal pain, vomiting, confusion, purging, salivation, skin cold and clammy, muscular weakness, disordered vision, pupils dilated, pulse slow and irregular, convulsions, coma.

TREATMENT.—Gastric lavage or an emetic. Artificial respiration and catheterisation as required. Quinidine or procainamide orally or intravenously for cardiac irregularities. Castor oil as purge to remove any unabsorbed drug.

D.N.O.C. Insecticides

SYMPTOMS.—Manifestations of poisoning are the result of stimulation of general metabolism and are aggravated by heat ; in acute poisoning death occurs within a few hours from heat stroke or cerebral oedema. Initial symptoms may be a feeling of well-being and abounding energy, and other early symptoms are excessive sweating, thirst and fatigue. Yellow staining of the sclerotics indicates absorption of, but not necessarily poisoning by, D.N.O.C. Early symptoms may be present as long as forty-eight hours before death. When the patient becomes acutely ill there is increased rate and depth of respiration, tachycardia, and rise in temperature. Death in coma follows rapidly.

TREATMENT.—The treatment of mild or moderately severe cases is expectant and symptomatic. Absolute rest must be ensured by the use of sedatives, oxygen, cold sponging, fluids for dehydration.

Ethylene Glycol (' Anti-freeze ')

SYMPTOMS.—Burning sensation in the throat, followed by malaise, sweating and vomiting; vertigo, drowsiness, coma, profuse sweating, acidosis, oliguria, anuria or haematuria. Death occurs from uraemia.

TREATMENT.—Gastric lavage with potassium permanganate solution 1 in 5000, repeated later; calcium gluconate intravenously. Treat for renal failure. Penicillin prophylactically.

Ferrous Sulphate

This substance is dangerous to very small children.

SYMPTOMS.—Pallor, coldness, vomiting, restlessness, low blood pressure, cyanosis, collapse, coma.

TREATMENT.—Emetics, gastric lavage with sodium bicarbonate solution, leaving some solution in the stomach. Supportive treatment for shock. Desferrioxamine (Desferal), orally and by injection. Desferrioxamine is a chelating agent and combines with iron to form a non-toxic water-soluble complex. Rapid treatment is essential, and is begun with a dose of 2 G. by intramuscular injection, followed by gastric lavage, then 5 G. orally in 50 to 100 ml. of water. Intravenous drip infusion of desferrioxamine at the rate of 15 mg./kg. hourly up to a maximum dose of 80 mg./kg. in twenty-four hours. Apparent recovery may be followed by relapse.

Food Poisoning

Salmonella Infection. Headache, abdominal pain, nausea, vomiting, diarrhoea, collapse, prostration.

TREATMENT.—Gastric lavage with a warm solution of sodium bicarbonate, chloramphenicol for systemic treatment; paromomycin orally for intestinal antibacterial action, dextrose-saline solution by intravenous infusion, stimulants.

Staphylococcus Enterotoxin. Vomiting occurs between one and six hours after ingestion of food. Illness rarely lasts more than twenty-four hours and in healthy persons there are no common complications or sequelae; energetic treatment will rarely be required.

Poisonous Fungi. Two main types of poisoning by fungi occur, the rapid type and the delayed type. In the rapid type symptoms include lacrimation, salivation, sweating, cardiovascular collapse, confusion, coma. The delayed type of poisoning occurs up to fifteen hours after ingestion of the fungus, and is characterised by the sudden onset of severe abdominal pains, nausea, vomiting and diarrhoea, dehydration and thirst. Jaundice, and oliguria or anuria from involvement of the liver and kidneys may occur.

TREATMENT.—In all cases of fungus poisoning gastric lavage or an emetic may be used together with symptomatic and supportive therapy; morphine or pethidine for pain, and the inhalation of oxygen if required.

The rapid type of poisoning may be caused by *Amanita muscaria* which contains muscarine, to which atropine is a specific antidote, and provided it is administered early the prognosis is good. Delayed poisoning may be due to *A. phalloides* and allied species such as *A. verna*, and in these the prognosis is grave. Antiphallinic serum should be given if available.

Iodine

SYMPTOMS.—Burning pain in throat and stomach, vomiting, purging (stools may be bloody), intense thirst, skin cold and clammy, cyanosis, giddiness, faintness, convulsions, coma.

TREATMENT.—Gastric lavage with a solution of sodium thiosulphate. This combines with iodine to form a colourless solution. A suspension of starch or flour in water may be given, as iodine forms an insoluble blue complex with starch. A saline purge may also be given, and demulcents and morphine or pethidine for pain.

Kerosene, Paraffin, Turpentine Substitute, Petrol, Tractor Vaporising Oil (T.V.O.)

SYMPTOMS.—Restlessness, coughing and choking of rapid onset, with nausea, vomiting and diarrhoea; drowsiness. In severe cases dyspnoea, cyanosis and pyrexia, especially if inhalation as well as ingestion has occurred; feeble and rapid pulse with failing respiration, convulsions, coma.

TREATMENT.—In mild cases no active measures need be taken. In more severe cases emetics should be avoided, owing to the risk of inhaling some of the poison, and gastric lavage should be carried out only in cases where large amounts of kerosene are known to have been ingested. Antibiotics in full doses prophylactically owing to the risk of bronchopneumonia. For respiratory symptoms oxygen inhalations and atropine.

Laburnum (seeds, leaves and bark)

SYMPTOMS.—Burning in mouth and abdomen, thirst, nausea, severe vomiting, diarrhoea, prostration, irregular pulse and respiration, delirium, twitching and unconsciousness, oliguria.

TREATMENT.—Gastric lavage or emetics, followed by sodium sulphate, 30 G. in 500 ml. of water, as cathartic; copious fluids, dextrose intravenously, oxygen.

Lead Compounds

SYMPTOMS.—Metallic taste, dry throat, intense thirst, abdominal colic, occasional diarrhoea (black stained), vomiting (may be bloody), muscular weakness, giddiness and stupor, convulsions, coma.

TREATMENT.—Gastric lavage with magnesium or sodium sulphate solutions followed by saline purge. Demulcents, pethidine or morphine for pain. Calcium disodium edetate intravenously for five days, also orally; calcium gluconate, atropine for colic.

Mercury Compounds (including corrosive sublimate, white precipitate, red precipitate, vermilion, cinnabar)

SYMPTOMS.—Metallic taste, burning pain in mouth and throat, choking sensation, tongue may be white and swollen, colic, vomiting, bloody diarrhoea, temperature subnormal, pulse rapid, irregular and feeble, skin cold and clammy, acute kidney inflammation, urine scanty or suppressed, restlessness, shock.

TREATMENT.—Gastric lavage, after giving large quantities of white of egg or charcoal water, leaving a quantity of white of egg in the stomach; for soluble mercuric salts, 5 to 10 per cent. solution sodium formaldehyde sulphoxylate; the stomach should be emptied again after a few hours and once more later. Give pethidine or morphine for pain; demulcents, stimulants. Dimercaprol by intramuscular injection in doses of 2 c.c. four-hourly is specific if injected early, but is of no value against the tissue damage that occurs after absorption of mercury compounds. Dimercaprol, also known as B.A.L., and calcium disodium edetate, also known as calcium disodium versenate, are chelating agents. Such compounds have the power of combining with heavy metals and blocking their toxic action. They are useful in the early stages of heavy metal poisoning, but are less effective, as might be expected, when the metal has already damaged the tissue cells.

Methyl Bromide

Frequently used in fire extinguishers either alone or mixed with carbon tetrachloride. Also employed for fumigation.

SYMPTOMS.—Systemic effects occur four to forty-eight hours after inhalation of the gas; diplopia, headache, vertigo, vomiting, dilated pupils; cerebral irritation characterised by epileptiform convulsions and delirium.

TREATMENT.—No specific antidote. Intramuscular paraldehyde or intravenous thiopentone sodium for convulsions; oxygen.

Metaldehyde

Used as a solid fuel and for poisoning slugs.

SYMPTOMS.—Abdominal pain, vomiting, diarrhoea, unconsciousness, cramp, convulsions, coma.

TREATMENT.—No known antidote. Immediate gastric lavage with sodium bicarbonate solution; purgative, repeated frequently; administration of alkalis to prevent acidosis; intravenous injection of caffeine or other stimulant; calcium gluconate. The convulsions and cramps may be controlled by intravenous thiopentone sodium.

Methyl Alcohol

SYMPTOMS.—Nausea, vomiting, severe gastric pain, mental confusion, visual disturbances which may cause blindness, prolonged coma. These symptoms are often slow in onset, and may take thirty-six hours to appear.

TREATMENT.—Keep patient warm and protect his eyes from light. Intravenous sodium bicarbonate or sodium lactate may be given to combat the severe acidosis. Morphine for pain. Delirium or convulsions can be controlled by injections of hyoscine or thiopentone.

Methyl Salicylate

SYMPTOMS.—Nausea, vomiting, mental confusion, profuse sweating, thirst and diarrhoea. Pulse and respiration are rapid at first but later dyspnoea may be evident. Bile pigments may be present in the urine, and jaundice with a toxic nephritis and oliguria may develop.

TREATMENT.—Immediate gastric lavage. Fluids should be given to overcome dehydration and promote urinary excretion of salicylic acid. The acidosis which is present may be relieved by intravenous sodium lactate, oral or intravenous sodium bicarbonate. Blood transfusion; vitamin K_1 if prothrombin is low.

Nicotine

Present in various horticultural pesticide products. It is one of the most toxic compounds, and in severe poisoning death may occur in a few minutes owing to respiratory paralysis.

SYMPTOMS.—Giddiness, nausea, vomiting, diarrhoea, confusion, convulsions, respiratory depression and collapse.

TREATMENT.—Gastric lavage with weak potassium permanganate or tannic acid solution. Remove any nicotine contaminated clothing and wash skin. Oxygen and artificial respiration. Intravenous thiopentone for convulsions.

Opium (including morphine, codeine, heroin, chlorodyne, etc.)

SYMPTOMS.—Preliminary mental excitement followed by headache, dizziness, nausea, ' pin-point ' pupils, skin cold and clammy, face cyanosed, muscular relaxation, pulse slow and feeble, respiration slow and shallow, temperature subnormal.

TREATMENT.—Gastric lavage with 0·2 per cent. solution of potassium permanganate, leaving 250 ml. in stomach at conclusion; saline purgative; hot coffee and stimulants ; nikethamide; amphetamine sulphate or methylamphetamine sulphate intravenously; frequent catheterisation.

Nalorphine (Lethidrone) is a specific antagonist of morphine and related alkaloids and also of synthetic analgesics such as pethidine, methadone, etc.; give 5 to 10 mg. intravenously to a total of 40 mg.

Phenol (including phenols in general, lysol and other cresols, creosote, etc.)

SYMPTOMS.—Characteristic odour of breath; whitened lips and mouth; burning pain from mouth to stomach at first, which may become dulled later owing to local anaesthetic effect; rapid collapse, temperature subnormal, feeble pulse, stomach contracted and rigid. Reflexes may be abolished, and the urine may turn black on standing. Accidental poisoning may occur by absorption through the skin.

TREATMENT.—Gastric lavage with a copious quantity of water, lime water or magnesium sulphate solution, followed by lavage with arachis or olive oil. Then copious sodium bicarbonate drinks for acidosis; by injection in coma. Milk, egg albumen or other demulcents later; artificial respiration; stimulants. Remove contaminated clothing and wash phenol from the skin.

Phosphorus Insecticides (Organic)

SYMPTOMS.—Tightness in the chest, slight twitching of eyelid and tongue muscles and contraction of the pupils; headache, anorexia and nausea aggravated by smoking; giddiness, anxiety, restlessness. Second-stage symptoms are respiratory distress, sweating, salivation, contraction of pupils, vomiting, abdominal cramps. Final stage characterised by great respiratory distress, ' pin-point ' pupils, muscular twitchings, incontinence, coma.

TREATMENT.—Atropine is a specific antidote and should be given (i.v. or i.m.) in doses of 2 mg. to be repeated every thirty to sixty minutes until the patient is obviously fully atropinised or improving. PAM or P2S are special antidotes, and should be administered intravenously as soon as possible in doses of 1 G., repeated after thirty minutes if no real improvement has occurred. Emergency supplies of these drugs are available from many regional distributing centres throughout Great Britain. Supportive measures include intravenous or intramuscular barbiturates for intense excitement or restlessness, postural drainage for bronchial hypersecretion and oxygen for respiratory distress.

Silver Nitrate

SYMPTOMS.—Burning pain in throat and stomach, vomiting, purging, dizziness, weak pulse, shallow respiration.

TREATMENT.—Give two tablespoonfuls of sodium chloride in a pint of water. This precipitates the silver as insoluble silver chloride, which may be removed by gastric lavage, or less effectively by an emetic. Repeat as necessary, then follow with milk in quantity, and a castor-oil purge. Morphine for pain, stimulants if necessary.

Snake Bite

SYMPTOMS.—Snake venoms are composed mainly of two constituents, a haemotoxin and a neurotoxin; the former destroys red blood cells and tissues, while the latter, which has a curare-like action, attacks the nerve centres. The only poisonous snake in Great Britain is the adder, but the poison is unlikely to prove fatal in an adult. Adder-bite antivenom is no longer freely available, and its use is said to be more dangerous than the snake-bite.

Viper Bite. Principally haemotoxin. Immediate swelling

and discoloration, oozing of blood from mouth and conjunctiva, haematuria, bloody vomiting, collapse and coma. Death may occur within twenty-four hours.

Cobra Bite. Principally neurotoxin. Slow moderate swelling, little or no discoloration, paralysis of respiratory and vasomotor centre, asphyxia.

TREATMENT.—Ligature the part above the bite; make deep cross-shaped incisions over the bite; suction—mechanically or by mouth—wash mouth and bite with 1 per cent. potassium permanganate, repeat suction for fifteen minutes every hour for several hours; specific antivenom serum, first dose should be given intravenously, later doses by subcutaneous injection around the bite. Give fluids by mouth or intravenously; stimulants and cortisone may be given for shock, and penicillin or other antibiotic to control infection.

Strychnine (including nux vomica)

Strychnine is used in certain vermin killers.

SYMPTOMS.—Feeling of suffocation, face livid, tetanic convulsions, sweating and exhaustion, staring eyeballs, rigid abdominal muscles. The jaw muscles are not affected till late (differentiation from tetanus).

TREATMENT.—Short-acting barbiturate intravenously to control or prevent convulsions. Gastric lavage (after the barbiturate) with weak solution of potassium permanganate, iodine or tannic acid. Protect from all possible stimuli. Further doses of barbiturate as required together with muscle relaxants. Oxygen. Recovery is usual if convulsive stage is survived.

CHAPTER XXIII

POISONS AND DANGEROUS DRUGS

IT has long been accepted that some legal control over the supply, storage and use of poisons is necessary, but with the extensive use of new and increasingly potent drugs, close control is more essential than ever.

The use of poisons is now regulated by the Pharmacy and Poisons Act, the Poisons List and Rules and the Pharmacy and Medicines Act. Habit-forming narcotic drugs or drugs of addiction are further controlled by the Dangerous Drugs Act and certain other potent drugs are controlled by the Therapeutic Substances Act. The Poisons List has two main divisions (Parts I and II). Part II refers to a number of common poisons, such as household disinfectants, which should be easily available to the public. Poisons in this group may be sold by registered suppliers, provided certain requirements governing labels and containers are observed. Poisons in Part I of the List include the more potent poisons, and can be supplied to the public only by pharmacists. The Poisons Act requires a strict control of Part I poisons, and specifies the records to be kept, the information and cautionary notices that must appear on the label, the type of container to be used, and conditions of storage and transport.

The poisons in Part I of the Poisons List are further divided into several sections, termed Schedules, of which the most important to nurses are Schedule I and Schedule IV. Schedule I poisons include many drugs, and also other substances which can be purchased when the purchaser is known to the pharmacist as a person to whom the poison may properly be sold (as for trade or manufacturing purposes), and signs a written record of the purchase, indicating the purpose for which the poison is required. Schedule IV poisons are medicinal substances, and can be obtained only on the prescription of a registered medical practitioner. Such prescriptions must bear the name and address of the patient, the name and amount of the poison to be dispensed, the date and signature of the doctor.

In hospitals, poisons in Schedules I and IV are supplied from the pharmacy for individual patients on medical prescriptions, and for ward stocks on the production of an order signed by the sister or nurse-in-charge.   When issued from the pharmacy the container must indicate by a label that the drugs are scheduled poisons, and when received in the ward must be stored in a locked poison cupboard, and the key kept *on the person* of the ward sister or deputy.   Poisons for external use are supplied in fluted bottles, distinguishable as such by touch, and must bear a label indicating that they are intended for external use.   These poisons must be stored in a separate poison cupboard.   All ward poison cupboards and dangerous drug cupboards are subject to inspection at intervals by the hospital pharmacist.

Dangerous Drugs

These are habit-forming drugs, and are subject to stricter control than Schedules I and IV poisons.   The drugs concerned include opium, morphine and related compounds, cocaine, diamorphine (heroin), cannabis indica (Indian hemp), pethidine, methadone (Physeptone), levorphanol (Dromoran), dextromoramide (Palfium), phenazocine (Narphen) and other synthetic, morphine-like compounds. (Certain standard preparations of some dangerous drugs, which contain only small amounts of active substances, *e.g.*, Kaolin and Morphine Mixture, are exempted from D.D.A. restrictions.)

These drugs can be obtained by the public only on prescription, and full records of every supply must be kept by the pharmacist. The use of dangerous drugs in hospitals is also rigidly controlled, and the strictly legal requirements are often extended.   Extensions of this kind are a protection to both staff and patient, and all records should be regarded as important legal documents.   The basic requirements can be summarised as follows :—

1. Prescriptions for individual patients must state the full amount or number of doses of the drug to be dispensed, and bear the signature of a registered medical practitioner.

2. Ward stocks of dangerous drugs must be ordered in the special D.D.A. book supplied for the purpose, and the order must be signed by the sister or her deputy.   The duplicate copies of the orders must be kept by the sister for at least two years.

3. All supplies of dangerous drugs must be signed for when received, and stored away from other poisons in a special locked cupboard, or locked inner compartment of a Schedule poison

cupboard, and the key must be kept *on the person* of the ward sister or deputy. No doctor has right of access to ward stocks of dangerous drugs, as the responsibility for their storage and use rests with the sister-in-charge.

4. A written record must be made of every amount of a dangerous drug received by a ward, and a detailed record kept of each dose given. Records of the administration of these drugs should be signed by the nurse who gives the dose, as well as by the nurse who checks the drug and dose.

5. A running record of stocks of all dangerous drugs must be kept, and any wastage or loss must be recorded immediately, countersigned and reported.

The following list indicates most of the drugs now subject to full D.D.A. control. It should be noted that most of these substances are also included in Schedule I of the Poisons List, but have been omitted from the list of such poisons on page 305 in order to make clear the distinction between the two groups. In general, the restrictions also apply to the salts, derivatives and preparations of the drug in question, but in order to simplify the list, the names of many preparations *i.e.* morphine tablets, have been omitted.

Acetyldihydrocodeine
Acetyldihydrocodeinone
Akolethe
Alidine
Allylprodine
Alphacetylmethadol
Alphameprodine
Alphaprodine
Amidone
Anileridine
Benzethidine
Benzoylmorphine
Benzylmorphine
Betacetylmethadol
Betameprodine
Betamethadol
Betaprodine
C.B. 11
Cannabis, extracts or tinctures or resins
Cetobemidone
Chloroform and Morphine Compound Tincture B.P.C., 1949
Clonitazene
Coca leaves
Cocaine and its salts and preparations unless diluted below o·1 per cent.

cocaine in a base from which the drug cannot be readily extracted
Codeine ; except preparations containing less than 2·5 per cent. in a base from which the drug cannot be readily extracted.
Codrenine
Desomorphine
Dextromoramide
Diacetylmorphine
Diamorphine hydrochloride
Diamorphine Linctus B.P.C.
Diampromide
Dicodid
Diconal
Diethylthiambutene
Dihydrocodeinone
Dihydrodesoxymorphine
Dihydrohydroxycodeinone
Dihydromorphine
Dihydromorphinone
Dilaudid preparations
Dimenoxadole
Dimepheptanol
Dimethylthiambutene
Dimotane Expectorant-DC
Dioxaphetyl butyrate

Diphenoxylate
Dipipanone
Dolantal
Dolantin
Dromoran
Duromorph
Ecgonine
Ethylmethylthiambutene
Etonitazene
Etoxeridine
Eucodal
Fentanyl
Ferrier's snuff
Furethidine
Gall and Opium Ointment
Genomorphine
Heptalgin
Heroin
Hydrocodone
Hydromorphinol
Hydromorphone
Hydroxypethidine
Isoamidone
Isomethadone
Indian Hemp
Ketobemidone
Laudanum
Levomethorphan
Levomoramide
Levophenacylmorphan
Levorphanol
Linseed, Liquorice and Chlorodyne Lozenges
Locosthetic
Lomotil Liquid
Metazocine
Methadone
Methadyl acetate
Methyldesomorphine (Methyldesorphine)
Methyldihydromorphine
Metopon
Morpheridine
Morphine ; its salts and preparations unless diluted below 0·2 per cent. morphine or its equivalent in a base from which the drug cannot be readily extracted.
Mortha
Myrophine

Narphen
Nepenthe
Nicomorphine
Noracymethadol
Norlevorphanol
Normethadone
Normorphine
Norpipanone
Numorphan
Numorphan Oral
Omnopon
Omnopon-Scopolamine
Operidine
Opium unless diluted below 0·2 per cent. morphine in a base from which the drug cannot be readily extracted.
Opoidine
Oxycodone
Oxymorphone
Palfium
Pamergan preparations
Papaveretum
Permonid
Pethidine
Pethilorfan
Phenadoxone
Phenampromide
Phenazocine
Phenomorphan
Phenoperidine
Pholcodine esters and ethers
Physeptone
Piminodine
Pinheroin
Pipadone
Proheptazine
Proladone
Properidine
Racemethorphan
Racemoramide
Racemorphan
Somnigen
Sublimaze
Sterilocaine
Thebacon
Thebaine
Themalon
Trimeperidine
Trivalin

The strictly legal restrictions governing the use of dangerous drugs should be regarded as the minimum, and in most hospitals a greater degree of control is exercised. The actual stock and the recorded stock of dangerous drugs should be checked at frequent intervals, and any loss reported and investigated. Such a system reminds users of the need for care when dealing with dangerous drugs, and could be extended with advantage to include many other potent drugs.

SCHEDULE I POISONS

The following list includes most of the
drugs in the official Schedule I Poisons List.

The following alkaloids and their salts.

Acetyldihydrocodeinone
Aconite alkaloids, except substances containing less than 0·02 per cent.
Apomorphine, except substances containing less than 0·2 per cent.
Atropine, except substances containing less than 0·15 per cent.
Belladonna alkaloids except substances containing less than 0·15 per cent.
Brucine, except substances containing less than 0·2 per cent.
Calabar bean and its alkaloids
Codeine, except substances containing less than 1·5 per cent.
Colchicum alkaloids, except substances containing less than 0·5 per cent.
Coniine, except substances containing less than 0·1 per cent.
Cotarnine, except substances containing less than 0·2 per cent.
Curare alkaloids, curare bases
Emetine, except substances containing less than 1 per cent.
Ethylmorphine, except substances containing less than 0·2 per cent.
Gelsemium alkaloids, except substances containing less than 0·1 per cent.
Homatropine, except substances containing less than 0·15 per cent.
Hyoscine, except substances containing less than 0·15 per cent.
Hyoscyamine, except substances containing less than 0·15 per cent.
Jaborandi alkaloids, except substances containing less than 0·5 per cent.
Lobelia alkaloids, except substances containing less than 0·5 per cent.
Nicotine
Papaverine, except substances containing less than 1 per cent.
Pomegranate alkaloids, except substances containing less than 0·5 per cent.
Quebracho alkaloids
Sabadilla alkaloids, except substances containing less than 1 per cent.
Solanaceous alkaloids, not otherwise included in the Schedule, except substances containing less than 0·15 per cent.
Stavesacre alkaloids, except substances containing less than 0·2 per cent.
Strychnine, except substances containing less than 0·2 per cent.
Veratrum alkaloids, except substances containing less than 1 per cent.
Yohimba alkaloids

Acetarsol
Acetylarsan
Allylisopropylacetylurea
Anthiomaline
Antihistamines
Astiban
Antimonial poisons, except substances containing less than the equivalent of 1 per cent. of antimony trioxide
Apomorphine and its salts, except substances containing less than 0·2 per cent.
Arsenical poisons, except substances containing less than the equivalent of 0·01 per cent. of arsenic trioxide and except dentrifices containing less than 0·5 per cent. of acetarsol
Barium, salts of, other than sulphate, carbonate or silicofluoride
Buscopan
Calcium cyanide, except substances containing less than 0·1 per cent.
Cantharidin, except substances containing less than 0·01 per cent.
Carbachol
Carbarsone
Carperidine, and its salts
Cedilanid
Chlormerodrin
Chloroform
Choleflavin
Cinchocaine (Nupercaine)
Cocculin
Combiquine
Corangil
Crystodigin
Cyanides, except substances containing less than 0·1 per cent.
D.F. 118
Dextromethorphan ; its salts, except substances containing less than 1·5 per cent.
Dextropropoxyphene
Dextrorphan ; its salts
Diacetyl-N-allylnormorphine ; its salts
Diamethine
Digitalis, glycosides and other active principles of, except substances containing less than 1 unit of activity in 2 G. of the substance
Digoxin
Di-isopropyl fluorophosphonate
Distalgesic
Doloxene capsules
Dover's powder
Dyflos
Ecothiopate iodide
Ephedrine
Eumydrin
Fluoroacetamide ; fluoroacetanilide

Hydrocyanic acid except substances containing less than 0·15 per cent ; cyanides, except substances containing less than the equivalent of 0·1 per cent. of hydrocyanic acid (HCN) ; double cyanides of mercury and zinc

Hydroxycinchoninic acid and its derivatives, except substances containing less than 3 per cent.

Lanatoside C.

Lanoxin

Laudexium ; its salts

Laudolissin

Lead, compounds of, with acids from fixed oils

Lethidrone

Leucarsone

Levopropoxyphene

Mapharside

Melarsoprol

Memine

Mercardan

Mercloran

Mercuric chloride, except substances containing less than 1 per cent.; mercuric iodide, except substances containing less than 2 per cent.; nitrates of mercury, except substances containing less than the equivalent of 3 per cent., of mercury (Hg) ; potassiomercuric iodides, except substances containing less than the equivalent of 1 per cent. of mercuric iodide ; organic compounds of mercury, except substances, not being aerosols, containing less than the equivalent of 0·2 per cent. of mercury (Hg)

Mersalyl

Metanitrophenol ; orthonitrophenol ; paranitrophenol

Monofluoroacetic acid ; its salts

Mycozol

Nalorphine ; its salts

Nebadrene

Neostam

Neptal

Noradran

Novarsenobillon

Nupercaine

Nux Vomica, except substances containing less than 0·2 per cent. of strychnine

Oradon

Ouabain

Oxycinchoninic acid, derivatives of ; their salts ; their esters

Pamine

Pentostam

Pholcodine, except preparations containing less than 1·5 per cent.

Picrotoxin

Procaine, its salts, except substances containing less than 10 per cent.

Romilar tablets

Savin ; oil of
Skopyl
Stovarsol
Strophanthus, glycosides of
Surfacaine
S.V.C. tablets
Thallium, salts of
Tigloidine, except preparations containing less than 0·15 per cent.
Tiglyssin
Trasentin
Triostam
Trophenium
Tryparsamide
Zinc and mercury cyanide

SCHEDULE IV POISONS

The poisons in this Schedule are divided into two parts, A and B, which differ mainly in certain points of detail necessary on prescriptions concerning these drugs. These differences are of little significance to nurses, and do not merit further description in this book. This Schedule is of increasing size and importance, and the following list of drugs, although not a complete survey of Schedule IV poisons, gives most of those in general use.

Substances that are controlled by the Therapeutic Substances Act are given separately on page 312.

The names in parenthesis in the following list are those of some brand products of the drug concerned :—

Part A—
  Alcuronium chloride (Alloferin)
  Allylisopropylacetylurea (Sedormid)
  Azathioprine (Imuran)
  Barbituric acid ; its salts ; derivatives of barbituric acid ; their salts ; compounds of barbituric acid, its salts, its derivatives, their salts, with any other substance
  Busulphan (Myleran)
  Chlorambucil (Leukeran)
  Cyclophosphamide (Endoxana)
  Demecarium bromide (Tosmilen)
  Dinitrocresols (DNOC) ; their compounds with a metal or a base, except preparations for use in agriculture or horticulture
  Dinitronaphthols ; dinitrophenols ; dinitrothymols
  Disulfiram (Antabuse)

Dithienylallylamines; dithienylalkylallylamines; their salts; except diethylthiambutene, dimethylthiambutene and ethylmethylthiamiambutene

Gallamine (Flaxedil)

Hydroxyurea (Hydrea)

Mannomustine (Degranol)

Melphalan (Alkeran)

Mercaptopurine (Puri-Nethol)

Mustine and any other N-substituted derivatives of di-(2-chloroethyl)-amine; their salts

Phenacemide (Phenurone)

Phenylcinchoninic acid ; salicylcinchoninic acid ; their salts ; their esters

Polymethylenebistrimethylammonium salts

Tretamine ; its salts

Triaziquone (Trenimon)

Part B

Acetanilide ; alkyl acetanilides

Acetohexamide (Dimelor)

Acetylcarbromal (Abasin)

Adrenaline, except inhalations and topical preparations

Amidopyrine ; its salts ; amidopyrine sulphonates ; their salts

Amitriptyline (Laroxyl, Saroten, Tryptizol)

Amphetamines and any related compounds (except ephedrine) and derivatives (Benzedrine, Dexedrine, Methedrine, Mephine)

Androgens

Azacyclonol (Frenquel)

Benactyzine

Benzhexol (Artane, Pipanol)

Benztropine (Cogentin)

Bromvaletone (Bromural)

Captodiame (Covatin)

Caramiphen

Carbromal (Adalin)

Carisoprodol (Carisoma)

Chloral ; its addition and its condensation products (Welldorm, Tricloryl, Somilan)

Chlordiazepoxide (Librium)

Chlormethiazole (Heminevrin)

Chlorothiazide, and related diuretics

Chlorotrianisene (Tace)

Chlorphenoxamine (Clorevan)

Chlorphentermine (Lucofen)

Chlorpropamide (Diabinese)

Chlorprothixene (Taractan)

Chlorthalidone (Hygroton)

Clopamide (Brinaldix)

Clorexolone (Nefrolan)

Cyclarbamate (Casmalon)
Cycrimine ; its salts
Dehydrobenzperidine (Droperidol)
Desipramine (Pertofran)
Diazepam (Valium)
Dichlorphenamide (Daranide)
Dimethothiazine (Banistyl)
Diphenoxylate and its salts contained in (a) pharmaceutical prep-
    arations in solid or liquid form containing not more than 2·5 mg.
    of diphenoxylate calculated as base and not less than 25 mg. of
    atropine (Lomotil)
Droperidol (Droleptan)
Ectylurea (Nostyn)
Emylcamate (Striatran)
Ephedrine aerosols
Ergot and its alkaloids and related substances
Ethacrynic acid (Edecrin)
Ethchlorvynol (Arvynol, Serenesil)
Ethinamate (Valmidate)
Ethionamide (Trescatyl)
Ethoheptazine (Zactane)
Fencamfamin (Euvitol)
Fenfluramine (Ponderax)
Flufenamic acid (Arlef)
Flugesterone
Fluphenazine (Moditen, Modecate)
Glutethimide (Doriden)
Gonadotrophic hormones (Gestyl, Pregnyl)
Glymidine (Gondafon)
Haloperidol (Serenace)
Hexapropymate (Merinax)
Hydrazines, benzyl phenethyl or phenoxyethyl and their deriva-
    tives (Actomol, Cavodil, Marplan, Marsilid, Nardil, Niamid,
    Parnate)
Hydroxyzine (Atarax)
Imipramine (Tofranil)
Indomethacin (Indocid)
Iprindole (Prondol)
Isoetharine aerosols
Isoprenaline aerosols
Mebutamate (Capla)
Meclofenoxate (Lucidril)
Mefenamic acid (Ponstan)
Mephenesin (Myanesin, Tolseram)
Meprobamate (Equanil, Mepavlon, Miltown)
Metaxalone
Metformin (Glucophage)
Methaqualone (Mandrax, Melsedin, Paxidorm)
Methenolone (Primobolan)

Methixene (Tremonil)
Methocarbamol (Robaxan)
Methoxsalen
Methylpentynol (Atempol, Oblivon, Somnesin)
Methyl Phenidate (Ritalin)
Methyprylone (Nodular)
Methysergide (Deseril)
Metoclopramide (Maxolon)
Nitrazepam (Mogadon)
Nortriptyline (Allegron, Aventyl)
Oestrogens
Orciprenaline aerosols
Orphenadrine (Disipal, Norflex)
Oxazepam (Serenid-D)
Oxethazaine
Oxymetholone (Anapolon)
Oxyphenbutazone (Tanderil)
Paraldehyde
Paramethadione (Paradione)
Pargyline (Eutonyl)
Pemoline (Kethamed, Ronyl)
Pentazocine (Fortral)
Phenaglycodol (Ultran)
Phenbutrazate
Phencyclidine (Sernyl)
Phenetidylphenacetin
Phenformin (Dibotin)
Phenmetrazine (Preludin)
Phenothiazine compounds; except dimethoxanate and prometha-
    zine
Phenylbutazone (Butazolidin)
Phenytoin (Epanutin)
Pituitary gland, the active principles of ; except when contained in
    preparations intended for external application
Procainamide (Pronestyl)
Procarbazine (Natalan)
Procyclidine ; its salts (Kemadrin)
Progestogens
Prothionamide (Trevintix)
Prothipendyl (Tolnate)
Quinethazone (Aquamox)
Quinine, except substances containing less than 10 per cent.
Rautrax
Rauwolfia, alkaloids and derivatives (Serpasil, Rauwiloid, Raudixin,
    Decaserpyl, Harmonyl, Hypertane)
Salbutamol (Ventolin)
Styramate (Sinaxar)
Sulphinpyrazone (Anturan)
Sulphonal ; alkyl sulphonals

Sulphonamides, except when contained in ointments or surgical dressings

Suprarenal gland products, except when contained in preparations intended for external application only or in inhalants, rectal preparations or preparations intended for use in the eye

Syrosingopine (Isotense, Singoserp)

Tetrabenazine (Nitoman)

Thalidomide ; its salts

Thiocarlide (Isoxyl)

Thyrocalcitonin

Thyroid gland products

Tolbutamide (Artosin, Rastinon)

Tranylcypromine (Parnate)

Tribromethyl alcohol (Avertin)

Trimeprazine (Vallergan)

2, 2, 2-Trichloroethyl alcohol, esters of ; their salts

Trimipramine (Surmontil)

Troxidone (Tridione)

Tybamate (Benvil, Solacen)

Verapamil (Cordilox)

Zoxazolamine (Flexin)

THERAPEUTIC SUBSTANCES ACT, 1956

A number of drugs are now in use which are not poisons, yet have a degree of potency or a type of activity which on rational grounds should be subject to some control. These drugs, of which the largest single group is the antibiotics, are controlled by the Therapeutic Substances Act, and may be obtained only on the prescription of a registered medical practitioner. Such prescriptions are valid for one supply (with certain specific exceptions), and must be dispensed within three months of the date of the prescription.

The most important of the drugs subject to the provisions of the Therapeutic Substances Act (T.S.A.) are the following :—

ACTH	Chlortetracycline	Griseofulvin
Amphomycin	Corticotrophin	Hydrocortisone and
Amphotericin	Cortisone and	related substances
Aureomycin	related substances	Isoniazid
Bacitracin	Cycloserine	Kanamycin
Capreomycin	Erythromycin	Lincomycin
Cephalexin	Framycetin	Nalidixic acid
Cephaloridine	Fusidic acid	Neomycin
Chloramphenicol	Gentamicin	Novobiocin

Nystatin
Oleandomycin
Oxytetracycline
Paromomycin
Penicillin
Polymyxins
Prednisolone

Prednisone
Rifamycins
Ristocetins
Spiramycin
Streptomycin
Tetracycline and
    related substances

Triacetyloleando-
    mycin
Vancomycin
Viomycin

APPENDIX I

APPROVED AND BRAND NAMES OF DRUGS

NEW drugs are usually introduced under a brand or proprietary name, which represents the product of a single manufacturer. If the drug gains general acceptance, it may receive official recognition by being described in the British Pharmacopoeia (B.P.) or the British Pharmaceutical Codex (B.P.C.), but the use of brand names in official publications can cause difficulties. The Pharmacopoeia Commisssion has therefore devised a list of non-proprietary or 'approved' names for many new drugs. These names are intended for official use should the drug concerned eventually reach B.P. or B.P.C. status, but they are also used generally as alternative names for proprietary products not yet official. The following lists give both the Approved Name and Proprietary Name of drugs :—

Approved Name	*Proprietary Name*
Acetazolamide	Diamox
Acetohexamide	Dimelor
Acetylcarbromal	Abasin
Acetylcysteine	Airbron
Alcuronium	Alloferin
Aldosterone	Aldocorten
Allopurinol	Zyloric
Allyloestrenol	Gestanin
Aloxiprin	Palaprin
Amantadine	Symmetrel
Ambenonium	Mytelase
Aminocaproic Acid	Epsikapron
Amiphenazole	Daptazole
Amitriptyline	Laroxyl ; Saroten ; Tryptizol
Amodiaquine	Camoquin
Amphotericin B	Fungizone ; Fungilin
Ampicillin	Penbritin
Ancrod	Arvin
Antazoline	Antistin
Azathioprine	Imuran
Azuresin	Diagnex Blue
Bamethan	Vasculit
Bamifylline	Trentadil

Approved Name	*Proprietary Name*
Beclamide	Nydrane
Beclomethazone	Propaderm
Bemegride	Megimide
Bendrofluazide	Aprinox ; Centyl ; Neo-Naclex
Benzalkonium Chloride	Roccal
Benzathine Penicillin	Penidural
Benzhexol	Artane ; Pipanol
Benzilonium Bromide	Portyn
Benzphetamine	Didrex
Benztropine	Cogentin
Bephenium Hydroxynaphthoate	Alcopar
Betahistine	Serc
Betamethasone	Betnelan ; Betnesol ; Betnovate
Bethanidine	Bethanid ; Esbatal
Biperidon	Akineton
Bisacodyl	Dulcolax
Bretylium Tosylate	Darenthin
Bromhexine	Bisolvon
Bromodiphenhydramine	Ambodryl
Brompheniramine	Dimotane
Buclizine	Vibazine
Buclosamide	Jadit
Buphenine	Perdilatal
Bupivacaine	Marcain
Busulphan	Myleran
Calcium Benzamidosalicylate	Calcium B-PAS ; Therapas
Carbamazepine	Tegretol
Carbenicillin	Pyopen
Carbenoxolone	Biogastrone ; Duogastrone
Carbimazole	Neo-Mercazole
Carisoprodol	Carisoma
Cephalexin	Ceporex; Keflex
Cephaloridine	Ceporin
Chloral Betaine	Somilan
Chlorambucil	Leukeran
Chloramphenicol	Chloromycetin
Chlorcyclizine	Di-paralene ; Histantin
Chlordiazepoxide	Librium
Chlorhexidine	Hibitane
Chlormethiazole	Heminevrin
Chlormezanone	Trancopal
Chloroquine	Avloclor; Nivaquine; Resochin
Chlorothiazide	Saluric
Chlorotrianisene	TACE
Chlorphenesin	Mycil
Chlorpheniramine	Piriton
Chlorphenoxamine	Clorevan
Chlorproguanil	Lapudrine

11*

Approved Name	*Proprietary Name*
Chlorpromazine	Largactil
Chlorpropamide	Diabinese
Chlorprothixene	Taractan
Chlortetracycline	Aureomycin
Chlorthalidone	Hygroton
Cholestyramine	Cuemid; Questran
Choline Theophyllinate	Choledyl
Cinchocaine	Nupercaine
Cinnarizine	Mitronal
Clemizole	Allercur
Clindamycin	Dalacin C
Clioquinol	Vioform
Clofazimine	Lamprene
Clofibrate	Atromid-S
Clomiphene	Clomid
Clomocycline	Megaclor
Clonidine	Catapres
Clopamide	Brinaldix
Clorexolone	Nefrolan
Cloxacillin	Orbenin
Colaspase	Crasnitin
Colistin	Colomycin
Corticotrophin	ACTH
Cortisone	Adreson; Cortelan; Cortistab; Cortisyl
Crotamiton	Eurax
Cyanocobalamin	Cobalin ; Cytacon ; Cytamen
Cyclandelate	Cyclospasmol
Cyclizine	Marzine ; Valoid
Cyclobarbitone	Phanodorm
Cyclopenthiazide	Navidrex
Cyclopentolate	Cyclogyl ; Mydrilate
Cyclophosphamide	Endoxana
Cyproheptadine	Periactin
Cytarabine	Cytosar
Dapsone	Avlosulfon
Daunorubicin	Cerubidin
Debrisoquine	Declinax
Demecarium Bromide	Tosmilen
Demethylchlortetracycline	Ledermycin
Dequalinium Chloride	Dequadin
Deserpidine	Harmonyl
Desferrioxamine	Desferal
Desipramine	Pertofran
Dexamethasone	Decadron ; Dexacortisyl ; Oradexon
Dexamphetamine	Dexedrine ; Dexamed
Dextriferron	Astrafer

Approved Name	Proprietary Name
Dextromethorphan	Romilar
Dextromoramide	Palfium
Dextropropoxyphene	Doloxene
Dextrothyroxine	Choloxin
Diamthazole	Asterol
Diazepam	Valium
Diazoxide	Eudemine
Dichloralphenazone	Welldorm
Dichlorophen	Anthiphen
Dichlorphenamide	Daranide
Dicyclomine	Merbentyl ; Wyovin
Diethylcarbamazine	Banocide
Diethylpropion	Tenuate
Dihydrocodeine	D.F. 118
Dihydromorphinone	Dilaudid
Dihydrotachysterol	A.T.10
Di-iodohydroxyquinoline	Diododoquin ; Embequin ; Floraquin
Diloxanide	Furamide
Dimenhydrinate	Dramamine
Dimercaprol	B.A.L.
Dimethisoquin	Quotane
Dimethisterone	Secrosteron
Diphenhydramine	Benadryl
Diphenoxylate	Lomotil
Diphenylpyraline	Histryl
Dipipanone	Pipadone
Diprophylline	Neutraphylline ; Silbephylline
Distigmine	Ubretid
Disulfiram	Antabuse
Domiphen Bromide	Bradosol
Dothiepin	Prothiaden
Doxepin	Sinequan
Doxycycline	Vibramycin
Droperidol	Droleptan
Dydrogesterone	Duphaston
Dyflos	DFP
Ecothiopate Iodide	Phospholine Iodide
Edrophonium Chloride	Tensilon
Embramine	Mebryl
Emepronium bromide	Cetiprin
Enoxolone	Biosone
Epioestriol	Actriol
Erythromycin	Erythrocin ; Ilotycin
Ethacrynic Acid	Edecrin
Ethambutol	Myambutol
Ethamivan	Vandid
Ethamsylate	Dicynene

Approved Name	Proprietary Name
Ethchlorvynol	Arvynol, Serensil
Ethebenecid	Urelim
Ethinamate	Valmidate
Ethionamide	Trescatyl
Ethoglucid	Epodyl
Ethoheptazine	Zactane
Ethopropazine	Lysivane
Ethosuximide	Emeside ; Zarontin
Ethotoin	Peganone
Ethyl Biscoumacetate	Tromexan
Ethyloestrenol	Orabolin
Fenfluramine	Ponderax
Fentanyl	Sublimaze
Flucloxacillin	Floxapen
Fludrocortisone	Florinef ; Fludrocortone
Flufenamic acid	Arlef
Flumethasone	Locorten
Fluocinolone	Synalar
Fluocortolone	Ultralanum
Fluopromazine	Vespral ; Vesprin
Fluoxymesterone	Ultandren
Fluphenazine	Moditen
Flurandrenolone	Drenison
Framycetin	Framygen ; Soframycin
Frusemide	Lasix
Furazolidone	Furoxone
Gallamine	Flaxedil
Gentamicin	Cidomycin ; Genticin
Glibenclamide	Daonil ; Euglucon
Glutethimide	Doriden
Glymidine	Gondafon
Griseofulvin	Fulcin, Grisovin
Guaiphenesin	Respenyl
Guanethidine	Ismelin
Guanoclor	Vatensol
Guanoxan	Envacar
Halethazole	Episol
Haloperidol	Serenace
Halothane	Fluothane
Heptabarbitone	Medomin
Hyaluronidase	Hyalase
Hydrallazine	Apresoline
Hydrargaphen	Penotrane
Hydrochlorothiazide	Direma ; Esidrex ; Hydrosaluric
Hydrocortisone	Corlan ; Cortril ; Ef-Cortelan ; Hydro-Adreson ; Hydrocortistab ; Hydrocortisyl ; Hydrocortone ; Pabracort

Approved Name	*Proprietary Name*
Hydroflumethiazide	Hydrenox ; Naclex ; Rontyl
Hydromorphone	Dilaudid
Hydroxocobalamin	Neo-Cytamen
Hydroxychloroquine	Plaquenil
Hydroxyprogesterone	Primulot Depot
Hydroxyzine	Atarax
Hyoscine Methobromide	Pamine
Ibuprofen	Brufen
Idoxuridine	Kerecid ; Dendrid
Imipramine	Berkomine ; Tofranil
Indomethacin	Indocid
Inositol Nicotinate	Hexopal
Iobenzamic Acid	Osbil
Iodipamide	Biligrafin
Iopanoic Acid	Telepaque
Iophendylate	Myodil
Iothalamic Acid	Conray
Iprindole	Prondol
Iproniazid	Marsilid
Isoaminile	Dimyril
Isocarboxazid	Marplan
Isoniazid	Nicetal ; Nydrazid ; Pycazide ; Rimifon
Isophane Insulin	NPH Insulin
Isoprenaline	Aleudrin ; Neo-Epinine ; Norisodrine ; Saventrine
Isopropamide Iodide	Tyrimide
Isothipendyl	Nilergex
Isoxsuprine	Duvadilan
Kallikrein	Glumorin
Kanamycin	Kannasyn ; Kantrex
Ketamine	Ketalar
Lactulose	Duphalac
Levallorphan	Lorfan
Levodopa	Brocadopa ; Larodopa
Levorphanol	Dromoran
Lignocaine	Duncaine; Lidocaine; Lignostab; Xylocaine ; Xylotox
Lincomycin	Lincocin, Mycivin
Liothyronine	Tertroxin
Lymecycline	Armyl, Tetralysal
Lysuride	Lysenyl
Mannomustine	Degranol
Mebanazine	Actomol
Mebeverine	Colafac
Mebhydrolin	Fabahistin
Mecamylamine	Inversine
Meclofenoxate	Lucidril

Approved Name	*Proprietary Name*
Meclozine	Ancolan
Medroxyprogesterone	Provera
Mefenamic Acid	Ponstan
Melphalan	Alkeran
Mepenzolate	Cantil
Mephenesin	Myanesin
Mephentermine	Mephine
Meprobamate	Equanil ; Mepavlon ; Miltown
Mepyramine	Anthisan
Mercaptopurine	Puri-Nethol
Mestanolone	Androstalone
Metaraminol	Aramine
Metformin	Glucophage
Methacycline	Rondomycin
Methadone	Physeptone
Methallenoestril	Vallestril
Methandienone	Dianabol
Methaqualone	Mandrax ; Melsedin
Methdilazine	Dilosyn
Methenolone	Primobolan
Methicillin	Celbenin
Methisazone	Marboran
Methixene	Tremonil
Methocarbamol	Robaxin
Methohexitone	Brietal
Methoin	Mesontoin
Methoserpidine	Decaserpyl
Methotrimeprazine	Veractil
Methoxamine	Vasoxine
Methoxyflurane	Penthrane
Methoxyphenamine	Orthoxine
Methsuximide	Celontin
Methyclothiazide	Enduron
Methyldopa	Aldomet
Methylergometrine	Methergin
Methylpentynol	Oblivon
Methyl Phenidate	Ritalin
Methylprednisolone	Medrone
Methyprylone	Nodular
Methysergide	Deseril
Metoclopramide	Maxolon
Metronidazole	Flagyl
Metyrapone	Metopirone
Nalidixic Acid	Negram
Nalorphine	Lethidrone
Nandrolone	Deca-Durabolin ; Durabolin
Naphazoline	Privine
Natamycin	Pimafucin

Approved Name	*Proprietary Name*
Nealbarbitone	Censedal
Neostigmine	Prostigmin
Nialamide	Niamid
Niclosamide	Yomesan
Nicotinyl Alcohol	Ronicol
Nicoumalone	Sinthrome
Nikethamide	Coramine
Niridizole	Ambilhar
Nitrazepam	Mogadon
Nitrofurantoin	Furadantin
Nitrofurazone	Furacin
Noradrenaline	Levophed
Norethandrolone	Nilevar
Norethisterone	Norlutin-A ; Primolut N
Nortriptyline	Allegron, Aventyl
Noscapine	Coscopin
Nystatin	Nystan
Opipramol	Insidon
Orciprenaline	Alupent
Orphenadrine	Disipal
Oxazepam	Serenid
Oxprenolol	Trasicor
Oxycodone	Proladone
Oxymesterone	Oranabol
Oxymetholone	Adroyd ; Anapolon
Oxyphenbutazone	Tanderil
Oxyphencyclimine	Daricon
Oxyphenonium Bromide	Antrenyl
Oxytetracycline	Terramycin ; Imperacin
Pancuronium	Pavulon
Paracetamol	Calpol ; Panadol ; Tabalgin
Paramethadione	Paradione
Paramethasone	Haldrate ; Metilar
Pargyline	Eutonyl
Paromomycin	Humatin
Pemoline	Kethamed ; Ronyl
Pempidine	Perolysen
Penicillamine	Distamine
Penicillinase	Neutrapen
Pentaerythritol Tetranitrate	Mycardol ; Peritrate
Pentagastrin	Peptavlon
Pentazocine	Fortral
Pethienate	Monodral
Pentolinium Tartrate	Ansolysen
Pericyazine	Neulactil
Perphenazine	Fentazin
Phenacemide	Phenurone
Phenazocine	Narphen

Approved Name	Proprietary Name
Phenazopyridine	Pyridium
Phenelzine	Nardil
Phenethicillin	Broxil
Phenformin	Dibotin
Phenglutarimide	Aturbane
Phenindamine	Thephorin
Phenindione	Dindevan
Pheniramine.	Daneral
Phenmetrazine	Preludin
Phenobutiodil	Biliodyl
Phenoperidine	Operidine
Phenoxybenzamine	Dibenyline
Phenoxymethylpenicillin	Compocillin-VK ; Crystapen V; Distaquaine V-K ; Icipen V ; Penavlon V; V-Cil-K
Phenprocoumon	Marcoumar
Phensuximide	Milontin
Phentolamine	Rogitine
Phenylbutazone	Butazolidin
Phenylephrine	Neophryn
Pholcodine	Ethnine
Phytomenadione	Konakion
Pipazethate	Selvigon
Pipenzolate	Piptal
Piperazine	Antepar ; Entacyl
Poldine	Nacton
Polymyxin B	Aerosporin
Polynoxylin	Anaflex
Practolol	Eraldin
Prednisolone	Codelcortone ; Delta-Cortef ; Delacortril ; Delta-Stab ; Di-Adreson-F ; PreCortisyl ; Prednelan ; Predsol
Prednisone	DeCortisyl ; Deltacortone ; Di-Adreson ; Ultracortenol
Prenylamine	Synadrin
Prethcamide	Micoren
Prilocaine	Citanest
Primidone	Mysoline
Probenecid	Benemid
Procainamide	Pronestyl
Procarbazine	Natulan
Prochlorperazine	Stemetil
Procyclidine	Kemadrin
Promazine	Sparine
Promethazine	Phenergan
Promethazine Theoclate	Avomine
Propanidid	Epontol

Approved Name	*Proprietary Name*
Propantheline Bromide	Pro-Banthine
Propatyl Nitrate	Gina
Propicillin	Brocillin ; Ultrapen
Propiomazine	Indorm
Propranolol	Inderal
Propylhexedrine	Benzedrex
Propyliodone	Dionosil
Prothionamide	Trevintix
Prothipendyl	Tolnate
Protriptyline	Concordin
Proxyphylline	Brontyl
Pyrazinamide	Zinamide
Pyridostigmine	Mestinon
Pyrimethamine	Daraprim
Pyrrobutamine	Pyronil
Quinalbarbitone Sodium	Seconal Sodium
Quinethazone	Aquamox
Reserpine	Serpasil
Rifampicin	Rifadin ; Rimactane
Salbutamol	Ventolin
Salinazid	Nupa-sal
Sodium Acetrizoate	Diaginol
Sodium Antimonylgluconate	Triostam
Sodium Cromoglycate	Intal
Sodium Diatrizoate	Hypaque
Sodium Fusidate	Fucidin
Sodium Iothalamate	Conray
Sodium Ipodate	Biloptin
Sodium Iron Edetate	Sytron
Sodium Metrizoate	Triosil
Sodium Stibogluconate	Pentostam
Sorbide Nitrate	Vascardin
Spiramycin	Rovamycin
Spironolactone	Aldactone-A
Stanolone	Anabolex
Stanozolol	Stromba
Styramate	Sinaxar
Sulphacetamide	Albucid ; Ocusol
Sulphadimethoxine	Madribon
Sulphadimidine	Sulphamezathine
Sulphafurazole	Gantrisin
Sulphamethizole	Urolucosil
Sulphamethoxazole	Gantanol
Sulphamethoxydiazine	Durenate
Sulphamethoxypyridazine	Lederkyn ; Midicel
Sulphaphenazole	Orisulf
Sulphasalazine	Salazopyrin
Sulphinpyrazone	Anturan

Approved Name	*Proprietary Name*
Sulthiame	Ospolot
Superinone	Alevaire
Suxamethonium Bromide	Brevidil M
Suxamethonium Chloride	Scoline
Suxethonium Bromide	Brevidil E
Tetrabenazine	Nitoman
Tetracycline	Achromycin ; Steclin ; Tetracyn
Tetrahydrozoline	Tyzanol
Thiabendazole	Mintezol
Thialbarbitone	Kemithal
Thiethylperazine	Torecan
Thiocarlide	Isoxyl
Thiomersal	Merthiolate
Thiopropazate	Dartalan
Thioproperazine	Majeptil
Thioridazine	Melleril
Thurfyl Nicotinate	Trafuril
Thymoxamine	Opilon
Tigloidine	Tiglyssin
Tolazamide	Tolanase
Tolazoline	Priscol
Tolbutamide	Artosin ; Rastinon
Tranylcypromine	Parnate
Triacetyloleandomycin	Evramycin
Triamcinolone	Adcortyl ; Ledercort
Triamterene	Dytac
Triaziquone	Trenimon
Triclofos	Tricloryl
Triethanomelamine	Tretamine
Trifluoperazine	Stelazine
Trifluperidol	Triperidol
Trimeprazine	Vallergan
Trimetaphan	Arfonad
Trimipramine	Surmontil
Tripelennamine	Pyribenzamine
Triprolidine	Actidil
Troxidone	Tridione
Tybamate	Benvil
Vancomycin	Vancocin
Vinblastine	Velbe
Vincristine	Oncovin
Viomycin	Viocin ; Vionactane
Viprynium Embonate	Vanquin
Warfarin	Marevan
Zoxazolamine	Flexin

Anti notics — Fridge

Trolly -clean & clean Drying clo[...]

Damp. Sey clott x2. +1 at hanc[...]
for wiping botttes.

<u>CDA</u>   <u>NT</u>   DOA

Break Nicky's tablet befre hand,
insure she swallows it !

Proprietary Name	*Approved Name*
ACTH	Corticotrophin
A.T.10	Dihydrotachysterol
Abasin	Acetylcarbromal
Achromycin	Tetracycline
Actidil	Triprolidine
Actomol	Mebanazine
Actriol	Epioestriol
Adcortyl	Triamcinolone
Adreson	Cortisone
Adroyd	Oxymetholone
Aerosporin	Polymyxin-B
Airbron	Acetylcysteine
Akineton	Biperidon
Albamycin	Novobiocin
Albucid	Sulphacetamide
Alcopar	Bephenium
Aldactone-A	Spironolactone
Aldocorten	Aldosterone
Aldomet	Methyldopa
Aleudrin	Isoprenaline
Alevaire	Superinone
Alkeran	Melphalan
Allegron	Nortriptyline
Allercur	Clemizole
Alloferin	Alcuronium
Alupent	Orciprenaline
Ambilhar	Niridizole
Ambodryl	Bromodiphenhydramine
Anabolex	Stanolone
Anaflex	Polynoxylin
Anapolon	Oxymetholone
Ancolan	Meclozine
Androstalone	Mestanolone
Ansolysen	Pentolinium
Antabuse	Disulfiram
Antepar	Piperazine
Anthiphen	Dichlorophen
Anthisan	Mepyramine
Antistin	Antazoline
Antrenyl	Oxyphenonium Bromide
Anturan	Sulphinpyrazone
Apresoline	Hydrallazine
Aprinox	Bendrofluazide
Aquamox	Quinethazone
Aramine	Metaraminol
Arfonad	Trimetaphan

Proprietary Name	*Approved Name*
Arlef	Flufenamic acid
Artane	Benzhexol
Artosin	Tolbutamide
Arvin	Ancrod
Arvynol	Ethchlorvynol
Asterol	Diamthazole
Astrafer	Dextriferron
Atarax	Hydroxyzine
Atromid-S	Clofibrate
Aturbane	Phenglutarimide
Aureomycin	Chlortetracycline
Aventyl	Nortriptyline
Avloclor	Chloroquine
Avlosulfon	Dapsone
Avomine	Promethazine Theoclate
B.A.L.	Dimercaprol
Banocide	Diethylcarbamazine
Benadryl	Diphenhydramine
Benemid	Probenecid
Benvil	Tybamate
Benzedrex	Prophylhexedrine
Benzedrine	Amphetamine
Berkomine	Imipramine
Bethanid	Bethanidine
Betnelan	Betamethasone
Betnesol	Betamethasone Disodium Phosphate
Betnovate	Betamethasone
Biligrafin	Iodipamide
Biliodyl	Phenobutiodil
Biloptin	Sodium Ipodate
Biogastrone	Carbenoxolone
Biosone	Enoxolone
Bisolvon	Bromhexine
Bradosol	Domiphen
Brevidil E	Suxethonium Bromide
Brevidil M	Suxamethonium Bromide
Brietal	Methohexitone
Brinaldix	Clopamide
Brocadopa	Levodopa
Brocillin	Propicillin
Brontyl	Proxyphylline
Broxil	Phenethicillin
Brufen	Ibuprofen
Butazolidin	Phenylbutazone
Calcium B-PAS	Calcium Benzamidosalicylate
Calpol	Paracetamol
Camoquin	Amodiaquine

Proprietary Name	*Approved Name*
Cantil	Mepenzolate
Carisoma	Carisoprodol
Catapres	Clonidine
Celbenin	Methicillin
Celontin	Methsuximide
Censedal	Nealbarbitone
Centyl	Bendrofluazide
Ceporex	Cephalexin
Ceporin	Cephaloridine
Cerubidin	Daunorubicin
Cetiprin	Emepronium
Chloromycetin	Chloramphenicol
Choledyl	Choline Theophyllinate
Choloxin	Dextrothyroxine
Cidomycin	Gentamicin
Citanest	Prilocaine
Clomid	Clomiphene
Clorevan	Chlorphenoxamine
Cobalin	Cyanocobalamin
Codelcortone	Prednisolone
Cogentin	Benztropine
Colofac	Mebeverine
Colomycin	Colistin
Compocillin-VK	Phenoxymethylpenicillin
Concordin	Protriptyline
Conray 280	Iothalamic Acid; Meglumine salt
Conray 420	Sodium Iothalamate
Coramine	Nikethamide
Corlan	Hydrocortisone
Cortelan	Cortisone
Cortistab	Cortisone
Cortisyl	Cortisone
Cortril	Hydrocortisone
Cortrophin	Corticotrophin
Coscopin	Noscapine
Crasnitin	Colaspase
Cuemid	Cholestyramine
Crystapen V	Phenoxymethylpenicillin
Cyclogyl	Cyclopentolate
Cyclospasmol	Cyclandelate
Cytacon	Cyanocobalamin
Cytamen	Cyanocobalamin
Cytosar	Cytarabine
D.F.118	Dihydrocodeine
Dalacin C	Clindamycin
Daneral	Pheniramine
Daonil	Glibenclamide
Daptazole	Amiphenazole

Proprietary Name	*Approved Name*
Daranide	Dichlorphenamide
Daraprim	Pyrimethamine
Darenthin	Bretylium Tosylate
Daricon	Oxyphencyclimine
Dartalan	Thiopropazate
Decadron	Dexamethasone
Deca-Durabolin	Nandrolone
Decaserpyl	Methoserpidine
Declinax	Debrisoquine
Decortisyl	Prednisone
Degranol	Mannomustine
Delta-Cortef	Prednisolone
Deltacortone	Prednisone
Deltacortril	Prednisolone
Delta-Stab	Prednisolone
Dendrid	Idoxuridine
Dequadin	Dequalinium
Deseril	Methysergide
Desferal	Desferrioxamine
Dexacortisyl	Dexamethasone
Dexamed	Dexamphetamine
Dexedrine	Dexamphetamine
Diabinese	Chlorpropamide
Di-Adreson	Prednisone
Di-Adreson-F	Prednisolone
Diaginol	Sodium Acetrizoate
Diagnex Blue	Azuresin
Diamox	Acetazolamide
Dianabol	Methandienone
Dibenyline	Phenoxybenzamine
Dibotin	Phenformin
Dicynene	Ethamsylate
Didrex	Benzphetamine
Dilaudid	Hydromorphone
Dilosyn	Methdilazine
Dimelor	Acetohexamide
Dimotane	Brompheniramine
Dimyril	Isoaminile
Dindevan	Phenindione
Diodoquin	Di-iodohydroxyquinoline
Dionosil	Propyliodone
Di-paralene	Chlorcyclizine
Direma	Hydrochlorothiazide
Disipal	Orphenadrine
Distamine	Penicillinase
Distaquaine V-K	Phenoxymethylpenicillin
Doloxene	Dextropropoxyphene
Doriden	Glutethimide

Proprietary Name	*Approved Name*
Dothiepin	Prothiaden
Doxepin	Sinequan
Dramamine	Dimenhydrinate
Drenison	Flurandrenolone
Droleptan	Droperidol
Dromoran	Levorphanol
Dulcolax	Bisacodyl
Duncaine	Lignocaine
Duogastrone	Carbenoxolone
Duphalac	Lactulose
Duphaston	Dydrogesterone
Durabolin	Nandrolone
Durenate	Sulphamethoxydiazine
Duvadilan	Isoxsuprine
Dytac	Triamterene
Edecrin	Ethacrynic Acid
Ef-Cortelan	Hydrocortisone
Embequin	Di-iodohydroxyquinoline
Emeside	Ethosuximide
Endografin	Iodipamide
Endoxana	Cyclophosphamide
Enduron	Methyclothiazide
Entacyl	Piperazine
Envacar	Guanoxan
Episol	Halethazole
Epodyl	Ethoglucid
Epontol	Propanidid
Epsikapron	Aminocaproic Acid
Equanil	Meprobamate
Eraldin	Practolol
Erythrocin	Erythromycin
Esbatal	Bethanidine
Esidrex	Hydrochlorothiazide
Ethnine	Pholcodine
Eudemine	Diazoxide
Euglucon	Glibenclamide
Eurax	Crotamiton
Eutonyl	Pargyline
Evramycin	Triacetyloleandomycin
Fabahistin	Mebhydrolin
Fentazin	Perphenazine
Flagyl	Metronidazole
Flaxedil	Gallamine
Flexin	Zoxazolamine
Floraquin	Di-iodohydroxyquinoline
Florinef	Fludrocortisone
Floxapen	Flucloxacillin
Fluothane	Halothane

Proprietary Name	*Approved Name*
Fortral	Pentazocine
Framygen	Framycetin
Fucidin	Sodium Fusidate
Fulcin	Griseofulvin
Fungilin	Amphotericin-B
Fungizone	Amphotericin-B
Furacin	Nitrofurazone
Furadantin	Nitrofurantoin
Furamide	Diloxanide
Furoxone	Furazolidone
Gantanol	Sulphamethoxazole
Gantrisin	Sulphafurazole
Genticin	Gentamicin
Gestanin	Allyloestrenol
Gina	Propatyl Nitrate
Glucophage	Metformin
Glumorin	Kallikrein
Gondafon	Glymidine
Grisovin	Griseofulvin
Haldrate	Paramethasone
Harmonyl	Deserpidine
Heminevrin	Chlormethiazole
Hexopal	Inositol Nicotinate
Hibitane	Chlorhexidine
Histantin	Chlorcyclizine
Histryl	Diphenylpyraline
Honvan	Stilboestrol Diphosphate
Humatin	Paromomycin
Hyalase	Hyaluronidase
Hydrenox	Hydroflumethiazide
Hydril	Hydrochlorothiazide
Hydro-Adreson	Hydrocortisone
Hydrocortistab	Hydrocortisone
Hydrocortisyl	Hydrocortisone
Hydrocortone	Hydrocortisone
Hydrosaluric	Hydrochlorothiazide
Hygroton	Chlorthalidone
Hypaque	Sodium Diatrizoate
Icipen V	Phenoxymethylpenicillin
Ilosone	Erythromycin Estolate
Ilotycin	Erythromycin
Inderal	Propranolol
Indocid	Indomethacin
Indorm	Propiomazine
Insidon	Opipramol
Insulin Lente	Insulin Zinc Suspension
Insulin Semilente	Insulin Zinc Suspension (Amorphous)

Proprietary Name	*Approved Name*
Insulin Ultralente	Insulin Zinc Suspension (Crystalline)
Intal	Sodium Cromoglycate
Inversine	Mecamylamine
Ismelin	Guanethidine
Isoxyl	Thiocarlide
Jadit	Buclosamide
Kannasyn	Kanamycin
Kantrex	Kanamycin
Keflex	Cephalexin
Kemadrin	Procyclidine
Kemithal	Thialbarbitone
Kerecid	Idoxuridine
Ketalar	Ketamine
Kethamed	Pemoline
Konakion	Phytomenadione
Lamprene	Clofazimine
Lapudrine	Chlorproguanil
Largactil	Chlorpromazine
Larodopa	Levodopa
Laroxyl	Amitriptyline
Lasix	Frusemide
Ledercort	Triamcinolone
Lederkyn	Sulphamethoxypyridazine
Ledermycin	Demethylchlortetracycline
Lethidrone	Nalorphine
Leukeran	Chlorambucil
Levophed	Noradrenaline
Levorphan	Levorphanol
Librium	Chlordiazepoxide
Lignostab	Lignocaine
Lincocin	Lincomycin
Locorten	Flumethasone
Lomotil	Diphenoxylate
Lorfan	Levallorphan
Lucidril	Meclofenoxate
Lysenyl	Lysuride
Lysivane	Ethopropazine
Madribon	Sulphadimethoxine
Majeptil	Thioproperazine
Mandrax	Methaqualone
Marboran	Methisazone
Marcain	Bupivacaine
Marcoumar	Phenprocoumon
Marevan	Warfarin
Marplan	Isocarboxazid
Marsilid	Iproniazid
Marzine	Cyclizine

Proprietary Name	*Approved Name*
Maxolon	Metoclopramide
Mebryl	Embramine
Medomin	Heptabarbitone
Medrone	Methylprednisolone
Megaclor	Clomocycline
Megimide	Bemegride
Melleril	Thioridazine
Melsedin	Methaqualone
Mepavlon	Meprobamate
Mephine	Mephentermine
Merbentyl	Dicyclomine
Merthiolate	Thiomersal
Mesontoin	Methoin
Mestinon	Pyridostigmine
Methergin	Methylergometrine
Methscopolamine Bromide	Hyoscine Methobromide
Metilar	Paramethasone
Metopirone	Metyrapone
Micoren	Prethcamide
Midicel	Sulphamethoxypyridazine
Milontin	Phensuximide
Miltown	Meprobamate
Mintezol	Thiabendazole
Mitronal	Cinnarizine
Moditen	Fluphenazine
Mogadon	Nitrazepam
Monodral	Penthienate
Myambutol	Ethambutol
Myanesin	Mephenesin
Mycardol	Pentaerythritol Tetranitrate
Mycil	Chlorphenesin
Mycivin	Lincomycin
Mydrilate	Cyclopentolate
Myleran	Busulphan
Myodil	Iophendylate
Mysoline	Primidone
Mytelase	Ambenonium
NPH Insulin	Isophane Insulin
Naclex	Hydroflumethiazide
Nacton	Poldine
Narcotine	Noscapine
Nardil	Phenelzine
Narphen	Phenazocine
Natulan	Procarbazine
Navidrex	Cyclopenthiazide
Nefrolan	Clorexolone
Negram	Nalidixic Acid
Neo-Cytamen	Hydroxocobalamin

Proprietary Name	*Approved Name*
Neo-Epinine	Isoprenaline
Neo-Mercazole	Carbimazole
Neo-Naclex	Bendrofluazide
Neophryn	Phenylephrine
Neosynephrine	Phenylephrine
Nephril	Polythiazide
Neulactil	Pericyazine
Neutrapen	Penicillinase
Neutraphylline	Diprophylline
Niamid	Nialamide
Nicetal	Isoniazid
Nilergex	Isothipendyl
Nilevar	Norethandrolone
Nitoman	Tetrabenazine
Nivaquine	Chloroquine
Nivemycin	Neomycin
Noludar	Methyprylone
Norflex	Orphenadrine
Norisodrine	Isoprenaline
Norlutin-A	Norethisterone
Nupa-sal	Salinazid
Nupercaine	Cinchocaine
Nydrane	Beclamide
Nystan	Nystatin
Oblivon	Methylpentynol
Ocusol	Sulphacetamide
Oncovin	Vincristine
Operidine	Phenoperidine
Opilon	Thymoxamine
Orabolin	Ethyloestrenol
Oradexon	Dexamethasone
Oranabol	Oxymesterone
Orbenin	Cloxacillin
Orisulf	Sulphaphenazole
Orthoxine	Methoxyphenamine
Osbil	Iobenzamic Acid
Ospolot	Sulthiame
Pabracort	Hydrocortisone
Palaprin	Aloxiprin
Palfium	Dextromoramide
Pamine	Hyoscine Methobromide
Panadol	Paracetamol
Paradione	Paramethadione
Parnate	Tranylcypromine
Pavulon	Pancuronium
Peganone	Ethotoin
Penavolon V	Phenoxymethylpenicillin
Penbritin	Ampicillin

Proprietary Name	*Approved Name*
Penicillin V	Phenoxymethylpenicillin
Penidural	Benzathine Penicillin
Penotrane	Hydrargaphen
Penthrane	Methoxyflurane
Pentostam	Sodium Stibogluconate
Peptavlon	Pentagastrin
Perdilatal	Buphenine
Periactin	Cyproheptadine
Peritrate	Pentaerythritol Tetranitrate
Perolysen	Pempidine
Pertofran	Desipramine
Phanodorm	Cyclobarbitone
Phenergan	Promethazine
Phenurone	Phenacemide
Phospholine	Ecothiopate
Physeptone	Methadone
Pimafucin	Natamycin
Pipadone	Dipipanone
Pipanol	Benzhexol
Piptal	Pipenzolate
Piriton	Chlorpheniramine
Plaquenil	Hydroxychloroquine
Ponderax	Fenfluramine
Ponstan	Mefenamic Acid
Portyn	Benzilonium Bromide
Precortisyl	Prednisolone
Prednelan	Prednisolone
Predsol	Prednisolone
Preludin	Phenmetrazine
Primobolan	Methenolone
Primulot Depot	Hydroxyprogesterone
Primolut N	Norethisterone
Priscol	Tolazoline
Privine	Naphazoline
Pro-Banthine	Propantheline Bromide
Proladone	Oxycodone
Promethazine Chlorotheo- phyllinate	Promethazine Theoclate
Prondol	Iprindole
Pronestyl	Procainamide
Propaderm	Beclomethasone
Prostigmin	Neostigmine
Provera	Medroxyprogesterone
Puri-Nethol	Mercaptopurine
Pycazide	Isoniazid
Pyopen	Carbenicillin
Pyribenzamine	Tripelennamine
Pyridium	Phenazopyridine

Proprietary Name	*Approved Name*
Pyronil	Pyrrobutamine
Questran	Cholestyramine
Quotane	Dimethisoquin
Rastinon	Tolbutamide
Resochin	Chloroquine
Respenyl	Guaiphenesin
Rimifon	Isoniazid
Ritalin	Methyl Phenidate
Robaxin	Methocarbamol
Roccal	Benzalkonium
Rogitine	Phentolamine
Romilar	Dextromethorphan
Rondomycin	Methacycline
Ronicol	Nicotinyl Alcohol
Ronyl	Pemoline
Rovamycin	Spiramycin
Salazopyrin	Sulphasalazine
Salicylazosulfapyridine	Sulphasalazine
Saluric	Chlorothiazide
Saroten	Amitriptyline
Saventrine	Isoprenaline
Scoline	Suxamethonium Chloride
Scopolamine Methobromide	Hyoscine Methobromide
Seconal Sodium	Quinalbarbitone Sodium
Secrosteron	Dimethisterone
Selvigon	Pipazethate
Serc	Betahistine
Serenace	Haloperidol
Serenesil	Ethchlorvynol
Serenid	Oxazepam
Serpasil	Reserpine
Silbephylline	Diprophylline
Sinaxar	Styramate
Sinthrome	Nicoumalone
Soframycin	Framycetin
Somilan	Chloral Betaine
Sparine	Promazine
Steclin	Tetracyline
Stelazine	Trifluoperazine
Stemetil	Prochlorperazine
Stromba	Stanozolol
Sublimaze	Fentanyl
Sulphamezathine	Sulphadimidine
Surmontil	Trimipramine
Symmetrel	Amantadine
Synadrin	Prenylamine
Synalar	Fluocinolone
Sytron	Sodium Iron Edetate

12

Proprietary Name	Approved Name
Tabalgin	Paracetamol
TACE	Chlorotrianisene
Tanderil	Oxyphenbutazone
Taractan	Chlorprothixene
Tegretol	Carbamazepine
Telepaque	Iopanoic Acid
TEM	Tretamine
Tensilon	Edrophonium
Tenuate	Diethylpropion
Terramycin	Oxytetracycline
Tertroxin	Liothyronine
Tetracyn	Tetracycline
Tetralysal	Lymecycline
Thephorin	Phenindamine
Therapas	Calcium Benzamidosalicylate
Thioparamizone	Thiacetazone
Thiosporin	Sulphomyxin
Thytropar	Thyrotrophin
Thytrophin	Thyrotrophin
Tiglyssin	Tigloidine
Tofranil	Imipramine
Tolanase	Tolazamide
Tolnate	Prothipendyl
Torecan	Thiethylperazine
Tosmilen	Demecarium Bromide
Trafuril	Thurfyl Nicotinate
Trancopal	Chlormezanone
Transithal	Buthalitone
Trasicor	Oxprenolol
Tremonil	Methixene
Trenimon	Triaziquone
Trentadil	Bamifylline
Trescatyl	Ethionamide
Tretamine	Triethanomelamine
Trevintix	Prothionamide
Tricloryl	Triclofos
Tridione	Troxidone
Triethanomelamine	Tretamine
Triethylene Melamine	Tretamine
Triflupromazine	Fluopromazine
Trihexyphenidyl	Benzhexol
Trillekamin	Trimustine
Triosil	Sodium Metrizoate
Triostam	Sodium Antimonylgluconate
Triperidol	Trifluperidol
Tromexan	Ethyl Biscoumacetate
Tryptizol	Amitriptyline
Tyrimide	Isopropamide

Proprietary Name	*Approved Name*
Tyzanol	Tetrahydrozoline
Ubretid	Dystigmine
Ultandren	Fluoxymesterone
Ultracortenol	Prednisolone
Ultralanum	Fluocortolone
Ultrapen	Propicillin
Urelim	Ethebenecid
Urolucosil	Sulphamethizole
V-Cil-K	Phenoxymethylpenicillin
Valium	Diazepam
Vallergan	Trimeprazine
Vallestril	Methallenoestril
Valmid	Ethinamate
Valmidate	Ethinamate
Valoid	Cyclizine
Vancocin	Vancomycin
Vandid	Ethamivan
Vanquin	Viprynium Embonate
Vascardin	Sorbide Nitrate
Vasculit	Bamethan
Vasoxine	Methoxamine
Vasylox	Methoxamine
Vatensol	Guanoclor
Velbe	Vinblastine
Ventolin	Salbutamol
Veractil	Methotrimeprazine
Veroxil	Piperazine
Vespral	Fluopromazine
Vesprin	Fluopromazine
Vibazine	Buclizine
Vibramycin	Doxycycline
Viocin	Viomycin
Vioform	Clioquinol
Vionactane	Viomycin
Vitamin K_1	Phytomenadione
Welldorm	Dichloralphenazone
Wyovin	Dicyclomine
Xylocaine	Lignocaine
Xylotox	Lignocaine
Yomesan	Niclosamide
Zactane	Ethoheptazine
Zarontin	Ethosuximide
Zinamide	Pyrazinamide
Zyloric	Allopurinol

APPENDIX II

WEIGHTS AND MEASURES

Metric System

Microgram (mcg.)=0·001 mg.
Milligram (mg.) =0·001 G.
Centigram (cg.) =0·01 G. ·
Decigram (dg.) =0·1 G.
Gram(me) (G.) =1 G.
Kilogram (kg.) =1000 G.

The abbreviation ' G.' is preferred for gram(me) in prescriptions, to avoid confusion with the abbreviation ' gr.' for grain in the Imperial System.

The common metric measures of volume are the millilitre (ml.), which is almost identical with the cubic centimetre (c.c.), and the litre (1000 ml. or c.c.).

The British National Formulary now gives all doses and formulations in the metric system. The standard dose for mixtures is 10 ml., for linctuses and children's mixtures the dose is 5 ml. Special 5-ml. medicine spoons are available, and the use of domestic teaspoons and tablespoons for measuring medicines should be abandoned. Some weights and measures of the old Imperial System are included for guidance where the change-over to the metric system is still incomplete.

Imperial System

Grain
Drachm=60 gr.
Ounce =437·5 gr.
Pound =16 oz.=7000 gr.

Volume

Minim
Drachm=60 min.
Ounce =480 min.
Pint   =20 fl. oz.

Approximate Metric and Imperial Equivalents

0·1 mg.	$\frac{1}{600}$ gr.
0·25 mg.	$\frac{1}{240}$ gr.
0·4 mg.	$\frac{1}{150}$ gr.
0·6 mg.	$\frac{1}{100}$ gr.
1 mg.	$\frac{1}{60}$ gr.
2·5 mg.	$\frac{1}{25}$ gr.
5 mg.	$\frac{1}{12}$ gr.
10 mg.	$\frac{1}{6}$ gr.
15 mg.	$\frac{1}{4}$ gr.
25 mg.	$\frac{2}{5}$ gr.
30 mg.	$\frac{1}{2}$ gr.
60 mg.	1 gr.
100 mg.	$1\frac{1}{2}$ gr.
250 mg.	4 gr.
450 mg.	$7\frac{1}{2}$ gr.
500 mg.	8 gr.
600 mg.	10 gr.
1 G. (1000 mg.)	15 gr.
4 G.	60 gr. (1 dr.)
15 G.	$\frac{1}{2}$ oz.
1 kg. (1000 G.)	2·2 lb.
0·5 ml.	8 min.
0·6 ml.	10 min.
1 ml.	15 min.
4 ml.	60 min. (1 dr.)
15 ml.	$\frac{1}{2}$ fl. oz.
100 ml.	$3\frac{1}{2}$ fl. oz.
300 ml.	10 fl. oz.
500 ml.	17 fl. oz.
600 ml.	20 fl. oz. (1 pint)
1 litre (1000 ml.)	35 fl. oz.

Domestic measures have the following nominal capacities, but in fact vary widely, and they should not be used for medicines :—

One teaspoonful	1 dr. (4 ml.)
One dessertspoonful	2 dr.
One tablespoonful	4 dr.

INDEX

340